Nutritional Management
of Diabetes Mellitus

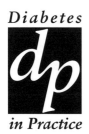

Diabetes

in Practice

Nutritional Management of Diabetes Mellitus

Edited by

Gary Frost

Hammersmith Hospital and Imperial College School of Medicine, London, UK

Anne Dornhorst

Imperial College School of Medicine, London, UK

Robert Moses

Illawarra Area Health Service, NSW, Australia

WILEY

Copyright © 2003 John Wiley & Sons Ltd, The Atrium, Southern Gate, Chichester,
West Sussex PO19 8SQ, England

Telephone (+44) 1243 779777

Email (for orders and customer service enquiries): cs-books@wiley.co.uk
Visit our Home Page on www.wileyeurope.com or www.wiley.com

Other Wiley Editorial Offices

John Wiley & Sons Inc., 111 River Street, Hoboken, NJ 07030, USA

Jossey-Bass, 989 Market Street, San Francisco, CA 94103-1741, USA

Wiley-VCH Verlag GmbH, Boschstr. 12, D-69469 Weinheim, Germany

John Wiley & Sons Australia Ltd, 33 Park Road, Milton, Queensland 4064, Australia

John Wiley & Sons (Asia) Pte Ltd, 2 Clementi Loop #02-01, Jin Xing Distripark, Singapore
129809

John Wiley & Sons Canada Ltd, 22 Worcester Road, Etobicoke, Ontario, Canada
M9W 1L1

Wiley also publishes its books in a variety of electronic formats. Some content that
appears in print may not be available in electronic books.

Library of Congress Cataloging-in-Publication Data

Nutritional management of diabetes mellitus / edited by Gary Frost, Anne Dornhorst,
   Robert Moses.
      p. ; cm
   Includes bibliographical references and index.
   ISBN 0 471 49751 7 (alk. paper)
      1. Diabetes--Diet therapy. I. Frost, Gary, 1959–   II. Dornhorst, Anne.
   III. Moses, Robert, 1946–
      [DNLM: 1. Diabetes Mellitus--diet therapy.   2. Diabetic Diet. WK 818 N9768 2003]
   RC662.N89 2003
   616.4′620654--dc21
                                                                           2003049741

British Library Cataloguing in Publication Data

A catalogue record for this book is available from the British Library

ISBN 0 471 49751 7

Typeset in 10/12pt Times by Dobbie Typesetting Ltd, Tavistock, Devon
Printed and bound in Great Britain by Biddles Ltd, Guildford and Kings Lynn
This book is printed on acid-free paper responsibly manufactured from sustainable forestry
in which at least two trees are planted for each one used for paper production.

A032276

WK810

Contents

List of Contributors

BOYLE, JOANNE

Nutrition and Dietetic Department, Charing Cross Hospital, Fulham Palace Road, London W6 8RF, UK

BRAND-MILLER, JANETTE C.

Human Nutrition Unit, Department of Biochemistry, University of Sydney, NSW 2006, Australia

BRYNES, AUDREY

Research Dietitian, Hammersmith Hospital, Du Cane Road, London W12 0HS, UK

CARTER, LINDA

Nutrition and Dietetic Department, Charing Cross Hospital, Fulham Palace Road, London W6 8RF, UK

CLEATOR, JACQUELINE

Diabetes and Endocrinology Clinical Research Group, Clinical Sciences Centre, University Hospital Aintree, Longmoor Lane, Liverpool L9 7AL, UK

DASSANAYAKE, THUSHARA

Senior Renal Dietitian, Nutrition and Dietetic Department, Hammersmith Hospital, Du Cane Road, London W12 0HS, UK

DORNHORST, ANNE

Nutrition and Dietetic Research Group, Department of Metabolic Medicine and Nutrition and Dietetics, Division of Investigational Science, Hammersmith Hospital Campus, Faculty of Medicine, Imperial School of Medicine, Du Cane Road, London W12 0NN, UK

DYSON, PAMELA

Diabetes Specialist Dietitian, Oxford Centre for Diabetes, Endocrinology and Metabolism, Churchill Hospital, Headington, Oxford OX3 7LJ, UK

ENGEL, BARBARA

Senior Renal Dietitian, Department of Nutrition and Dietetics, Charing Cross Hospital, Fulham Palace Road, London W6 7RS, UK

FOOTE, DEBORAH

Senior Dietitian, Diabetes Centre, Level 10 Queen Mary Building, Royal Prince Alfred Hospital, Grose Street, Camperdown, NSW 2050, Australia

FROST, GARY

Nutrition and Dietetic Research Group, Department of Metabolic Medicine and Nutrition and Dietetics, Division of Investigational Science, Hammersmith Hospital Campus, Faculty of Medicine, Imperial School of Medicine, Du Cane Road, London W12 0NN, UK

HICKSON, MARY

Research Dietitian, Hammersmith Hospitals NHS Trust, Dietetic Department, Charing Cross Hospital, Fulham Palace Road, London W6 8RF, UK

HOLT, SUSANNA H. A.

Human Nutrition Unit, Department of Biochemistry, University of Sydney, NSW 2006, Australia

KELLY, MARIE

Chief Dietitian, Nutrition and Dietetic Department, Hammersmith Hospital, Du Cane Road, London W12 0HS, UK

MCGOUGH, NORMA

Freelance Dietitian, The Auction Room, 20 Temple Street, Aylesbury, Bucks HP20 2RQ, UK

MOSES, ROBERT

Director of Diabetes Services, Illawarra Area Health Service, 4/393 Crown Street, Wollongong, NSW, 2500, Australia

OLIVER, LINDSAY

Lead Diabetes Dietitian for Northumbria Trust, Diabetes Resource Centre, North Tyneside General Hospital, Rape Lane, North Tyneside, UK

PARKIN, TRACEY — *Diabetes Specialist Dietitian, Diabetes Centre, Queen Alexandra Hospital, Cosham, Portsmouth, Hants PO6 3LY, UK*

PEAKE, HILARY — *Dietetic Department, Hammersmith Hospital, 150 Du Cane Road, London W12 0HS, UK*

REAVEN, GERALD M. — *Department of Medicine, Stanford University School of Medicine, Stanford, CA 94305, USA*

SLEVIN, KAREN — *Diabetes and Endocrinology Clinical Research Group, Clinical Sciences Centre, University Hospital Aintree, Longmoor Lane, Liverpool L9 7AL, UK*

SUTTON, JO — *Consultant Dietitian, PO Box 780, Knaphill, Woking, Surrey GU21 2TL, UK*

SWIFT, PETER — *Consultant Paediatrician, Leicester Royal Infirmary, Leicester LE1 5WW, UK*

WALDRON, SHERIDAN — *Diabetes Specialist Dietician (Paediatric), 49 Swithland Lane, Rothley, Leics LE7 7SG, UK*

WILDING, JOHN — *Diabetes and Endocrinology Clinical Research Group, Clinical Sciences Centre, University Hospital Aintree, Longmoor Lane, Liverpool L9 7AL, UK*

WRIGHT, LUCY — *Charing Cross Hospital, Fulham Palace Road, London W6 8RF, UK*

Introduction

The Ancient Greeks were the first to advocate diet and lifestyle management for people with diabetes. Until the discovery and use of insulin in the 1920s and suphonylureas in the 1940s, diet and lifestyle intervention were the only treatment options available. For people with Type 1 diabetes this was woefully ineffective and consisted of near starvation diets imposed on already severely malnourished individuals. While such diets may have prolonged life by a few months, an inevitable early death from ketoacidosis was all too often replaced with death from infections due to the severe malnutrition and other co-morbidities. The introduction of insulin radically reduced the death rates from ketoacidosis and problems associated with malnutrition, however, survival brought other lethal problems in the form of microvascular and macrovascular disease.

The dietary management of Type 1 diabetes over the last 80 years has had to adapt to the many changes in insulin formulations as well as changes in staple foods and eating patterns. Over the years the premise for the dietary advice given, of optimising growth while minimising diabetes associated complications, has not changed. By contrast the dietary advice given has radically changed in response to advances in our understanding of the biochemical and physiological mechanisms involved in diabetic complications. Today the dietary advice offered for people with Type 1 diabetes has little resemblance to the advice given by R. D. Lawrence three-quarters of a century ago. R. D. Lawrence's diet advocating a high-fat and low-carbohydrate intake has been replaced by the more healthy low-fat and high-carbohydrate diets of today. To what extent today's dietary advice will resemble that in 75 years time, will, we believe, reflect the quality of the scientific evidence behind this advice.

Since the advent of insulin and oral agents, other changes to the dietary management of diabetes have included the way dietary advice is imparted. There has been a move away from prescriptive diets given by authoritarian

Nutritional Management of Diabetes Mellitus. Edited by G. Frost, A. Dornhorst and R. Moses
© 2003 John Wiley & Sons, Ltd. ISBN 0 471 49751 7

physicians towards trying to achieve the necessary dietary and lifestyle changes through educating individuals to a level such that they can make their own informed choices regarding their management. However, a greater under-standing of the factors that influence the uptake of lifestyle advice is required if more effective dietary management for people with diabetes is to be achieved in the future.

Despite the availability of several different classes of oral hypoglycaemic agents for the management of Type 2 diabetes, dietary and lifestyle manage-ment remains crucial for the optimal effectiveness of these drugs. It might at first appear strange that this book contains only a summary chapter dealing with Type 2 diabetes. This is because the lifestyle messages for the management of people with Type 2 diabetes are covered in other chapters throughout the book, including those addressing guidelines, exercise, counselling and obesity. Lifestyle and dietary changes for people with Type 2 diabetes are required, not only for glycaemic control but also for reducing important cardiovascular risk factors.

The aim of this book is to provide a practical guide for the dietary management of diabetes based on basic physiological principles as well as nutritional and clinical evidence. We hope this book will aid health professionals to provide their patients with informed evidence-based advice in a way most likely to achieve the meaningful nutritional changes that will improve their quality of life.

Acknowledgement

We wish to thank Dr Louise Goff for her help in proof reading this book.

1

Nutritional Recommendations in Diabetes Management

NORMA MCGOUGH BSc SRD
Aylesbury, Buckinghamshire, UK

INTRODUCTION

The first position statement on diet in diabetes care was made by Diabetes UK, formerly the British Diabetic Association, 20 years ago (1). The recommendations liberalised the diet for people with diabetes. Previous advice had focused specifically on carbohydrate intake and sugar restriction. The new recommendations promote a diet in line with healthy eating recommendations for the general population and compatible with dietary advice for people at high cardiovascular risk. Further review, 10 years later, resulted in an update that re-enforced the high-carbohydrate, low-fat diet (2). These recommendations have now been superseded by recommendations from other parts of the world including Europe (3) and America (4). A more recent technical review of the nutritional management of patients with diabetes also helps to put a clear perspective on dietary education in diabetes care (5).

CURRENT POSITION

Recommendations will change in time as new data becomes available and consensus and views on emphasis differ. Any recommendations require careful interpretation and communication for the maximum benefit of those individuals with diabetes.

Nutritional Management of Diabetes Mellitus. Edited by G. Frost, A. Dornhorst and R. Moses
© 2003 John Wiley & Sons, Ltd. ISBN 0 471 49751 7

The biggest change in emphasis of the recommendations currently in use compared to previous recommendations focuses on a greater flexibility between the proportion of energy from carbohydrate and fat, with promotion of the use of monounsaturated fat. Diets rich in monounsaturated fat reduce total and low-density lipoprotein cholesterol without adverse effects on high-density lipoprotein cholesterol or triglyceride levels (6). It is necessary to restrict the total fat content of the diet where obesity is an issue and calorie intake needs to be limited. Otherwise, a range of carbohydrate (45–60%) and fat (25–35%) intakes is compatible with good diabetes control provided that low glycaemic index carbohydrates and foods high in monounsaturated fat are promoted.

Other significant changes in the recommendations include:

- There is less emphasis on the benefits of cereal fibre other than for gastrointestinal health and its satiety value.
- The precise effects of antioxidant nutrients with regard to being potential cardio-protective factors is still uncertain and so clear guidance is not possible in the light of the evidence available.
- In most European countries, the average intake of protein is in excess of the recommended intake and for those people with Type 1 diabetes, especially in those with hypertension, intakes of protein should not exceed 10–20% total energy because of the increased risk of nephropathy.
- The benefits of physical activity for people with diabetes are becoming increasingly evident. Regular, moderate intensity exercise is associated with a reduced risk of developing Type 2 diabetes in men, women and individuals who are overweight (7,8). Exercise can produce a reduction in plasma triglycerides, increases HDL and can also aid weight loss (9). The overall impact of exercise on blood pressure is also beneficial (10).

AIMS OF THE NUTRITIONAL RECOMMENDATIONS

The goals of dietary advice are to achieve and maintain good health and quality of life, with avoidance and management of short-term symptoms, including hypoglycaemia and freedom from the long-term complications of the disease, for as long as possible. Evidence available from America from the Diabetes Control and Complications Trial in Type 1 diabetes (11) and also from the United Kingdom Prospective Diabetes Study in Type 2 diabetes (12) suggests that normalisation of metabolic markers like blood glucose levels and management of blood pressure constitute key aims. There needs to be a balance between the attainment of objectives of care and the demands that they may impose on the individual person with diabetes.

The recommendations should be adapted to an individual's lifestyle, culture and socio-economic status. Personalised targets, based on the recommendations, need to be negotiated, clearly defined and communicated. There should be regular review and on-going dietary education.

The Practice Guidelines for Medical Nutrition Therapy developed in the USA for Type 1 diabetes have been shown to result in significant improvements in glycaemic control, and require more frequent and longer contacts between dietitians and patients (13). Patients from UKPDS, in centres with a greater availability of dietetic advice, lost more weight than those with less advice and also tended to have a greater decrease in plasma glucose (14), thus showing the need for more intensive care of diabetic patients.

APPLICATION OF THE NUTRITIONAL GUIDELINES

Since diabetes is a life-long disease that affects all groups of the population, irrespective of age, culture or socio-economic status, it is vitally important to identify the most appropriate approach to the application of the nutritional guidelines, from the outset. Dietetic intervention requires an appropriate level of knowledge, experience and skill if dietary habits and eating behaviour are to be adjusted, effectively (15). The Clinical Standards Advisory Group (CSAG) in the UK recommended that all newly diagnosed patients should be offered a dietetic consultation within four weeks of diagnosis and that non-crisis dietetic review should be available, annually, to all people with diabetes (16). UKPDS showed that the first three months were vitally important in determining response to dietary intervention (14). Currently in the UK one current issue of dietary management in diabetes care is the under-provision of dietetic services in diabetes care (17).

PROVISION OF SERVICES IN DIABETES CARE

In 1997, Diabetes UK, formerly the British Diabetic Association, investigated the provision of dietetic services in diabetes care. They carried out a postal survey to dietitians in the UK to assess level of provision and current practices including application of nutritional guidelines, audit and evaluation. The survey showed that 85% of dietitians worked in situations where dietetic provision was less than the current recommendation of 22.5 hours per 100 000 of the population, made by Diabetes UK, in 1999 (18). One of the outcomes of this situation is that people with diabetes may not receive dietary education from a State Registered Dietitian. Dietary education may be part of an education package offered in general practice by the practice nurse. The evolution of the nutritional guidelines for people with diabetes to a status which is in line with healthy eating recommendations for the general population may have 'de-mystified' the diet in diabetes care to the extent that it was perceived as being a package that could be relayed without the expertise of a dietitian.

There is a need for a consistent approach from health care professionals. Co-ordination of training of all health care professionals involved in diabetes education on nutrition and diabetes as well as overall management of dietary education in diabetes care is essential to ensure a high-quality service to all people with diabetes. Continuing professional development is essential to update knowledge and skills.

THE ROLE OF THE DIETITIAN IN DIABETES CARE

Ideally, it is the role of the dietitian to provide the dietetic intervention. A vital part of the dietetic consultation is the assessment of readiness to change eating behaviour (19). Exploration of barriers to change and awareness of psycho-social issues form part of the dietary consultation process. In the short term, food intake needs to be regulated and balanced against medication, in order to optimise blood glucose control. This also includes assessment of whether current medication matches the meal pattern and therefore whether it is appropriate, as well as the management and prevention of hypoglycaemia and hyperglycaemia. Long-term dietary control can offer protection against cardiovascular disease with weight management and modification of other lifestyle factors being essential. Dietary counselling should be innovative and specific to the requirements of the individual, rather than being rigid, prescriptive and restricted to a particular system of teaching, as may be the case when knowledge, experience and skills in diet therapy are limited.

AUDIT AND EVALUATION

Since the 1970s, the success or failure of diet in diabetes care has been based on compliance (20). The most important consideration being whether or not a patient was deemed to have modified their dietary intake and achieved a particular dietary prescription. Evaluation needs to consider the impact of diet on clinical outcomes like body weight, lipid levels and HbA_1C. Application of the nutritional guidelines is not about achieving the gold standard but about the modification of an individual's dietary intake to shift the balance in the direction of the gold standard and at the same time, maximise health benefits and quality of life for that individual.

Findings of the Diabetes UK survey in 1997 show that a quantitative method of dietary prescription is no longer applied in practice. The survey also shows that most dietitians reported, at the time, following the 1992 nutritional guidelines. The nutritional recommendations in the UK are under review and the more up-to-date guidelines from Europe and America should be applied until updated recommendations are published in the UK.

RECOMMENDATIONS: TYPE 1 AND TYPE 2 DIABETES

Although the nutritional recommendations for people with Type 1 and Type 2 diabetes are in essence the same, there may be a difference in emphasis. Cardiovascular disease is the main cause of mortality in both Type 1 and Type 2 diabetes, so restriction of saturated fat is a prime aim for all people with diabetes. However, there should be greater emphasis on modification of fat intake for people with Type 2 diabetes where lipid abnormalities are more common.

People with diabetes who are overweight or obese have a wide range of complications of their obesity: more symptoms can be related to BMI (body mass index) than can be related to blood glucose, so weight management is a fundamental aspect of treatment in Type 2 diabetes.

For Type 1 diabetes greater emphasis should be placed on attempts to modify the progression of microvascular disease, especially nephropathy, by restricting protein intake.

The ultimate goals of management depend on the priorities relevant to the individual person with diabetes.

ENERGY BALANCE AND BODY WEIGHT

Obesity is recognised as a leading cause of insulin resistance (21). It therefore contributes to the development of Type 2 diabetes. This is particularly true for a central distribution of body fat, associated with a range of metabolic disturbances. Weight management is crucial in controlling blood glucose levels in people with Type 2 diabetes, although from UKPDS there is evidence that to normalise glucose tolerance usually requires major weight loss. Studies suggest that at least 80% of newly diagnosed patients with Type 2 diabetes are overweight and weight loss in people with Type 2 diabetes who are overweight increases life expectancy. Obesity is an additional risk factor for coronary heart disease and stroke. All cardiac risk factors (glycaemia, hypertension, lipids) are improved with weight management (22). This is true for individuals with Type 1 diabetes as well as Type 2 diabetes. However, it is also important to make sure that energy requirements are adequate in children and adolescents with Type 1 diabetes.

Dietary strategies for weight management should be based on realistic target weights. Assessment of target weights and the appropriate level of energy

Table 1.1

Age range (yr)	BMR (kcal/day)	Activity level	24-h Energy expenditure (kcal/day)
Men			
10–18	$17.5W + 651$	Inactive	$BMR \times 1.30$
18–30	$15.3W + 679$	Light	$BMR \times 1.55$
30–60	$11.6W + 879$	Moderate	$BMR \times 1.78$
> 60	$13.5W + 487$	Heavy	$BMR \times 2.10$
Women			
10–18	$12.2W + 746$	Inactive	$BMR \times 1.30$
18–30	$14.7W + 496$	Light	$BMR \times 1.56$
30–60	$8.7W + 829$	Moderate	$BMR \times 1.64$
> 60	$10.5W + 596$	Heavy	$BMR \times 1.82$

W = weight (kg).

restriction is not a precise science. Equations are available for estimating basal metabolic rate and daily energy expenditure from body weight in kilograms and activity level, when prescribing calorie-controlled diets (23), see Table 1.1.

In general, long-term lifestyle changes and strategies are more likely to result in sustained weight loss. Realistic calorie deficits of 500 kcal/day usually produce better end results than very restrictive diets (24). Strategies to support individuals trying to lose weight may range from individual counselling to group therapy. The use of very low calorie diets (VLCDs) in people with diabetes has however been shown to have positive effects on plasma lipids, lowering triglyceride levels and raising HDL cholesterol (25). Most of the benefits relate to energy restriction not weight loss (26). Although more weight is lost over a 3–6 month period than using conventional diets there is no evidence that in the long term (1–2 years) the continued benefit of using VLCDs is maintained. VLCDs should only be used in a specialist setting as complications of VLCD therapy can include alterations in body composition including bone loss and possibly loss of cardiac muscle (27). As a generalisation the use of anti-obesity drugs should be restricted to specialist medical centres in the absence of large-scale studies of their application in diabetes. The Royal College of Physicians (28) produced guidelines for the use of anti-obesity drugs for obesity treatment.

Individuals who are overweight should have the necessary advice and support to reduce their calorie intake and to increase their energy expenditure in order to shift their energy balance and weight in the direction of a more ideal BMI. Sustained weight loss and prevention of weight regain are important goals which are preferable to more rapid weight loss which usually results in excessive loss of lean body mass. Even modest weight loss confers benefits to health (29). Whenever possible those people who are overweight should be offered a multi-disciplinary structured approach to weight management. Dietary advice should take into account an increase in physical activity, which may also facilitate weight loss and help to maintain muscle mass. Normally, people's appetites increase with exercise automatically. However, for those with Type 1 diabetes adequate or additional carbohydrate before, during and after exercise as well as insulin adjustment needs to be anticipated, see Chapter 2. For those people with Type 2 diabetes on oral hypoglycaemic therapy, adjustment of medication is usually not necessary unless on sulphonylureas where hypoglycaemia may be a risk with sustained exercise. The level of activity will depend on age and degree of fitness but moderate activity (walking) for at least 20–30 min a day will be beneficial. Adjustment of medication for both Type 1 and Type 2 may be necessary if weight loss occurs and is maintained in the long term.

MACRONUTRIENT COMPOSITION OF THE DIET

The main dietary components of the diet for an individual with diabetes should be carbohydrate-containing foods with a low glycaemic index and *cis*-monounsaturated fat.

Although it is important to give people with diabetes advice to modify their dietary intakes so that they shift the balance of their nutritional intake in the direction of the recommendations, the relative proportions of macronutrients may vary depending on the markers of diabetes control for the individual.

A combination of carbohydrate and *cis*-monounsaturated fatty acids should provide 60–70% total daily energy intake. Total fat intake should be restricted to 35% total energy. *Cis*-monounsaturated fatty acids should provide between 10 and 20% total energy. Saturated and *trans*-fatty acids should provide under 10% total energy. Polyunsaturated fatty acids should not exceed 10% total energy. Protein intake should range between 10 and 20% total energy. Protein intake should not go below 0.6 g/kg normal body weight/day but should be at the lower end of the range (0.8 g/kg body weight/day) in cases of nephropathy or where abnormal microalbuminuria has been identified.

The relative proportions of macronutrients recommended in diabetes:

Protein (10–20%)
Carbohydrate (45–60%)
Cis-monounsaturated fat (10–20%)
Polyunsaturated fat (< 10%)
Saturated/*trans* fat (< 10%)

CARBOHYDRATE

The proportion of energy derived from carbohydrate is related to the level of fat intake. Recommendations in the past have tended to be narrow and precise with regard to fat and carbohydrate intake. Although good diabetes control can be achieved with a range of carbohydrate intake (45–60%), it can be difficult to maintain a high-carbohydrate/low-fat balance in practical terms. The current emphasis is on a more flexible approach dependent upon the individual's lifestyle, habits and diabetes management.

To minimise the risk of hypertriglyceridaemia and an associated increased risk for cardiovascular disease, high-carbohydrate diets for people with diabetes should incorporate a high intake of soluble fibre and resistant starch (30).

In cases where a lower carbohydrate intake is optimal for control and lifestyle, intake of energy from monounsaturated fat can be increased, as long as calorie control is monitored.

GLYCAEMIC INDEX

The glycaemic index (GI), see Chapter 11, was proposed as a method to guide food selection in the early 1980s by Jenkins and colleagues. It is based on the assessment of carbohydrate foods in terms of glycaemic response compared to the same amount of a standard carbohydrate-containing food (usually bread or glucose) (31).

The GI of a food is determined by a number of factors, including the rate of digestion and absorption. The soluble fibre content as well as the structure of the food and other meals and foods consumed as part of the overall diet are all significant influences on the glycaemic index of a particular food (32).

FIBRE

Dietary fibre or non-starch polysaccharides may broadly be classed as soluble fibre (gums, gels and pectins) and insoluble fibre (cellulose and lignin).

There is epidemiological evidence that low intakes of insoluble fibre are associated with an increased risk of Type 2 diabetes (33). In general, the benefits of insoluble fibre are limited to promoting healthy gut functioning. The intake of soluble fibre is however beneficial to glycaemic and lipid control (34).

SUGAR AND SWEETENERS

SUCROSE

The diabetic diet has in the past been referred to as the sugar-free diet but many studies have shown that consuming iso-caloric amounts of other carbohydrates can raise blood glucose levels and aggravate hyperglycaemia more than sucrose itself (35,36). The consensus view is that sucrose may be consumed in the diet of people with diabetes at the same level, 10% of total calories, as that recommended for the general population.

FRUCTOSE

Fructose has been shown to invoke a lower glucose and insulin response compared to other carbohydrates (37). However, dietary fructose in amounts comparable to those of sugars in Western diets (7.5–20% daily energy) can result in raised fasting triglycerides and LDL concentrations. There may also be a greater risk of gastrointestinal disturbances with large doses (38). There is no reason to believe that fructose either confers special benefits for people with diabetes or that it is detrimental to health in the amounts found in everyday foods.

NUTRITIVE SWEETENERS

Polyols or sugar alcohols like sorbitol, xylitol, mannitol and isomalt are bulk or nutritive sweeteners which contain calories and raise blood glucose levels. They must still be accounted for in meal planning. They have a slightly lower glycaemic response than sucrose and a slightly lower calorie value (2.4 kcal/g) because they are not completely digested and absorbed. Polyols may therefore cause diarrhoea, particularly if consumed in large amounts (> 25 g). Although they have a lower cardiogenic effect compared to sucrose, polyols offer no special benefit to people with diabetes.

NON-NUTRITIVE SWEETENERS

Intense or non-nutritive sweeteners are sugar-free and calorie-free. Permitted sweeteners in the UK and Europe include aspartame, saccharin, acesulfame potassium, cyclamate, sucralose and alitame. These substances are very often used in combination as table-top sweeteners or in food products in order to produce a better flavour synergy or heat stability. There has been ongoing public debate about the safety of these substances, but there is no conclusive evidence to suggest that particular health problems are implicated by their use. In the UK the government Food Standards Agency (FSA) (formerly the

Ministry of Agriculture, Foods and Fisheries (MAFF)) monitors consumption of sweeteners and provides guidelines to the food industry regarding levels of intense sweeteners permitted in foods. In this way there is deemed to be control over intake.

ALCOHOL

Recommendations regarding alcohol consumption and diabetes currently relate to a number of different sources but focus on two main issues, hypoglycaemia for Type 1 diabetes and the increased cardiovascular risks with Type 2 diabetes, see Chapters 9 & 12. The Nutrition Subcommittee of Diabetes UK produced a paper in 1985 which refers to a maximum safe intake of 30 g (3 units) per day for men and 20 g (2 units) per day for women (39). The government's report, Sensible Drinking, published in 1997 (40), refers to a maximum intake of 3 units per day for women and 4 for men. Precautions which apply to the general population also apply to people with diabetes. However, for people on insulin therapy and sulphonylureas, alcohol should always be consumed with carbohydrate-containing foods. This is because of the increased risk of hypoglycaemia as alcohol suppresses gluconeogenesis (41). Alcohol can also interfere with the action of glucagon in insulin-induced hypoglycaemia (42). People taking sulphonylureas can experience facial flushing with alcohol.

Daily alcohol intake has been associated with cataract development which is independent of the effects of diabetes itself.

Alcohol contributes 7 kcal/g and so may contribute to calorie intake and impact on weight control in people with Type 2 diabetes as well as aggravate hypertriglyceridaemia.

More recent studies on people with Type 2 diabetes suggest that people with well-controlled diabetes can safely consume 21–28 g/d alcohol with no change in glycaemic control (43). There are possible beneficial effects of alcohol on blood lipids and coagulability. Moderate intake of wine (one or two glasses per day) which contains flavonoids and phenolic compounds may confer benefits by virtue of antioxidant properties (44).

DIETARY FATS

People with diabetes have a two- to fourfold increased risk of coronary heart disease, and an increased risk of mortality due to the low HDL with high triglyceride syndrome that is seen in Type 2 diabetes, even when well treated (45). Epidemiological evidence suggests that populations of people with diabetes who consume a low-fat diet have a lower mortality rate, see Chapters 9 & 12 (46).

SATURATED FAT

Reducing intake of saturated fat can lower levels of total and LDL cholesterol, risk factors for coronary heart disease (47). The recommended level is less than 10% energy from saturated fat. Although there are no large studies of diabetic populations it is considered appropriate to base the prevention and management of heart disease on the same principles as in non-diabetic populations.

Individual fatty acids have different effects, with lauric, myristic and palmitic having a hypercholesterolaemic effect and stearic being neutral.

TRANS FATTY ACIDS

Most *trans* fatty acids are formed during partial hydrogenation of vegetable oils to produce margarine and certain baked foods including biscuits and pastries. *Trans* fatty acids have a similar impact on lipid levels as saturated fat, decreasing HDL and increasing LDL (48). Specific information relating to people with diabetes is lacking but there are some large studies that show the evidence is not conclusive regarding coronary risk and *trans* fatty acid intake. The Nurses Health Study (49) shows that high intakes of foods that are a significant source of *trans* fat may be associated with a risk of coronary heart disease. The EURAMIC study (50) however found no significant effect.

POLYUNSATURATED FATS (n-6)

The WHO recommendation for the general population is a maximum intake of 3–7% dietary energy. This is because polyunsaturated fats are more susceptible to oxidation and therefore more atherogenic. In addition, a reduction in HDL may occur when larger amounts are consumed.

FISH OILS (n-3)

The general recommendation with regard to fish oils for the population as a whole is not to take therapeutic doses but to consume one helping of oily fish per week. Increasing fish intake in the non-diabetic population is associated with reduced mortality from coronary heart disease. However, despite available evidence showing that fish oils can reduce plasma triglycerides and VLDL concentrations in the diabetic population (51), as well as reducing blood pressure (52), there are also potential deleterious effects of fish oils on LDL cholesterol and glycaemic control in people with diabetes (53).

MONOUNSATURATED FATS

In the Mediterranean, where the prevalence of coronary heart disease is lower, the typical diet is high in monounsaturated fatty acids (54). The beneficial effects of monounsaturated fats include the fact that they are more resistant to lipid peroxidation and increased MUFA intakes have also been associated with lower daytime blood pressures. There have been studies in both diabetic and non-diabetic populations which show falls in total cholesterol with no changes in HDL levels or triglyceride levels. The choice of MUFA as the prime source of dietary fat is therefore recommended.

CHOLESTEROL

Restriction of saturated fat will also limit intake of cholesterol. The EASD recommendations refer to a maximum intake of 300 mg/day.

PROTEIN

There is a need for more long-term studies on protein intake for people with diabetes in order to be able to make evidence-based recommendations. The WHO (55) recommendation for intake of protein for adults is 0.8 g/kg/day (56) but most European populations consume more than this. There is epidemiological evidence to suggest that diets rich in protein may contribute to the pathogenesis of early nephropathy (57). There are also studies which indicate that protein intakes at the lower end of the recommendation may have advantages in people with diabetes with renal changes. In people with evidence of clinical diabetic nephropathy a protein restriction to < 0.6 g/kg/day can reduce the elevated GFR and albuminuria (55). In people with persistent proteinuria a similar protein restriction has been shown to modify the progression of the disease (58). There is no conclusive evidence about the different properties of animal or vegetable proteins and their effect on diabetic renal disease. The recommendation for protein intake for people with diabetes is that it should range between 10 and 20% of total energy.

VITAMINS AND ANTIOXIDANTS

There is a need for more conclusive evidence on the benefits of vitamins and antioxidant nutrients in terms of protection from cardiovascular disease and general health benefits for the diabetic and non-diabetic population. Pharmacological doses of supplements are therefore not advised. However, it is recommended that a diet rich in foods which naturally contain significant quantities of antioxidants, especially fruit and vegetables, is followed.

MINERALS

SALT

The general population has been recommended to restrict intake of salt to 6 g/day. Normal intake in Northern Europe is twice this amount. Dietary sodium restriction can reduce systolic blood pressure in mild hypertension in Type 2 diabetes (59). However, there is still debate about the efficacy of sodium restriction with regard to hypertension. In addition, the impact of weight loss in treating people who are overweight with hypertension also makes it difficult to distinguish between the benefits of salt restriction and energy restriction.

People with diabetes should be advised to eat plenty of fruit and vegetables and other fresh, rather than processed, foods, which contribute to a significant proportion of the sodium in the diet, in order to cut down on salt intake.

CHROMIUM

There has been a lot of media hype over chromium and its ability to improve glycaemic control in people with Type 2 diabetes. Chromium is an essential trace element that has a role in glucose, insulin and lipid metabolism. Suboptimal dietary intake of chromium is related to increased risk factors associated with diabetes and cardiovascular disease. There are a number of small clinical trials which show supplements of chromium have been related to improvement in glucose tolerance in Type 1, Type 2 and steroid-induced diabetes. However, these studies are very small and carried out over a short period of time. There is an urgent need for properly powered research before the reported benefits of chromium supplementation can be assessed (60).

MEAL PLANNING

There are a number of teaching systems available for meal planning but they are all subject to limitations. The emphasis should be on appropriate advice conveyed in the most appropriate way for a particular individual. There should not necessarily be a focus on one specific teaching system.

In the past, the main educational tool in the dietary education of people with diabetes, particularly for Type 1 diabetes, was the exchange system. Measurement of carbohydrate intake by using an exchange system devised by R. D. Lawrence was considered to be essential for good blood glucose control. The exchange system was devised to ensure that carbohydrate was included with meals and snacks but it resulted in a restriction of carbohydrate.

People with diabetes were advised on the amount of carbohydrate they should consume by the prescription of a number of exchanges per meal or snack, over the day. The exchanges were based on units of 10 g carbohydrate and lists of foods containing 10 g were used to swap foods and vary dietary intake.

Another tool, the plate model, can be used to assess and convey the proportions of the different foods that make up the appropriate macronutrient composition of the diet. There are various adaptations including the Balance of Good Health, a national teaching model for food selection, launched in 1993 in the UK, by the Department of Health, Ministry of Agriculture, Fisheries and Food and the Health Education Authority.

REFERENCES

1. Nutrition Subcommittee, British Diabetic Association. Dietary recommendations for diabetics for the 1980s. *Human Nutr: Appl Nutr* 1982; 36A: 378–394.
2. Nutrition Subcommittee, British Diabetic Association. Dietary recommendations for people with diabetes: an update for the 1990s. *Diabetic Med* 1992; 9: 189–202.
3. The Diabetes and Nutrition Study Group (DSNG) of the European Association for the Study of Diabetes (EASD) 1999. Recommendations for the nutritional management of patients with diabetes mellitus. *Eur J Clin Nutr* 2000; 54: 353–355.
4. American Diabetes Association. Evidence-Based Nutrition Principles and Recommendations for the Treatment and Prevention of Diabetes and Related Complications. *Diabetes Care* 2003 (Suppl 1): Vol 26, S51–S61.
5. Ha TKK, Lean MEJ. Technical review: recommendations for the nutritional management of patients with diabetes mellitus. *Eur J Clin Nutr* 1998; 52: 467–481.
6. Kris-Etherton PM, Pearson TA, Wan Y, Hargrove RL, Moriarty K, Fishell V, Etherton TD. High-monounsaturated fatty acid diets lower both plasma cholesterol and triacylglycerol concentrations. *Am Manual Clin Nutr* 1999; 70: 1009–1015.
7. Helmrich SP, Ragland DR, Leung RW, Paffenbarger RS. Physical activity and reduced occurrence of insulin dependent diabetes. *New Engl J Med* 1991; 324: 147–152.
8. Manson JE, Rimm EG, Stampfer MJ, Colditz GA, Willett WC, Krolewski AS, Rosner B, Hennekens CH, Speizer FE. Physical activity and incidence of non insulin dependent diabetes in women. *Lancet* 1991; 338: 774–778.
9. Schwartz RS. Exercise training in treatment of diabetes mellitus in elderly patients. *Diabetes Care* 1990; 13: 77–85.
10. Barnard RJ, Ugianskis EJ, Martin DA, Inkeles SB. Role of diet and exercise in the management of hyperinsulinaemia and associated atherosclerotic risk factors. *Am J Cardiol* 1992; 69: 440–444.
11. The Diabetes Control and Complications Trial Research Group. The effect of intensive treatment of diabetes on the development and progression of long-term complications in insulin-dependent diabetes mellitus. *New Engl J Med* 1993; 329: 977–986.

12. UK Prospective Diabetes Study (UKPDS) Group. Intensive blood glucose control with sulphonylureas or insulin compared with conventional treatment and risk of complications in patients with Type 2 diabetes (UKPDS 33). *Lancet* 1998; 352: 837–853.

13. Delahanty LM. Clinical significance of medical nutrition therapy in achieving diabetes outcomes and the importance of process. *J Am Diet Assoc* 1998; 98: 28–30.

14. UK Prospective Diabetes Study Group. Response of fasting plasma glucose to diet therapy in newly presenting Type 2 diabetic patients (UKPDS 7). *Metabolism* 1990; 39: 905–912.

15. Purnell B. The role of the dietitian in diabetes care. *Diabetes Primary Care* 1999; 1: 84–87.

16. Clinical Standards Advisory Group. *Standards of Clinical Care for People with Diabetes*. Report of a CSAG committee and the government response. London: HMSO, 1994.

17. Nutrition Subcommittee, British Diabetic Association. Survey of dietetic provision for patients with diabetes. *Diabetic Med* 2000; 17: 565–571.

18. British Diabetic Association. *Recommendations for the Structure of Specialist Diabetes Care*. London: BDA, 1999.

19. Miller WR, Rollnick S. (1991) *Motivational Interviewing*. Guilford Press, New York.

20. West KM. Diet therapy of diabetes: an analysis of failure. *Ann Intern Med* 1973; 79: 425–434.

21. Krotkiewski M, Bjorntorp P, Sjostrom L, Smith U. Impact of obesity on metabolism in men and women: importance of regional adipose tissue distribution. *J Clin Invest* 1983; 72: 1150–1162.

22. Lean MEJ, Powrie JK, Anderson AS *et al.* Obesity, weight loss and prognosis in Type 2 diabetes. *Diabetic Med* 1990; 7: 29–133.

23. Lean MEJ, James WPT. Prescription of diabetic diets in the 1980s. *Lancet* 1986; I: 723–725.

24. Frost G. Comparison of two methods of energy prescription for obese non-insulin dependent diabetics. *Pract Diabetes* 1989; 6: 273–275.

25. Uusitupa MIJ, Laaksok M, Sarlund H, Majander H, Takala J, Penttila I. Effects of a very low calorie diet on metabolic control and cardiovascular risk factors in the treatment of obese non insulin dependent diabetics. *Am J Clin Nutr* 1990; 51: 768–773.

26. Henry RR, Guumbiner B. Benefits and limitations of very low calorie diet therapy in obese NIDDM. *Diabetes Care* 1991; 14: 802–823.

27. Avenell A, Richmond PR, Lean MEJ, Reid DM Bone loss associated with a high fibre weight reduction diet in post menopausal women. *Eur J Clin Nutr* 1994; 48: 561–566.

28. Report by the Royal College of Physicians of London. Clinical management of overweight and obese patients with particular reference to the use of drugs. *J R Coll Physicians London* 1999; 33: 1.

29. Golstein DJ. Beneficial health effects of modest weight loss. *Int J Obes* 1992; 16: 397–415.

30. Riccardi G, Rivellese A, Pacioni D, Genovese S, Mastanzo P, Mancini M. Separate influence of dietary carbohydrate and fibre on the metabolic control in diabetes. *Diabetologia* 1984; 26: 116–121.

31. Jenkins DJA, Wolever TMS, Taylor RH, Barker H, Fielden H, Baldwin JM, Bowling AC, Newman HC, Jenkins AL, Goff DV. Glycaemic index of foods. A physiological basis for carbohydrate exchange. *Am J Clin Nutr* 1981; 34: 362–366.

32. Hermansen K. Research methodologies in the evaluation of intestinal glucose absorption and the concept of glycaemic index. In: *Research Methodologies in Human Diabetes*, eds CE Morgensen and R Stahdl. Berlin: Walter de Gruyter, 1994: 205–218.
33. Salmeron J, Ascherio A, Rimm EB, Colditz GA, Spiegelman D, Jenkins DJ, Stamper MJ, Wing AL, Willet WC. Dietary fibre, glycaemic load and risk of NIDDM in men. *Diabetes Care* 1997; 20: 545–550.
34. Aro A, Uustitupa M, Voutilainen E, Hersio K, Korhoren T, Siitoner O. Improved diabetic control and hypercholesterolaemia effect induced by long term supplementation with guar in Type 2 diabetes. *Diabetologia* 1981; 20: 29–33.
35. Slama G, Jean-Joseph P, Goicolea I, Elgrably F, Haardt MJ, Costagliola D, Bornet F, Tchobroutsky G. Sucrose taken during a mixed meal has no additional hyperglycaemic action over iso-caloric amounts of starch in well-controlled diabetics. *Lancet* 1984; 2(8395): 122–125.
36. Mann JL, Truswell AS, Pimstone BL. The different effects of oral sucrose and glucose on alimentary lipaemia. *Clin Sci* 1971; 41: 123–129.
37. Anderson JW, Story LJ, Zettwoch NC, Gustafson NJ, Jefferson BS. Metabolic effects of fructose supplementation in diabetic individuals. *Diabetes Care* 1989; 12: 337–344.
38. Born P, Eimiller A, Paul F. High rate of gastrointestinal side effects in fructose consuming patients. *Diabetes Care* 1987; 10: 376–377.
39. Connor H, Marks V. Alcohol and Diabetes. *Diabetic Med* 1985; 2: 413–416.
40. Department of Health. (1995) *Sensible Drinking: the report of an inter-departmental working group*. London: Department of Health.
41. Lieber CS. Alcohol and the liver. *Gastroenterology* 1994; 106: 1085–1105.
42. Arky RA, Veverbrants E, Abramson EA. Irreversible hypoglycaemia: a complication of alcohol and insulin. *J Am Med Assoc* 1968; 206: 575–578.
43. Christansen C, Thomsen C, Rasmussen O, Glerup H, Bertelsen J, Hansen C, Orskov H, Hermansen K. Acute effects of graded alcohol intake on glucose, insulin and FFA levels in NIDDM subjects. *Eur J Clin Nutr* 1993; 47: 648–652.
44. Gronbaek M, Deis A, Sorensen TA, Bedier U, Schriohr P, Jensen G. Mortality associated with moderate intakes of wine, beer or spirits *Br Med J* 1995; 310: 1165–1169.
45. Stamler J, Vaccaro O, Neaton JD, Wentworth D. Diabetes, other risk factors, and 12-year cardiovascular mortality for men screened in the multiple risk factor intervention trial. *Diabetes Care* 1993; 16: 434–475.
46. Uusitupa MI, Niskanen LK, Siitonen O, Voutilainen E, Pyorala K. Ten year cardiovascular mortality in relation to risk factors and abnormalities in lipoprotein composition in type 2 (non insulin dependent) diabetic and non-diabetic subjects. *Diabetologia* 1993; 36: 1175–1184.
47. Laker M. Plasma lipids and lipoproteins in diabetes mellitus. *Diabetes Annual 3*, eds KGMM Alberti and L Krall. Amsterdam: Elsevier, 1987: 459–478.
48. Mensink RP, Zock PL, Katan MB, Hornstra G. Effect of dietary cis and trans fatty acids on serum lipoprotein (a) levels in humans. *J Lipid Res* 1992; 33: 1493–1501.
49. Willett WC, Stampfer MJ, Manson JE, Colditz GA, Speizer FE, Rosner BA, Sampson LA, Hennekens CH. Intake of trans fatty acids and risk of coronary heart disease among women. *Lancet* 1993; 341(8852): 1093–1094.
50. Aro A, Kardinaal AF, Salminen I, Kark JD, Riemersma RA, Delgado-Rodriguez M, Gomez-Aracena J, Huttunen JK, Kohlmeier L, Martin BC *et al*. Adipose tissue isomeric trans fatty acids and risk of myocardial infarction in nine countries: the EURAMIC study. *Lancet* 1995; 345 (8945): 273–278.

51. Mori TA, Vandongen R, Masarei JRL. Fish oil-induced changes in apolipoproteins in IDDM subjects. *Diabetes Care* 1990; 14: 725–732.
52. Appel LJ, Miller ER, Seidler AJ, Whelton PK. Does supplementation of diet with fish oil reduce blood pressure? A meta-analysis of controlled clinical trials. *Arch Intern Med* 1989; 153: 1429–1438.
53. Ascherio A, Rimm EB, Stampfer MJ, Giovannucci EL, Willett WC. Dietary intake of marine n-3 fatty acids, fish intake and the risk of coronary disease among men. *New Engl J Med* 1995; 332: 977–982.
54. Keys A, Menotti A, Karvonen MJ, Aravanis C, Blackburn H, Buzina R, Djordjevic BS, Dontas AS, Findanza F, Keys MH. The diet and death rate in the 7 countries study. *Am J Epidemiol* 1986; 124: 903–915.
55. WHO. *Energy and Protein Requirements.* WHO Technical Report Series 724. Geneva: World Health Organization, 1985.
56. Kupin WL, Cortes P, Dumler F, Feldkamp CS, Kilates MC, Levin NW. Effects on renal function of change from high to moderate protein intake in type 1 diabetic patients. *Diabetes* 1987; 36: 73–79.
57. Viberti GC. Low protein diet and progression of diabetic kidney disease. *Nephrol Dial Transplant* 1988; 3: 334–339.
58. Zeller KR, Katan MB. Low protein diets in renal disease. *Diabetes Care* 1991; 14: 856–866.
59. Dodson PM, Beevers M, Hallworth R, Webberley MJ, Fletchier RF, Taylor KG. Sodium restriction and blood pressure in hypertensive type 2 diabetics. *Br Med J* 1989; 298: 227–230.
60. Anderson RA. Chromium in the prevention and control of diabetes. *Diabetes Metab* 2000; 26: 22–27.

2

Diabetes and Physical Activity

PAMELA DYSON
Oxford Centre for Diabetes, Endocrinology and Metabolism, Oxford, UK

INTRODUCTION

It is now widely accepted that increasing physical activity leads to great health benefits whether or not people have diabetes (1). Increased physical activity has been associated with physical, mental and social benefits including the following:

- Reduction in all-cause mortality (2,3).
- Reduction in cardiovascular disease (CVD) including coronary heart disease (CHD), stroke and heart attack (4).
- Blood pressure reduction (5).
- Improved weight loss in the obese and weight maintenance in those of normal weight (6).
- Prevention of Type 2 diabetes and improved glycaemic control (7–10).
- Prevention of osteoporosis (11).
- Improved flexibility and strength (12).
- Increased self-esteem and confidence (13).

These benefits apply to all people whether they have diabetes or not, but the benefits of improved glycaemic control are especially appropriate to people with diabetes. In addition, a reduction in the incidence of CVD and the positive effect on body weight associated with physical activity can only benefit the health of people with diabetes.

Nutritional Management of Diabetes Mellitus. Edited by G. Frost, A. Dornhorst and R. Moses
© 2003 John Wiley & Sons, Ltd. ISBN 0 471 49751 7

PREVENTION OF TYPE 2 DIABETES

There is now unequivocal evidence that physically fit people are less likely to develop Type 2 diabetes and some intervention trials have shown that encouraging people with impaired glucose tolerance (IGT) to increase their physical activity significantly reduces their risk of developing diabetes (14–16). This benefit is independent of body mass index (BMI) and there is some evidence that physical activity has a greater protective effect as BMI increases (17). It may be of more importance for people at risk of Type 2 diabetes to increase their physical fitness rather than concentrate on weight reduction.

GLYCAEMIC CONTROL

The benefits associated with improved glycaemic control are related to changes in insulin sensitivity, and are more pronounced in people who have Type 2 diabetes (18) or who are overweight (19). For many people with Type 1 diabetes, who do not exhibit insulin resistance, the main benefits of exercise may be related to improvements in dyslipidaemia, enhanced cardiovascular function and blood pressure reduction (10).

CARDIOVASCULAR RISK FACTORS

The role of exercise and the prevention of coronary heart disease in the general population have been well documented, but there is less evidence of a similar effect in people with diabetes. Modification of risk factors for CHD, including decreased total and LDL (low-density lipoprotein) cholesterol and triglyceride concentrations, have been demonstrated in Type 1 diabetes (20). People with Type 2 diabetes have two to four times the cardiovascular risk of those without diabetes and low cardiorespiratory fitness has been shown to be a predictor of mortality in men with diabetes (21).

BODY WEIGHT MANAGEMENT

Physical activity has a role in weight reduction and aids weight maintenance in those of normal weight. As 80% of people with Type 2 diabetes are overweight, most individuals would benefit from weight reduction.

EXERCISE AND DIABETES

Despite the widespread beliefs of the benefits of physical activity and the promotion of exercise by many health professionals, people with diabetes are reluctant to increase their physical activity (22). This is not restricted to those with diabetes as it applies to the British population as a whole. A UK study in 1990 showed that only 15–30% of British adults are taking sufficient exercise for optimum health and that there is a large discrepancy between people's perception of their fitness and the amount of exercise they actually take (23). A recent Canadian study has shown that while 84% of people with diabetes thought they should be exercising, only 45% were actually doing so (24). Against this background of reluctance to exercise there is also a lack of knowledge of the physiology of exercise. In order to maximise the advice given to people with diabetes who wish to increase their physical activity, it is essential to gain an understanding of the physiology of physical activity, exercise and sport.

PHYSICAL ACTIVITY, EXERCISE AND SPORT

DEFINITIONS

Physical activity refers to any body movement made by the skeletal muscles and resulting in energy expenditure, e.g. walking, gardening, housework.

Exercise is planned, structured repetitive body movements usually taken as a leisure time pursuit, e.g. aerobics, jogging, swimming.

Sport is physical activity which involves competitive situations which are usually governed by rules, e.g. football, rugby, netball.

The effects of physical activity programmes depend upon the intensity, frequency and duration of exercise.

INTENSITY

Physical activity, exercise and sport can all be classified as either light, moderate or vigorous.

Light activities require little exertion and do not cause a significant change in breathing.

Moderate activities require sustained muscular movements and will result in heavier breathing and a feeling of warmth.

Vigorous activities require sustained muscular movements and result in a feeling of being sweaty or out of breath.

Examples of different activities and their intensity are shown in Table 2.1.

Table 2.1 Intensity of various activities

Intensity of activity	Examples
Light	Slow walking, light gardening (weeding, mowing with power mower), light housework (dusting, hoovering), light DIY (decorating), bowls, golf, snooker
Moderate	Brisk walking, heavy housework (scrubbing, spring cleaning), heavy gardening (digging), heavy DIY (sawing, mixing cement), football, tennis, cycling, swimming, aerobics, all at a level to produce some breathlessness and a feeling of warmth, working as a labourer, roofer or refuse collector
Vigorous	Sport and exercise at a level to induce sweating and breathlessness, e.g. squash, running, football, rugby, swimming, tennis, aerobics, cycling, gym work, any work or occupation involving frequent climbing, lifting, carrying, e.g. mining, forestry

FREQUENCY AND DURATION

The exercise guidelines issued by the American College of Sports Medicine (ACSM) in 1978 recommend at least three sessions of 20–40 min of vigorous activity each week. This was revised in 1990 and 30 min of moderate activity daily is now recommended (25).

In 1994, the UK Health Education Authority (HEA) adopted an international consensus statement and recommended the following:

moderate intensity activity;
of 30 minutes duration or more;
at a frequency of 5 or more days each week (1).

The majority of research has concentrated upon the effect of physical activity on CHD rates and as a result the emphasis has been on increasing aerobic or vigorous activity. Recent research has shown the benefit of moderate activity and for many people with diabetes the greatest health benefit may be in changing from a sedentary lifestyle to a moderately active lifestyle (26).

PHYSIOLOGY OF EXERCISE

In people without diabetes, a precise endocrine response ensures that the energy needs of the exercising muscle are met and glucose homeostasis is maintained. This metabolic response is ameliorated in Type 2 diabetes and lost in Type 1 diabetes and the challenge is to reproduce the physiological state of the non-diabetic individual. A brief review of the metabolic, hormonal and physiological responses to exercise is given below.

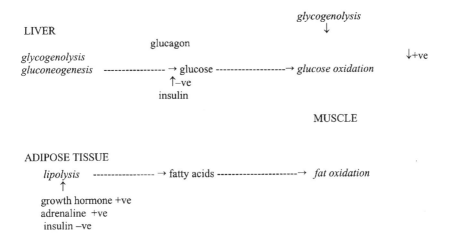

Figure 2.1

Metabolic changes provide the energy required for exercise. Glucose uptake by exercising muscle increases and at the onset of exercise, muscle glycogen is converted to lactate to provide the energy substrate. When muscle glycogen is exhausted, energy is provided by glucose from the liver following glycogenolysis and eventually from metabolism of free fatty acids in adipose tissue. The metabolic response depends on a number of factors:

- *Intensity and duration of exercise.* High intensity/short duration of exercise, e.g. sprinting, will utilise carbohydrate (glycogen) as energy substrate and low intensity/long duration, e.g. marathon running, will utilise carbohydrate (glycogen) initially, but predominately fat (FFA).
- *Exercise timing.* The amount of available glucose will depend upon whether exercise is taken in the fasting or post-prandial state.
- *Level of fitness.* Athletes who train for endurance events show reduced rates of glycogen breakdown and are able to utilise FFA more efficiently.
- *Dietary intake.* The amount and type of carbohydrate consumed routinely and pre- and post-events will affect performance.

Hormonal responses to exercise are characterised by the action of insulin and its counter regulatory hormones glucagon, cortisol and catecholamines. The key response to exercise is the suppression of insulin secretion, accompanied by a rise in catabolic hormones (Figure 2.1). This stimulates release of glucose from the liver and FFA from adipose tissue and maintains energy levels during exercise.

Physiological responses are shown by the increased heart rate, stroke volume and cardiac output which accompanies exercise and which facilitates increased oxygen delivery and removal of carbon dioxide.

At the end of a period of exercise, recovery takes place as hormone concentrations return to their pre-exercise levels and glycogen stores are replenished. There is continued oxidation of fat, which limits the use of glucose as an energy substrate and allows replenishment of liver and muscle glycogen. Muscle uptake of glucose is enhanced through increased glucose transporters (GLUT-4) and this process of glycogen storage can last up to 12–18 h after exercise. The speed of this process depends upon the type and duration of exercise.

People with Type 2 diabetes usually have sufficient circulating insulin to precipitate the normal metabolic response to exercise and any risk of hypoglycaemia is associated with the use of either insulin or oral hypoglycaemic agents.

People with Type 1 diabetes depend upon exogenous supplies of insulin and any exercise may pose some risk of hypoglycaemia. When a person with Type 1 exercises with too little insulin the counter-regulatory hormonal response may elevate both circulating glucose and ketone levels. On the other hand, too much insulin increases the risk of hypoglycaemia by blocking the exercise-induced increase in glycogenolysis and gluconeognesis. The risk of hypoglycaemia can continue for 6–14 h after strenuous exercise as glucose is synthesised to replace lost glycogen stores and insulin sensitivity is increased during the recovery period.

Advice to people with diabetes who wish to increase their physical activity or improve performance will cover the whole range of activities from a gentle stroll to competing at the top level. Advice should take into consideration the following:

- Perceptions and beliefs
- Type, intensity, frequency and duration of exercise
- Medication
- Contraindications to exercise
- Dietary intake

Perceptions and beliefs

Barriers to increasing physical activity include time constraints, usually linked to domestic or work commitments, health status, age, performance expectations and lack of will power. The emphasis should be on adapting advice to fit in with the individual's lifestyle and avoiding prescriptive advice, which may fail to address the individual's perceptions and beliefs.

People with Type 2 diabetes who wish to increase their levels of general activity will need encouragement, motivation and the choice of a physical activity or sport which matches their individual needs. For the majority of this middle-aged sedentary population, an increase in gentle exercise, e.g. walking, can be safely recommended. Exercise at this level has been shown to have health benefits for people with Type 2 diabetes (27). It is feasible for people with Type 2 to increase physical activity at a higher intensity, but recommendations should include checking with their physician before beginning a programme of vigorous exercise and exercising under supervision.

Type, Intensity, Frequency and Duration

Advice to people with diabetes will depend upon the type of exercise they wish to do. Gentle exercise at light or moderate intensity does not place the same demands upon diabetes management as that caused by vigorous exercise. People with Type 1 diabetes may be at risk of hypoglycaemia and it is important to consider the effect of the type, intensity, frequency and duration of exercise and its effect on blood glucose. Timing of meals and sessions of physical activity should be planned wherever possible and exercise should avoid the peak action of insulin as this has been shown to precipitate hypoglycaemia. The majority of people with Type 1 who take exercise find that they may have to adjust their insulin, their carbohydrate intake or a combination of both. People who are taking part in competitive sports or who wish to take part in endurance races or increase their activity to a vigorous level are strongly recommended to consult a specialist diabetes professional.

Medication

People with Type 2 diabetes who are controlled by diet alone, or who take metformin or acarbose, are able to exercise without risk of hypoglycaemia. They do not need to make any adjustment to their medication when increasing physical activity. Those taking insulin or oral hypoglycaemic agents will need to time exercise sessions to avoid peak action of agents and may need to take extra carbohydrate during training to prevent hypoglycaemia. It is difficult to adjust insulin for exercise in people taking an insulin mixture twice daily and in Type 2 diabetes this is further complicated by an inability to measure accurately insulin resistance. Because of the action of increasing insulin sensitivity, people with Type 2 diabetes who increase their physical activity may find that their insulin requirements decrease over time and that they may need less insulin. This is best measured on an individual basis and should be monitored by frequent blood glucose tests.

People with Type 1 diabetes will need to plan ahead for exercise and make appropriate insulin adjustment. One study has shown that moderately intensive exercise sessions lasting 45 min can lead to hypoglycaemia and this was effectively overcome by a reduction in insulin by 30–50% before exercise (28). The effects of exercise are mediated by the timing of exercise (pre- or post-prandial) and the blood glucose levels at the start of exercise. It is impossible to formulate precise guidelines for insulin adjustment for those with Type 1 wishing to exercise, but consultation and experimentation accompanied by frequent blood glucose tests can help to identify the most effective strategies in individuals with Type 1 diabetes.

The absorption of insulin injected subcutaneously can be accelerated by exercise and may precipitate hypoglycaemia. To prevent this, it is advised that insulin is injected away from the site of exercising muscle, e.g. into the abdomen in the case of runners and cyclists, and that exercise does not take place at the time of peak insulin action.

Contraindications to Exercise

Although the health benefits of exercise are well established, there are certain areas where caution must be observed. Encouragement to increase physical activity for people with diabetes will be affected by some underlying features and physical exercise is not without risk in diabetes. All people with diabetes are advised to have a medical examination prior to beginning an exercise programme to identify any complications which may be adversely affected by exercise. Those wishing to take part in strenuous activity will find the following are relative contraindications: poor glycaemic control, the presence of ketones, proliferative retinopathy, microangiopathy, neuropathy, nephropathy and cardiovascular disease. Although strenuous activity may be contraindicated, some individuals may be able to increase general everyday physical activity.

Practical implications of increasing physical activity include consideration of possible damage to the soft tissues and joints, especially in the feet, and it is recommended that those with diabetes consult a podiatrist and purchase good, supportive footwear.

Precipitation of cardiac events is possible, especially in those with Type 2 diabetes, and exercise should not be encouraged without giving the following guidelines: avoid irregular, strenuous exercise, do not exercise when unwell and stop exercise immediately if any pain, especially chest pain, is experienced. It is also important to warm up and cool down thoroughly before and after exercise sessions.

DIETARY ADVICE FOR EXERCISE

PRACTICAL MANAGEMENT

Dietary advice to people with diabetes wishing to increase physical activity is individual and will depend upon many factors including medication, type, frequency and duration of exercise and for many people it is a process of experimentation. For those taking insulin, there is more than one way to regulate blood sugar levels during exercise either by reducing insulin, increasing carbohydrate intake or a combination of the two. Advice should be tailored to the individual depending upon the following:

- Dietary intake
- Insulin regime
- Blood glucose levels
- Type of activity
- Timing of activity

Dietary Intake

It is now universally accepted that the best diet for maximising exercise tolerance and performance is one that is high in carbohydrate (50–60% energy from carbohydrate). Athletes routinely use high-carbohydrate diets when training. The Diabetes UK recommendations for all people with diabetes encourage a high-carbohydrate diet and this should apply whether people are exercising or not. This diet should help protect against the risk of hypoglycaemia during periods of increased physical activity.

There is some discussion about the type and amount of carbohydrate. The glycaemic index (GI) of carbohydrate foods has been shown to be a useful tool in maximising performance in athletes and sportsmen and women and there may be a role for it in people with diabetes who exercise at a strenuous level for more than 60 min (29). It is recommended that low GI foods are consumed at the meal or snack before exercise takes place and that high GI foods are consumed during endurance events and after exercise to replenish glycogen stores. Examples of low GI foods, which can be eaten before an exercise session and high GI foods/drinks, which can be taken during or after an event, are given in Table 2.2.

Table 2.2 Examples of high and low GI carbohydrate foods

GI	Examples of food	Timing
Low	Pasta, Basmati rice, couscous, instant noodles, barley, wholegrain products, porridge, muesli, All-Bran, oat-based cereal bars, lentils and pulses including baked beans, chick peas and kidney beans, dried apricots	2–3 h before exercise, especially endurance events
High	Isotonic sports drinks, fruit juice, ordinary squash, jelly beans, ripe bananas, honey sandwich	During an exercise session (if required)
High	Corn Flakes, Rice Krispies, sugared cereals, white bread, rice (other than Basmati), potatoes	Within 30–60 mins of completing an exercise session

It is recommended that people with diabetes eat before exercising and that they should exercise approximately 3 h after a large meal to ensure digestion and absorption of food. Additional carbohydrate may be needed immediately before exercise, during exercise and after exercise to replenish glycogen stores. The amount of carbohydrate will depend upon blood glucose levels.

Intake of sufficient fluid should be advised to avoid dehydration. Water, sugar-free squashes and sugar-free sports drinks are suitable for rehydration if fluid only is required. Fruit juice, ordinary squash and isotonic sports drinks are useful for replenishing fluid and carbohydrate. Hypertonic drinks, e.g. Lucozade, are not suitable for rehydration and should be used only to treat hypoglycaemia. Fizzy drinks and sodas may cause problems with bloating and wind and are best avoided.

Insulin Regime

For those who are on a basal/prandial regimen it may be necessary to reduce insulin by 30–50% before strenuous activity. Extra carbohydrate should be taken when engaging in unplanned activity where it is impossible to reduce insulin. It is advisable that people avoid periods of strenuous physical activity when short-acting insulin is peaking, i.e. within 2 h of use. People with Type 1 diabetes may find they can reduce their insulin after an endurance event, e.g. marathon running, and that it may take several days before they return to their pre-race insulin dose. This process should be supported by frequent blood glucose tests.

Blood Glucose Levels

It is recommended that people with diabetes monitor their blood glucose levels before, during and after exercise. Optimum blood glucose levels are those between 6–13 mmol/l before exercise begins. If blood glucose levels are < 6 mmol/l, people should be advised to take some carbohydrate with a high glycaemic index, e.g. isotonic sports drinks, ripe bananas. If blood glucose levels are above 13 mmol/l, then exercise should be delayed until blood glucose falls to the acceptable levels. If blood glucose drops below 5 mmol/l during exercise, fast-acting carbohydrate should be taken immediately to prevent hypoglycaemia.

Type of Activity

The amount of carbohydrate to be taken during exercise depends upon the type of activity. People with Type 2 diabetes who are increasing physical activity at low/moderate intensity by going for a walk often need to make no change to their medication or dietary intake. However, if they take insulin and are planning on taking up strenuous exercise, they may need to reduce their insulin dose. As they become physically fitter, insulin sensitivity will improve and overall insulin requirements may decrease. This can be judged by frequent blood glucose monitoring.

People with Type 1 diabetes are unlikely to require extra carbohydrate if blood glucose levels are above 10 mmol/l at the start of exercise and if they are taking part in light or moderate activity for 20–30 min. During moderate activity lasting 30–60 min, an additional 10–20 g carbohydrate may be required. During strenuous activity lasting 30–60 min, an extra 30–50 g carbohydrate may be required. A general rule of thumb is that 10–20 g carbohydrate should be taken every 30 min during moderate or strenuous exercise lasting more than 30 min.

Timing of Activity

It is important to consider the timing of exercise or physical activity sessions in order to reduce the risk of hypoglycaemia. For those taking oral hypogly-caemic agents exercise should be avoided at high-risk times, e.g. immediately before the mid-day meal. For those taking insulin, exercise should be avoided at peak action of short-acting insulin. The risk of hypoglycaemia appears to be lowest if exercise is taken in the morning, before taking any insulin or food. Conversely, late afternoon or early evening exercise may increase the risk of late hypoglycaemia during the night. The adjustment of diet and insulin for exercise is facilitated if the timing of exercise from day to day is consistent.

Summary of advice for people with diabetes wishing to exercise

Before exercise:

- Monitor blood glucose regularly – before, during and after exercise.
- Eat a low GI meal 2–3 h before an endurance event.
- Reduce insulin by 30–50% for strenuous or endurance training.
- Optimum blood glucose levels are 6–13 mmol/l.
- If blood glucose < 6 mmol/l, take 10–20 g fast-acting carbohydrate.
- If blood glucose > 13 mmol/l, delay exercise.

During exercise:

- 20–30 min of light/moderate activity should not require extra carbohydrate.
- 30–60 min of moderate activity may require an extra 10–20 g high GI carbohydrate.
- 30–60 min of strenuous activity may require an extra 30–50 g high GI carbohydrate.

- Endurance training may require an additional 10–20 g high GI carbohydrate for each 30 min of exercise.
- Remember to consume adequate fluid to prevent dehydration.

After exercise:

Replenish glycogen stores by consuming high GI carbohydrate-rich foods within 30–60 min of exercise. After endurance training, e.g. marathon running, cycling, monitor blood glucose levels, replenish glycogen stores with high GI carbohydrate and adjust insulin accordingly.

REFERENCES

1. Health Education Authority. *Health Update 5. Physical Activity*. London: Health Education Authority 1995.
2. Paffenbarger RS Jr, Hyde RT, Wing AL, Hsieh CC. Physical activity, all-cause mortality and longevity of college alumni. *New Engl J Med* 1986; 314: 605–613.
3. Paffenbarger RS Jr, Hyde RT, Wing AL, Lee IM, Jung DL, Kampert JB. The association of changes in physical activity levels and other lifestyle characteristics with mortality among men. *New Engl J Med* 1993; 328: 538–545.
4. Morris JN. The role of exercise in the prevention of coronary heart disease: today's best buy in public health. *Med Sci Sport Ex* 1994; 26: 807–813.
5. Fagard RH. Physical fitness and blood pressure. *J Hypertens* 1993; 11 Suppl 5: S47–S52.
6. Garrow J, Summerball C. Meta-analysis: effect of exercise, with and without dieting, on the body composition of overweight subjects. *Eur J Clin Nutr* 1995; 49: 1–10.
7. Manson JE, Rimm EB, Stampfer HJ, Colditz GA, Willett EC *et al*. Physical activity and incidence of non-insulin-dependent diabetes mellitus in women. *Lancet* 1991; 338: 774–778.
8. Helmrich SP, Ragland DR, Leung RW and Paffenbarger RS Jr. Physical activity and reduced occurrence of non-insulin-dependent diabetes. *New Engl J Med* 1991; 325: 147–152.
9. Wei M, Gibbons LW, Mitchell TL, Kampert JB, Lee CD, Blair SN. The association between cardiorespiratory fitness and impaired fasting glucose and Type 2 diabetes mellitus in men. *Ann Intern Med* 1999; 130: 89–96.
10. Pierce NS. Diabetes and exercise. *Br J Sports Med* 1999; 33: 161–172.
11. Wolman R. Osteoporosis and exercise. *Br Med J* 1994; 309: 400–403.
12. Young A, Dinan S. Fitness for older people. *Br Med J* 1994; 309: 331–333.
13. MacAuley E. Physical activity and psychosocial outcomes. In: *Physical Activity, Fitness and Health; International Proceedings and Consensus Statement*, ed. C Bouchard. Human Kinetics Publishers Inc., 1994.
14. Pan XR, Li GW, Hu YH, Wang WY, An ZW *et al*. Effects of diet and exercise in preventing NIDDM in people with impaired glucose tolerance. *Diabetes Care* 1997; 20: 537–544.

15. Bourn DM. The potential for lifestyle change to influence the progression of impaired glucose tolerance to non-insulin-dependent diabetes mellitus. *Diabet Med* 1996; 13: 938–945.
16. Eriksson J, Lindstrom J, Valle T, Aunola S, Hamalainen H *et al.* Prevention of Type 2 diabetes in subjects with impaired glucose tolerance: The Diabetes Prevention Study (DPS) in Finland. *Diabetologia* 1999; 42: 793–801.
17. Sato Y. Diabetes and life-styles: role of physical exercise in primary prevention. *Br J Nutr* 2000; 84: S187–S190.
18. Braun B, Zimmerman MB, Kretchmer M. Effects of exercise on insulin sensitivity in women with non-insulin-dependent diabetes mellitus. *J Appl Physiol* 1995; 78: 300–306.
19. Rice B, Janssen I, Hudson R, Ross R. Effects of aerobic or resistance exercise and/or diet on glucose tolerance and plasma insulin levels in obese men. *Diabetes Care* 1999; 22: 684–691.
20. Wasserman DH, Zinman B. Exercise in individuals with IDDM. *Diabetes Care* 1994; 8: 924–937.
21. Wei M, Gibbons FW, Kampert JB, Nichaman MZ, Blair SB. Low cardiorespiratory fitness and physical activity as predictors of mortality in men with Type 2 diabetes. *Ann Intern Med* 2000; 132: 605–611.
22. Hays LM, Clark DO. Correlates of physical activity in a sample of older adults with Type 2 diabetes. *Diabetes Care* 1999; 22: 706–712.
23. Health Education Authority and Sports Council. *Allied Dunbar National Fitness Survey: Main Findings.* London: Sports Council and HEA, 1992.
24. Plotnikoff RC, Brez S, Hotz SB. Exercise behavior in a community sample with diabetes: understanding the determinants of exercise behavioral change. *Diabetes Educ* 2000; 26: 450–459.
25. American College of Sports Medicine. The recommended quantity and quality of exercise for developing and maintaining cardiorespiratory and muscular fitness in healthy adults. *Med Sci Sports Ex* 1990; 22: 265–274.
26. Hu FB, Sigal RJ, Rich-Edwards JW, Colditz JA, Solomon CG *et al.* Walking compared with vigorous physical activity and Type 2 diabetes in women. *J Am Med Assoc* 1999; 282: 1433–1439.
27. Yamanouchi K, Shinozaki T, Chikada K, Nishikawa T, Ito K *et al.* Daily walking combined with diet therapy is a useful means for obese NIDDM patients to not only reduce body weight but also to improve insulin sensitivity. *Diabetes Care* 1995; 18: 775–778.
28. Schiffrin A, Pankh S. Accommodating planned exercise in Type 1 diabetic patients on intensive treatment. *Diabetes Care* 1985; 8: 337–343.
29 Leeds A, Brand Miller J, Foster-Powell K and Colagiri S. *The Glucose Revolution.* London: Hodder and Stoughton 2000.

3

Counselling in Diabetes

TRACEY PARKIN
Queen Alexandra Hospital, Portsmouth, UK

INTRODUCTION

The day-to-day management of diabetes includes appropriate use of medication, monitoring of blood or urine glucose levels and lifestyle issues such as exercise and diet. These self-care behaviours are all determined by the patient. Effectiveness of treatment will therefore be limited by the patient's actions.

The current culture of patient training tends to be strongly influenced by the medical model, an issue that was first raised in dietetic training in 1987. Evidence highlighted dissatisfaction with this method and non-compliance [1]. This predominant style is still often used by both dietitians and other health professionals to advise patients on diet. This model assumes that patients are ready and motivated to change because a credible professional has told them to. The traditional educational strategies employed have relied on the health professional's perception of what the patient with diabetes needs to know. A didactic process of persuasion is then entered into, in which the health professional attempts to persuade the patient to change his or her diet. The conversation is one-sided and based on information gathering to help the health care professional determine what the patient needs to be told to do. In practice this method of communication is only likely to work for a small number of patients, and this type of expert-led, confrontational counselling style could lead to resistance and a poor outcome [2,3].

Information overload is another common practice, and relates to the fear that the patient may not attend another session and hence must be given all the

Nutritional Management of Diabetes Mellitus. Edited by G. Frost, A. Dornhorst and R. Moses
© 2003 John Wiley & Sons, Ltd. ISBN 0 471 49751 7

information necessary in case this occurs. By doing this however there is a real danger of overloading the patient with information and thus demotivating them with the sheer volume of change that is required (4). It also carries the risk that the health care professional's own health beliefs and priorities will be involved in the changes dictated. This is unrealistic and counterproductive as patients' concerns are very different from those of health professionals, and unless we take these into account we will fail to meet their needs (5). The end result is frustration both on the part of the health care professional, who labels the patient as non-compliant or a failure, and on the part of the patient, who feels their needs are not being met (6).

The way we deliver our message therefore needs to change. If something is not working it is clearly ineffective to continue to practise in the same way. Most studies tend to review knowledge as an outcome, but there is ample evidence to indicate that although essential, knowledge alone is not sufficient to change behaviour or establish healthy eating (2,7–9). The information-giving and instructional aspects of dietary counselling must therefore be extended to incorporate motivational and behavioural components (9,10).

Reviews of available data on educational and psychosocial interventions for adults with diabetes, and other chronic illnesses, indicate that a 'patient-centred' approach is more effective in enhancing patient communication and their subsequent health (11–13). For example, interventions designed to increase patient participation and autonomy have resulted in improvements in self-care behaviour and glycosolated haemoglobin (HbA$_{1c}$) (14,15). Some studies however fail to clearly define what is meant by 'patient-centredness'. In diabetes care we can take the definition of 'patient-centredness' to mean a process that involves the health care professional being open and responsive to the concerns and needs of patients, including needs for information and participation in decision making (16). This definition encompasses the basis of the majority of counselling models currently used in behaviour change for diabetes care.

It has long been recognised that changing behaviour takes more than a directive approach of telling people what to do. Whole person care is important, and this involves identifying psychological issues which may influence how patients respond to the disease and its treatment. By identifying these issues we can help patients to find ways of coping more effectively with their diabetes. The ultimate aim is to improve the level of knowledge and health locus of control of the patient, as well as trying to help develop a positive attitude to active self-care (17). Not everyone with diabetes will require formal counselling, but exposure to the theories and ideas behind counselling can help everyday diabetes education (18,19).

To practise, we require a range of skills, which involve being able to give information where appropriate, teaching, counselling and advising (20). To practise effectively we must also review our basic skills in communication,

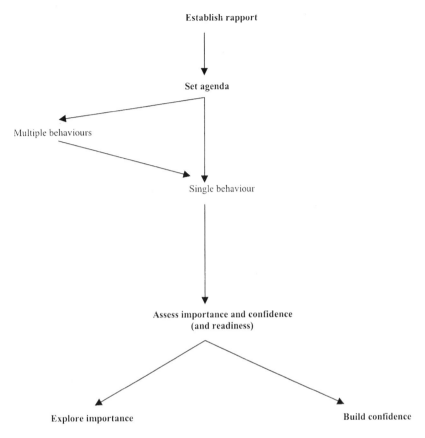

Figure 3.1 Key stages in the consultation
Reproduced from Rollnick *et al.* (21), p. 12.

although this would appear to be fundamental as it underpins the majority of the work that we do.

Key stages in the consultation are outlined in Figure 3.1.

ESTABLISH RAPPORT

The discussion should begin with open questions to get patients talking, and is an ideal opportunity to find out what it is they want to know and what they expect from the health care professional. Questions should begin with words like how, what and could you/can you. For example, *'How did you feel when you were told that you had diabetes?'*, *'What concerns you most about your diabetes?'*. Avoid phrases including words such as 'difficulties', 'problems' and 'help' as this implies that you perceive them as having problems when this may not be the way that they see things themselves. Closed questions require a yes or no response; they can be used once discussion has been initiated and are a useful way of checking your understanding of the conversation. *'Did you say that you have tried that diet five times before?'* Another useful opener to establish rapport would be to use a typical day (21). For example, *'Can you take me through a typical day in your life, so that I can understand in more detail what happens?'* or *'Can you think of a recent typical day? Take me through this from beginning to end'*.

Active listening is an essential skill for this process of communication and counselling to work effectively. It is hard work, as it includes attending to your own non-verbal and verbal behaviour as well as that of your patient. It uses minimal encouragements such as mmm's, aah's, nods and varying degrees of eye contact to encourage people to continue and to let them know that you are listening. Silence can be one of the most useful tools in this arsenal, but for many it proves to be difficult, as the urge to speak and fill the silence is so great. This is a greatly missed opportunity, as it allows patients time to collect their thoughts for a response rather than having them hijacked with your ideas or solutions. This can be very premature as you may not fully understand the real dilemma for the patient. Silence has long been noted to be a difficult tool for health providers, Rollnick *et al.* (21) suggest saying a rhyme to yourself to allow that passage of time before the patient speaks. Silence enables a period of reflection on what has passed and a guide to the direction of the conversation so far, and therefore helps you and the patient move forward.

Once a rapport has been established reflect back comments both to show that you are listening and to check that you have correctly understood what the patient is trying to say. A simple reflection could be *'You've tried many diets then'*.

Paraphrasing is another method to use, and is a way of summing up the essence of the conversation and providing more concrete information than simple reflection. It conveys to patients that you are with them, crystallises comments, checks accuracy and gives direction. It is aimed more at content rather than feeling. *'It sounds as if you have tried lots of diets in the past, one of which you found particularly good for you as it resulted in the 2 stone weight loss that you were after.'* Paraphrasing should always be applied tentatively to show that you are checking your understanding of the conversation so far. It is a way of clarifying the conversation for both of you, and can be a useful way of highlighting good and positive aspects of a patient's situation which can often be overlooked (22). For example, *'It sounds like you were really pleased with the way that you dealt with that hypo.'*

Being able to keep the conversation to the point is an essential skill when using this approach, and clarifying questions and paraphrasing concisely can help. *'It sounds as if you have a number of concerns about your eating and weight. Which would you like to talk about, or shall we talk about these one by one?'* Vague solutions to vague problems will never be effective, so clarify statements; *'You say that "it", that is the diet, always makes you feel bad'*. By drawing out these emotions and feelings it is possible to clarify exactly what the patient is trying to say. It is important to identify their concerns about diet, health, weight and diabetes as these will influence both their behaviour and outcomes, and determine the agenda for the discussion.

Reflecting feelings is important and needs to be dealt with as they arise. Recognising signs, verbal and non-verbal, will help with this. Watch out for giggling, tearfulness, fidgeting, wringing of hands, crying, etc. Feelings must be acknowledged and labelled; *'you seem to be angry with the way events have gone'*, ... *'I sense you're frustrated with your diabetes'*, ... *'it sounds like you felt let down'*, ... Acknowledging feelings as they arise is another way of indicating that you have heard what the patient said, and are able to empathise with the feelings that a certain situation or event has caused. It shows understanding and demonstrates active listening is taking place.

Open discussion provides valuable insight into the attitudes, beliefs and lifestyle that have influenced patients' eating behaviour. They may have encountered different messages, approaches and attitudes towards diabetes, weight and eating in the past. These will have influenced their behaviour and need exploring (23). While information-giving can improve confidence and reduce anxiety, be clear why information is being given, find out what the patient already knows, ask patients' views before giving your own (20). Patients need to be given the opportunity to talk and the environment should be conducive towards this. Acknowledge the patient's expectations and allay their anxieties. The key to any good discussion is an understanding of the patient's current situation. How are they coping with the diagnosis, are they ready to make changes, and what is the level of personal responsibility for the management of their diabetes (24)? These factors will determine the type of responses that are required, as well as the type of strategies that may be used (24,25).

In summary, to start the consultation:

- Use open questions
  - to establish rapport
  - to identify patients' concerns
  - to examine patients' beliefs, attitudes, values and understanding of diabetes, weight, eating and exercise
  - A typical day can help to open discussion
- Use closed questions to clarify points.
- Use silence to allow thoughts to be gathered.
- Reflect content to check understanding.

- Acknowledge and reflect emotions as they arise.
- Paraphrase and clarify points as they arise.

EXPLORING PROBLEMS WHICH PATIENTS PRESENT

Eating habits are intensely personal and are a result of nutritional, emotional and social components such as family pressures, lifestyles, beliefs about food and diet (26). Successful management means considering all of these factors. If only the nutritional component is taken into account, poor dietary compliance may be the result of a failure to adopt a comprehensive educational model that considers emotional and social dimensions (27–29).

Past problems may need exploring to enable patients to examine their understanding of previous events and help them identify what was difficult about the task that they had been set and how it could have been made easier. This is an essential step if they want to avoid similar pitfalls in the future. We learn from our mistakes and from our own life experiences, not from other people telling us what to do. This is probably the hardest lesson for health professionals, as we want them to get it right all the time. Letting go can be difficult.

Concreteness can be a way of interrupting long vague stories, with clarifying questions, concrete paraphrases and reflections. '*What happened exactly . . . what did you say . . . How did you react . . . Have I got this right, on the one hand you have had all these difficulties that have prevented you from doing the things that you want to do, and equally you have discovered an amazing ability to cope and get on with things?*'

Emotions experienced by the patient need to be explored and expressed by the patient. They form an important part of the picture of how the patient is coping in relation to food, weight and diabetes, and as such provide valuable insight. They can help to explain why people eat when they are not hungry.

In practice this can prove a dilemma, as responding to emotional issues and avoiding a problem-solving approach is difficult. Instead of providing answers we need to help patients draw from their own conclusions about how to manage or solve such issues for themselves. Dealing with emotions can be hard, and professionals can find it upsetting, or even frightening, and may worry that they will make things worse if people shout or cry. However, the reality is that people appreciate expressing their feelings or even simply having them labelled. Completely ignoring emotions, or belittling them by saying '*It's not that bad, everyone feels that*', is not helpful but it may serve to make you feel better and safe. Emotions have a major role to play in dietary education, and the link between emotions and eating is well established (28,30–32). So aim to get people thinking through their behaviour and reflecting on past experiences.

Empowerment is a philosophy of diabetes care that uses as its base a four-step counselling approach. Its use in diabetes care has been increasing over the last few years, and it encompasses a lot of the areas discussed in this chapter (33).

Useful questions from this work are '*What part of your diet is the most difficult or unsatisfying for you?*', '*How does that situation make you feel?*', '*How would this situation have to change for you to feel better about it?*'

In summary, to explore the issues raised:

- Use open questions.
- Explore the emotional aspect of issues raised.
- Aim to get people thinking through their behaviour and reflecting on past experiences.
- Clarify by paraphrasing and concreteness to check issues being addressed are the real concerns of the patient.

Agreeing goals

Having clarified a patient's concerns and focused on the emotions behind them it is now necessary to look at self-care management options available to the patient. What self-care behaviour are they willing to make and commit to? Remember that you are still facilitating the process and the patient should be fully instrumental in the decision process, so negotiation is vital (31).

If a patient suggests a change, they are far more likely to follow it through and to understand their responsibility for the solution and ultimate control of the diabetes lies with them. Inflexible advice can be negative as it will lower self-esteem and make the patient more resistant to change (34). By allowing the patient increased autonomy, on the other hand, you can identify those who are poorly motivated and find ways to increase their motivation and alter methods of care appropriately.

Rollnick *et al.* (21) describe two aspects to motivation or readiness to change. These are 'importance' and 'confidence'. Importance looks at the 'why' aspect of change, and confidence looks at the 'how' and 'what' aspect of change (see Figure 3.2). This can help to break down a difficult area of behaviour change by focusing on the aspect that, for the patient, is inhibiting or preventing change. For example, the patient may understand the importance of change but lack the understanding or skills to make the practical changes required. Alternatively, you may have a patient who is confident that they could change their diet as they have done so in the past. They have the necessary information to do this, but they do not perceive the change as important and so action has not been taken.

Decisional balance can also help, as weighing up the pros and cons with patients can assist them to focus on the issues around change. List factors that will support change and highlight how the proposed action will be beneficial.

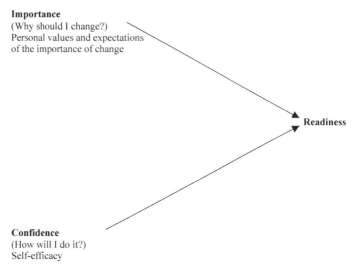

Importance
(Why should I change?)
Personal values and expectations
of the importance of change

Readiness

Confidence
(How will I do it?)
Self-efficacy

Figure 3.2 Readiness to change
Reproduced from Rollnick *et al.* (21), p. 22.

At the end of the discussion key concerns should have been identified, summarised and key points or individual goals negotiated and written down. A patient-centred personalised problem-solving educational process should have taken place where collaborative goals are set, and both barriers and supports in patients' social environments are identified. Useful empowerment questions to help this process would be:

'*Are you willing to take action to improve the situation for yourself?*', '*Are there some steps that you could take to bring you closer to where you want to be?*', '*Is there one thing you will do when you leave here to improve things for yourself?*'

In summary, when agreeing goals:

- Weigh up the pros and cons of change.
- Explore the patient's motivation, using Rollnick *et al.* (21).
- Allow the patient to identify and set their own goals.

FACILITATING CHANGE

EVALUATING EFFECTS OF DECISIONS AND ACTIONS

When focusing on dietary management of diabetes, discussions of issues other than food will achieve a clearer picture of the events or triggers related to certain eating behaviours, and allow better understanding of why the patient eats in a particular way. Exploring 'what if' situations helps to equip the patient with more life-management skills, especially once they have a greater understanding of their own behaviour. For patients, their real concerns are being listened to and knowing they are learning to cope with their diabetes.

PROFESSIONAL PRACTICE

In order to develop consultation skills effectively we need to evaluate the way that we practise as an individual; to let go of advice giving and let the patient take charge (33,35). Before we can practise differently we need to examine the way that we currently practise. We need to examine our own preconceptions first, and over time develop a less judgmental approach to our care. This means that behaviour change takes time both for the professional and the patient.

Rollnick *et al.* (21) state that all models of education are only as effective as the practitioners who use them. A review of their study on behaviour change in 2000 showed the model of education used, wasn't as effective as anticipated, as the professionals found it hard to change their behaviour and therefore lapsed into a previous consultation mode. Encouraging patients to make their own decisions and to set their own targets was harder than anticipated, especially when good diabetic control was not being achieved. This posed a number of questions, one of which was 'Do we need to reconsider the issue and extent of professional responsibility?' Further, 'Do we aim for the change in patient behaviour that the professional wants or facilitate informed choice by the patient?' Not all professionals will behave in the same way, and patients' perceptions of their condition, their coping strategies and the implications of these on their long-term health status, will also vary considerably (36). So although we may think that we have encountered a situation before, the solution will always vary as the patient's needs and drive will be different. More research is needed into professional perspectives on chronic care, the strategies used by professionals to manage patients and to cope with their own feelings, and the implications of these strategies for patients (16,37).

If you are trying to change your behaviour to enable you to work more effectively with patients, you need to constantly review the process. It will continuously evolve over time, and within the educational models you will adapt and find certain aspects that work best for certain patients – this is not a process set in stone. It does, however, require a core set of basic counselling skills, as all models require the application of these during their use. Videos of consultations and case reviews are an effective way to enrich and develop your practice and that of others. In Doherty's study in North Shields the most valuable training methods were individual supervision and video examples. Videos of consultations can be used as a teaching aid to illustrate certain techniques or as a way to assess current practice. Reflective practice is a vital part of personal development. This is essential in developing and supporting practice, as perceived and actual communication can vary (37).

You could use the following questions at the end of a consultation to reflect on your practice:

- How much was I able to accomplish by just asking questions?
- Was I tempted to jump in with advice and solutions?
- How did the patient respond to my questions?
- Was the session effective?
- Who did most of the talking?
- Did the patient express any concerns with regard to their diabetes and management, and were these acknowledged?
- Who set the agenda?
- Who set the goals?
- Did I listen?
- Do I feel that I understood what motivates the patient?
- Do I know how confident the patient feels to follow through the changes discussed?
- Do I know how competent the patient feels to follow through changes and the impact this will have on their life?

Giving patients a greater role in the management of their own condition corresponds to current views stressing the importance of being more patient-centred and developing an equal partnership with patients with a chronic illness. There is work starting to emerge that suggests behavioural counselling leads to improvements in healthy behaviour. It suggests that extended counselling to help patients sustain and build on behaviour changes may be required before differences in biological risk factors emerge. On the whole behaviours change simply, and it may be unrealistic to expect people to embrace a consistently healthy lifestyle in one fell swoop. Patient-centred empowerment and behavioural problem-solving skills training interventions produce results superior to both usual care and more traditional knowledge-based diabetes education (39). Interventions that help facilitate self-management have been proven to be effective, and sometimes even cost-effective (40).

There is still a need to provide additional strong data to support this work, as many educational models support its ideology but the evidence is sometimes lacking (41,42).

REFERENCES

1. Davidson C, Kowalska AZ, Nutman PN, Pearson GC. Dietitian–patient communication: a critical appraisal and approach to training. *Human Nutr: Appl Nutr* 1987; 41A: 381–389.
2. Vickery CE, Hodges PAM. Counselling strategies for dietary management: expanded possibilities for effecting behaviour change. *J Am Diet Assoc* 1986; 86: 924–928.
3. Rollnick S. Behaviour change in practice: targeting individuals. *Int J Obes* 1996; 20 (Suppl 1): S22–S26.
4. Coles C. Diabetes education: theories of practice. *Pract Diabetes* 1989; 6(5): 199–202.
5. Genev NM, Flack JR, Hoskins PL *et al.* Diabetes education: whose priorities are met? *Diabet Med* 1992; 9; 475–479.
6. Freeman J, Loewe R. Barriers to communication about diabetes mellitus. Patient's and physician's different view of the disease. *J Fam Pract* 2000; 49 (6): 507–512.
7. Padgett D, Mumford E, Hynes M, Carter R. Meta-analysis of the effects of educational and psychosocial interventions on management of diabetes mellitus. *J Clin Epidemiol* 1988; 41: 1007–1029.
8. Brown SA. Effects of educational interventions and outcomes in diabetic adults: a meta-analysis revisited. *Patient Educ Counsel* 1990; 16: 189–215.
9. Glanz K, Eriksen MP. Individual and community models for dietary behaviour change. *J Nutr Educ* 1993; 25 (2): 80–85.
10. Hunt P. Dietary counselling: theory into practice. *J Inst Health Educ* 1995; 33 (1): 4–8.
11. Stewart MA. Effective physician–patient communication and health outcomes: a review. *Can Med Assoc J* 1995; 152: 1423–1433.
12. Griffin S, Kinmouth AL, Skinner C, Kelly J. Educational and psychosocial interventions for adults with diabetes. British Diabetic Association Report, 1999, http://www.diabetes.org.uk
13. Golin CE, DiMatteo MR, Gelberg L. The role of patient participation in the doctor visit. Implications for adherence to diabetes care. *Diabetes Care* 1996; 19 (10): 1153–1164.
14. Greenfield S, Kaplan SH *et al.* Patient's participation in medical care: effects on blood sugar control and quality of life in diabetes. *J Gen Intern Med* 1998; 3: 448–457.
15. Anderson R, Funnell M *et al.* Learning to empower patients: results of professional education program for diabetes educators. *Diabetes Care* 1991; 14 (7): 584–590.
16. Mead N, Bower P. Measuring patient-centredness: a comparison of three observation-based instruments. *Patient Educ Counsel* 2000; 39: 71–80.
17. de Weerdt I, Visser AP, Kok G, van der Veen EA. Determinants of active self care behaviour of insulin treated patients with diabetes: implications for diabetes education. *Soc Sci Med* 1990; 30 (5): 605–615.
18. Dohety Y, Hall D, James PT, Roberts SH, Simpson J. Change counselling in diabetes: the development of a training programme for the diabetes team. *Patient Educ Counsel* 2000; 40 (**3**): 263–278.
19. Isselmann MC, Deubner LS, Hartman M. A Nutrition Counselling Workshop: Integrating Counselling Psychology into Nutrition Practice. 1993; 93 (3): 324–326.
20. Shillitoe R. *Counselling People with Diabetes.* Leicester: The British Psychological Society, 1994.
21. Rollnick S, Mason T, Butler C. *Health Behaviour Change: A Guide for Practitioners.* Edinburgh: Churchill Livingstone, 1999.

22. Shillitoe R. Carers should also be psychologists. *Pract Diabetes* 1993; 10 (4): 129.
23. Sutton MR, Gamsu DS, Killips JA, Ward JD. An overview of non-insulin dependent diabetes and weight: broadening the focus. *Pract Diabetes Int* 1997; 14 (5) 134–138.
24. Anderson RM, Genthner RW. *A Guide for Assessing a Patient's Level of Personal Responsibility for Diabetes Management.* Patient Education and Counselling, Vol. 16. Ireland: Elsevier Scientific, 1990; 269–279.
25. Hunt P, Hillsdon M. *Changing Eating and Exercise Behaviour. A Handbook for Professionals.* Oxford. Blackwell Science, 1996.
26. Currie C, Amos A, Hunt SM. The dynamics and processes of behavioural change in five classes of health related behaviour – findings from qualitative research. *Health Educ Res* 1991; 6 (4): 443–453.
27. Glasgow RE, Toobert DJ. Social environment and regimen adherence among Type II diabetic patients. *Diabetes Care* 1988; 11 (5): 377–386.
28. Travis T. Patient perceptions of factors that affect adherence to dietary regimens for diabetes mellitus. *Diabetes Educ* 1997; 23 (2): 152–156.
29. Delamater AM, Smith JA, Kurtz SM, White NH. Dietary skills and adherence in children with Type I diabetes mellitus. *Diabetes Educ* 1997; 14 (1): 33–36.
30. Peveler R. When diet is too much in mind. *Diabetes Care* 1995; 4 (2): 8–9.
31. Thomas D. Dietary care – negotiation or prescription? *Diabetes Care* 1994; 3 (3): 8–9.
32. Steele JM, Young RJ, Lloyd GG, Macintyre CCA. Abnormal eating attitudes in young insulin-dependent diabetics. *Br J Psychiatry* 1989; 155: 515–521.
33. Anderson RM, Funnell MM, Barr PA, Dedrick RF, Davis WK. Learning to empower patients: the results of a professional education program for diabetes educators. *Diabetes Care* 1991; 13: 584–590.
34. Street RL Jr, Priziak VK *et al.* Provider–patient communication and metabolic control. *Diabetes Care* 1993; 16 (6): 714–721.
35. Klawuhn G. Learning to empower patients: a journey in, a journey out. *Diabetes Educ* 1997; 23 (4): 457–462.
36. Murphy E, Kinmouth A-I Marteau T. General practice based surveillance: the views of patients. *Br J Gen Pract* 1992; 42: 279–283.
37. Roisin P, Rees ME, Stott NCH, Rollnick SR. Can nurses learn to let go? Issues arising from an intervention designed to improve patient's involvement in their own care. *J Adv Nursing* 1999; 29 (6): 1492–1499.
38. Roisin P, Stoot NCH, Rollnick SR, Rees M. A randomised controlled trial of an intervention designed to improve the care given in general practice to type II diabetic patients: patient outcomes and professional ability to change behaviour. *Fam Pract* 1998; 15 (3): 229–235.
39. Health Behaviour Change in Managed Care. A Status Report on Selected Evidence for Behavioural Risk Reduction in Clinical Settings: Dietary Practices. Florida: Centre for the Advancement of Health, 2000, http://www.cfah.org
40. McCann S, Weinman J. Encouraging patient participation in general practice consultations: effect on consultation length and content, patient satisfaction and health. *Psychol Health* 1996; 11: 857–869.
41. Bensing J. Bridging the gap. The separate worlds of evidence-based medicine and patient centred medicine. *Patient Educ Counsel* 2000; 39: 17–25.
42. Stewart MA. Effective physician–patient communication and health outcomes: a review. *Can Med Assoc J* 1995; 152: 1423–1433.

4

Dietitian and Diabetic: Thoughts on Working and Living with Diabetes

JO SUTTON
Knaphill, Surrey, UK

I have been invited to share with you some of my thoughts and experiences on working in and living with diabetes, so that you may gain another perspective in diabetes care. Through my professional knowledge and personal experience I hope to give you a greater insight into this condition, that will aid you in the education and support of people with diabetes. I have included various topics, not just food and nutrition, to emphasise the importance of taking a holistic approach to diabetes management, regardless of your specific role. These are my thoughts and experiences and I do not imply they are those of all people who live with diabetes. I start by telling you a little of my story.

I was diagnosed with insulin-dependent diabetes 20 years ago. Back then, I didn't know anything about diabetes, nor how much it would influence my life and ultimately determine my future career. My only understanding of diabetes then was that my great uncle injected himself daily, was not allowed sweet foods and was certainly not a picture of health. I can still remember how scared and anxious I felt, waiting for those final blood tests to confirm my, and my parents', worst fears. Injections frightened me, I didn't know what I was allowed to eat and I seriously thought I might die. Perhaps many people with diabetes share these feelings when they are first diagnosed.

- *Because of the well-intended advice given by family and friends, some of us may have preconceived ideas about what having diabetes means. Please clarify any misconceptions by ensuring you give us all the necessary information, regardless of how knowledgeable we may appear. This is*

Nutritional Management of Diabetes Mellitus. Edited by G. Frost, A. Dornhorst and R. Moses
© 2003 John Wiley & Sons, Ltd. ISBN 0 471 49751 7

- *particularly important when it comes to nutrition. Many believe people with diabetes should never eat sugar and this perception could mean we are unnecessarily restricting our diet.*
- *For young children newly diagnosed with diabetes, what you don't say can be just as frightening as what you do say. We usually need reassurance about all aspects of diabetes, including what we can and cannot eat.*
- *Be very careful how you word things and remember to talk to the children too, not just the parents.*

Following my diagnosis, I spent two weeks in hospital (how things have changed), getting better, but more importantly learning how to manage my diabetes. I realised that insulin injections were not that bad, there were still some things I *could* eat (more about this later) and that I wasn't going to die. When my blood sugars had finally returned to normal levels, I no longer felt lethargic and thirsty and I began to 'help' the nurses. Whether I was helping or not is questionable, I was probably more of a hindrance than a help. None the less, I diligently filled water jugs for patients, and felt an extremely important nine-year-old, handing patients their drugs with a glass of water during the drug rounds. For the most part I loved being in hospital and had lots of fun. The care and support I received from staff was invaluable in helping me to adjust to life with diabetes and planted a seed that would later grow into a passion and subsequent career in health care. Of course the love and support from friends and family was also extremely important and I would not have got through it without them. Meeting someone else who had diabetes while I was in hospital gave me hope and reassurance that I would be OK.

But it was not always smooth sailing during my hospital stay. I shed tears every night when Mum left the hospital, and the death of the elderly lady opposite me did nothing to reassure me. I was scared and worried. Although I seemed to handle my diagnosis with ease, perhaps I was putting on a brave face during an obviously traumatic time. Others must have done the same for me.

- *Support from family and friends helps us to cope with the transition of living with diabetes, but please do not underestimate the importance of having health professionals nearby. Your support can make all the difference.*
- *If possible, introduce us to other people who have diabetes, because this gives us a sense of normality and proof that there are other people successfully coping with diabetes. They may also be able to give us some practical tips on how they manage on a day-to-day basis.*

During my hospital stay health professionals taught me everything they thought I should know about living with diabetes. They were fantastic at demonstrating insulin injections, blood glucose monitoring and what I could and couldn't eat. They also taught me to fear the never-ending list of complications that would inevitably result if I didn't follow their never-ending list of advice. As a child, I had no idea what insulin injections, glucose monitoring and avoiding sugar had to do with my eyes, heart and kidneys, let alone my feet! All I knew was that from that point on my life would need to revolve around injecting, testing and eating.

- *Teach us how to manage our diabetes independently and encourage us to take responsibility for our* own *health.*
- *Don't underestimate our fear of diabetic complications, even when our behaviours don't reflect it.*
- But, *sometimes we need reminding of the complications that can result from poor lifestyle habits!*

What health professionals didn't prepare me for was the frustration I would experience in trying to achieve what I sometimes felt was the impossible: normal blood glucose levels. It sounded so easy in hospital, inject this, eat this, don't eat that, but in reality it became harder the older I got. Life became a choice between being different with normal blood sugars or sacrificing my health to fit in. The two rarely coincided. Occasionally I would do what was best for my diabetes, but more often than not I would ignore it and carry on regardless. Nobody prepared me for the emotional aspects of living with diabetes. Whether this was dealing with the guilt of missing blood sugar tests, eating things I was told not to or feeling like a failure when, despite following all the 'rules', my blood sugars seemed to have a mind of their own. What was the matter with me and *my* diabetes?

- *Diabetes does not always take first priority in our lives, just as looking after your own health is not always your first priority. We need your support and encouragement to help keep diabetes on our agenda.*
- *Often our inability to achieve normal blood sugars can make us feel like failures. Try not to reinforce this with your body language and the words you use. For example, referring to abnormal blood glucose results as 'bad' is often interpreted as 'I am bad because I cannot achieve normal sugar levels'.*
- *Most people with diabetes wouldn't mind performing blood glucose tests and injections every day, as long as they were guaranteed normal blood glucose results. If only diabetes was this simple!*
- *When you are frustrated with our blood glucose results, try to imagine how frustrated we may feel.*

Like life, living with diabetes has its ups and downs. Often, our lifestyle habits and those of our family are better than most, because of the information we have received from health professionals, particularly on diet and exercise. On a more serious note, the personal responsibility for blood glucose control can bring a rare level of maturity and dependability early on in life. Conversely, there are no holidays from diabetes and sometimes the juggling act of insulin, food, exercise and stress can feel draining, time-consuming and often difficult.

- *Occasionally we need reminding of the positive aspects of living with diabetes.*
- *Sometimes, living with diabetes can feel very serious – try to laugh with us once in a while.*
- *Try not to make assumptions about us – we may all have diabetes, but we may cope and manage things in very different ways.*

Since getting diabetes I have been privileged to meet some very talented health professionals. Sadly, I have also been disappointed by professionals who did little to help me. My first paediatrician literally jumped for joy and seemed more pleased than I was when my HbA_{1c}'s were near-normal. Occasionally I was lucky enough to see Joan, a paediatrician living some distance away, who I saw on and off into adulthood. She was very good at identifying the gaps in my diabetes management that other doctors never seemed to notice. For example, falsifying my blood glucose results when I didn't want anyone to know how 'bad' they were or when I simply wanted to pretend that I didn't have diabetes. Other doctors and dietitians appeared to be far removed from what it was like to live with diabetes, and I just couldn't connect with them. I don't doubt that they were fine professionals, but they seemed to operate to their own agenda without asking what was concerning me.

- *We like you to share our enthusiasm when we achieve our goals but we also need your understanding and empathy when things aren't going so well.*
- *If you feel you are not getting anywhere with us, put the ball in our court by asking us where we need you to help.*
- *Just because we don't ask for help doesn't mean we don't need it.*
- *It may sound obvious, but remember to keep probing and asking questions until we find the best solutions to our diabetes-related problems.*
- *With your help, managing our diabetes can feel achievable.*

Having diabetes and regular exposure to health professionals over the years has certainly fuelled my interest in nutrition and dietetics. From an early age, I learnt much about how my body worked and this fascinated me. I was amazed at how directly food could affect my blood glucose levels and overall feeling of well-being on a daily basis. I was sure that food and nutrition must also affect people without diabetes, perhaps in a less obvious way, and I wanted to learn more. My frustration with the ever-changing dietary advice given to people with diabetes was also instrumental in my decision to become a dietitian.

When I was diagnosed (with diabetes), I was told to totally exclude sugar from my diet and follow very strict carbohydrate exchanges, which was the advice given by dietitians at that time. I can remember drinking gallons of fruit juice at mealtimes to 'make up' my set exchanges because I couldn't fit another mouthful in. I was repeatedly forced to snack when not hungry to avoid hypos, often unable to eat with everyone else because it wasn't the right time for my set diabetes regime. Cakes, chocolates, biscuits, etc. were of course strictly forbidden, as was any food containing added sugar, including baked beans! This made parties, sleepovers and canteen lunches difficult and, although allowed the indulgence of ice cream, it was only once a week and *if* my blood glucose levels were well controlled. Thankfully things have now changed.

As a dietitian I have lived and worked in Australia, the USA and the UK and have noted variations in the nutritional recommendations given by dietitians and diabetes specialist nurses in their everyday practice. Essentially, the same dietary information is given, but the emphasis varies considerably. Speaking in very general terms, the nutritional focus in the UK is on very good but quite general 'healthy eating' advice using the plate model, such as reducing saturated fats, increasing fruit and vegetable intake, increasing fibre, moderating refined sugar and salt, and so on. Only small consideration is given to the carbohydrate content of foods, at least from the patient's perspective. In Australia, similar approaches are taken to healthy eating using the food pyramid, but with a much greater emphasis on glycaemic index. In many centres in the USA, more time is devoted to estimating the carbohydrate content of foods/carbohydrate exchanges and how this relates to the need for varying insulin doses at meal times. Although 'healthy eating' concepts are discussed, there is a much smaller emphasis given to the glycaemic index.

Although we are all clear on many aspects of diabetes nutrition guidelines, such as the need to reduce fat intake in relation to heart disease, there are still many aspects upon which the jury is still deliberating. For example, should we be teaching patients in depth about how to estimate the carbohydrate content of foods and hence deliver variable amounts of insulin based on what and how much is eaten. Here in the UK, the development of new insulins and insulin delivery systems such as pens and infusion pumps is fuelling a returned interest in the need to teach patients about the carbohydrate content of foods. An ongoing interest in the glycaemic index is also being seen, and how it can be applied in a practical way to the nutritional management of all types of diabetes. Further discussion of these issues is included elsewhere in this book.

The best way of course to achieve consistency in diabetes nutrition recommendations is to carry out research. I believe it is important to remember that demonstrating the effectiveness of nutritional advice by assessing improvements in diabetes outcomes is not enough. We need to go further and ask ourselves whether or not people with diabetes are willing and able to follow our recommendations in the long term. This is a subject which continues to fascinate me, as I know that I did not always follow the advice given to me when I was growing up with diabetes. Why? A scientifically proven approach may well deliver the desired outcomes in a controlled clinical environment, but is it simple to apply in the real world and does it make a notable difference to diabetes control and perhaps more importantly quality of life? Assuming that you do not have either the time or resources to carry out your own clinical research, the time-tested approach of talking and listening to your patients can provide you with valuable information. The point here is that dietary advice is not a 'one size fits all' approach. The type and complexity of information given, how and when it is delivered will depend on the individual, the resources available to you and your professional judgement.

- *Don't rattle off the same piece of information to all of us, based on your own agenda. Make sure it is relevant to us, otherwise we see little point in following your advice or returning to see you.*
- *Dietitians are often not very realistic or practical. Talk to us about our everyday foods and how we can still eat the things we enjoy every now and again while maintaining our diabetes control.*
- *Remember to listen.*
- *Question tradition.*

As a dietitian who also has diabetes, what nutritional guidelines do I now use to manage my own diabetes? I believe I have taken the best from all I have learnt about food and diabetes over the years. I have not always followed 'current thinking' on nutritional guidelines, but rather I have used what works for me. I started insulin pump therapy five years ago to improve my glycaemic control and introduce greater flexibility to my daily life. I have therefore moved away from the strict 'sugar-free' diet that I followed on diagnosis, to what I think is a much more healthy and balanced approach to food and nutrition. I generally follow 'healthy eating' guidelines but occasionally have a sugar and fat-loaded treat. I estimate the carbohydrate content of foods, which allows me to adjust my insulin doses according to what and how much I feel like eating. I also use the glycaemic index to fine tune the way I deliver my food bolus, such as split or extended boluses and during exercise.

I remember very clearly during my dietetic training an eight-year-old boy, Josh, who was admitted to the children's ward with ketoacidosis. I spoke in great detail with Josh and his mum about juggling diet and insulin doses and answered their many questions about what he would be able to eat. After spending some time with them, his mum became quite upset. I told her that I had diabetes and her attitude seemed to change. The next day, I returned to the ward to review what we had spoken about. As I walked onto the ward, I remember hearing Josh's mum say to her friend, proudly and with enthusiasm, 'There is Josh's dietitian – she also has diabetes'. I don't routinely tell all the patients I see that I have diabetes, but for many patients it can be beneficial. Having diabetes has allowed me to:

- Gain a greater understanding and acceptance of patients when they do not follow the advice I give them, e.g. testing blood sugars or following dietary advice. This makes it less frustrating for me, and the patient usually feels less judged and better understood.
- Recognise in patients what they do not always recognise in themselves, e.g. denial, fear, anger, etc.
- Empower and inspire patients, 'If you can do it, then I can too' (you don't need diabetes to prove this, try following your own dietary guidelines coupled with saline injections for a week).
- Address, in small and subtle ways when appropriate, the emotional aspects of living with diabetes.
- Do not forget that there are many aspects involved in managing diabetes and that for many patients food and nutrition is not always the first priority.
- Realise that patients not only need information, they also need support, even if they don't admit or show it.

I firmly believe that all health professionals without diabetes can achieve this kind of empathy by working towards understanding their patients and believing that they can make a valuable contribution to the quality of life of people with diabetes.

As someone who has lived with and cared for people with diabetes, I would encourage you to teach them the necessary knowledge and skills to manage their own diabetes on a day-to-day basis, so that they take responsibility for their own health. Consider all aspects of diabetes not just the nutritional issues, so that you give your patients the best possible care. Ask questions and listen. I have tried to share with you some of my ideas and I realise that my experience is not that of all people with diabetes, but I hope this has enhanced your understanding and inspired you to give your patients the information and care they need to live a long and healthy life with, not despite, their diabetes.

I wish you all the best in educating and caring for people with diabetes.

5

The Nutritional Management of Children's Diabetes

SHERIDAN WALDRON,[1] PETER SWIFT,[2]
LINDSEY OLIVER[3] AND DEBORAH FOOTE[4]

[1]Leicestershire Nutrition and Dietetic Service, Leicestershire, UK
[2]Leicester Royal Infirmary Children's Hospital, Leicester, Leicestershire, UK
[3]North Tyneside General Hospital, North Tyneside, UK
[4]Royal Prince Alfred Hospital, Camperdown, NSW, Australia

INTRODUCTION

There is considerable consensus on the nutritional management of children and adolescents with diabetes, which has been brought together in the ISPAD Consensus Guidelines 2000 (1), having initially evolved from adult nutritional recommendations (2,3). Effective nutritional management for children and adolescents with diabetes is important not only for glycaemic control but also for long-term cardiovascular risk prevention in a group particularly susceptible to future heart disease (4,5).

To achieve these nutritional objectives paediatrically trained dietitians with experience in diabetes are essential (1,6). The assessment and management of the nutritional needs of diabetic children is both skilled and complex, requiring an understanding of childhood and adolescent psychology and family dynamics alongside a detailed knowledge of diabetes care. Simply transferring knowledge is not enough as effective management requires motivating behavioural changes, which is more difficult in the young than other age groups, especially in adolescence, when adherence to all aspects of their diabetic care is poor (7). This makes negotiation and compromise essential tools.

Nutritional Management of Diabetes Mellitus. Edited by G. Frost, A. Dornhorst and R. Moses
© 2003 John Wiley & Sons, Ltd. ISBN 0 471 49751 7

The safety and quality of life of children and adolescents with diabetes must not be compromised while trying to achieve the nutritional objectives outlined above. Consideration therefore needs to be given to an individual's:

- age
- lifestyle
- culture and beliefs
- food preference
- eating patterns
- food availability
- financial circumstances

An understanding and appreciation of the family's dietary habits is paramount before nutritional advice and education can begin. Ideally a home visit around the time of diagnosis by the dietitian should be made as this provides an insight into the family way of life and highlights potential constraints upon future dietary compliance. Not only will foods vary within households but also the timing of meals and styles of eating. Special attention needs to be given to the level of psychological and social development of the child and any dietary advice given should be set in the context of the whole family as this helps to prevent psychosocial isolation and makes meal planning within the family easier. Peer pressure must be acknowledged and discussed as it can contribute to major nutritional changes, especially in adolescence.

Today it is necessary for the paediatric dietitian to be able to provide nutritional advice for an increasing variety of different types of diabetes. Up until recently childhood diabetes was almost exclusively Type 1 in origin, this however is changing as the incidence of Type 2 diabetes in adolescents is increasing and predicted to continue to increase with the rapid rise in childhood obesity (8–13). Diabetes secondary to chronic childhood disorders such as cystic fibrosis and haemoglobinopathies is also increasing, as more of these children live on into young adulthood (14,15). Other forms of diabetes due to specific monogenetic gene defects of insulin secretion (MODY) are being increasingly diagnosed (16).

There are numerous challenges ahead for the paediatric dietitian treating diabetes. Despite overwhelming evidence that tight metabolic control matters and can reduce the development of microvascular complications (17), the changes in the environment in which we strive to achieve this level of diabetic control are increasingly hostile to good lifestyle behaviour. The disestablishment of the family unit and with it set family meals has helped fuel the deteriorating diets and rise in consumption of fast foods, and these eating patterns have been confounded by the rise in levels of physical inactivity in young people.

MAIN NUTRITIONAL RECOMMENDATIONS

These are similar to nutritional recommendations for adults with diabetes (2,3). Children above 5 years should be encouraged to adopt these adult nutritional recommendations, while children under 5 years require a more energy-dense diet, see Table 5.1.

Table 5.1 Nutritional recommendations for childhood and adolescent Type 1 diabetes

1. Healthy eating principles applicable to the whole family

2. Distribution of energy and carbohydrate intake to balance insulin action profiles and exercise (and adjustment of insulin doses to varying food patterns)

3. Total energy needs to be sufficient for growth but to avoid overweight and obesity

4. Total daily energy intake should be distributed as follows:

    (i) Carbohydrate $> 50\%$
        mainly as complex unrefined higher fibre carbohydrate
        promote soluble fibre
        moderate sucrose intake
    (ii) Fat 30–35%
        $< 10\%$ saturated fat
        $< 10\%$ polyunsaturated fat
        $> 10\%$ monounsaturated fat
    (iii) Protein 10–15% (decreasing with age)

5. Fruit and vegetables (recommend five portions per day)

AIMS OF NUTRITIONAL MANAGEMENT OF CHILDHOOD AND ADOLESCENT TYPE 1 DIABETES

- Provide appropriate energy and nutrients for optimal growth, development and health
- Achieve and maintain ideal body weight
- Achieve and maintain optimal glycaemic control on an individual basis, balancing food intake with metabolic requirements, physical activity and insulin treatment
- Prevent hypo- and/or hyperglycaemia due to insulin, illness and exercise
- Reduce the risk of long-term micro- and macrovascular complications
- Preserve social and psychological well-being

'PROVIDE APPROPRIATE ENERGY AND NUTRIENTS FOR OPTIMAL GROWTH, DEVELOPMENT AND HEALTH'

Energy and Nutrients

Children with well-controlled diabetes have similar average energy intakes and nutrient requirements as their peers. As individual daily intakes and requirements vary due to growth, maturity and exercise, nutritional requirements need to be reviewed regularly with the use of height/weight growth charts. All advice should aim to achieve ideal body weight while meeting the recommendations specified in the Dietary Reference Values (DRVs) for the United Kingdom (18).

Growth in Relation to Energy Balance and Metabolic Control

Children's growth rate is continually changing but the phases of particularly rapid growth are in infancy and puberty. Health care professionals need to be made aware that for optimal growth between 6 and 12 years children with diabetes must double their energy intake. Total energy and protein intake needs to increase at this time. However after these rapid phases of growth, or cessation of growth, failure to reduce energy intake will lead to obesity. Adjusting dietary intake during these continually changing metabolic demands is central to the dietary management of childhood diabetes and requires ongoing regular review by a trained paediatric dietitian.

Growth potential may not be fulfilled when glycaemic control is poor, as glycosuria can cause significant urinary energy loss while insufficient insulin treatment can cause inadequate anabolism. Energy requirements, carbohydrate intake and insulin doses increase throughout childhood and rise markedly during puberty. Adolescents and parents need to be reassured that increasing carbohydrate intake is both normal and essential at this time and will not jeopardise overall metabolic control. Parents often compensate for the increased appetite of puberty by increasing inappropriate non-carbohydrate foods that are high in fat and/or protein. In boys, particularly, appetite can increase dramatically during the pubertal growth spurt and parents and adolescents need to appreciate that any increase in food intake should be accompanied by an increase in insulin dose.

Protein

The normal protein requirements are:

- 2 g/kg per day in early infancy
- 1 g/kg per day for a 10-year-old
- 0.8 g/kg in later adolescence towards adulthood

Children in Western countries however find it easy to exceed these requirements, obtaining 15–20% of their total energy intake as protein (19), while a safer level is nearer 10–15% (1,19,20).

Proteinuria (albumin excretion rate > 300 μg/min) is uncommon before puberty but microalbuminuria may start or accelerate during puberty. Sustained high protein loads may be detrimental to renal function, especially if there is renal disease (19,21), and this is particularly important in adolescents. However, any protein restriction should not be allowed to compromise normal growth and maturation and it is essential under these circumstances that careful nutritional and metabolic assessment is carried out.

Animal sources of protein are associated with higher fat intakes, especially saturated fat and therefore should not be consumed in large amounts. Vegetable protein is lower in fat, higher in fibre and complex carbohydrates and should therefore be encouraged. Until further evidence is available it is not necessary to decrease protein intake below that recommended for non-diabetic children and in the UK the national standard DRVs for Food Energy and Nutrients for the United Kingdom should be adhered to (18).

Carbohydrate

Children in the UK achieve 51% of total energy intake from carbohydrate (22); however, children with diabetes find it more difficult to achieve the recommended targets and have a lower reported carbohydrate intake of 49% (23). More practical suggestions may be useful to encourage larger amounts of carbohydrate to prevent excess protein and fat intakes.

Sucrose

Work in adults with diabetes has shown that sucrose has a lower glycaemic index than most starches (24,25). Studies in children have shown no correlation between glycaemic control and 'total' sucrose intake; however, if sucrose is eaten in isolation and excess this will affect control (26,27). These findings support a more liberal approach to sucrose intake when part of mixed meals or mixed with foods with a low glycaemic index, and this more flexible approach to sucrose can make food more palatable to children. It is reasonable to follow the recommendations for sucrose for the general population, that for many countries is less than 10% of total energy. In addition to glucose, sucrose can be used before exercise and for the treatment of hypoglycaemia. A reduction in sucrose must however also be considered in overweight children.

Dietary Fats

Dietary fat intake and the fatty acid composition are important in diabetes because of the associations with cardiovascular disease. The dietary recommendations for fat and fatty acids have been formulated for adults (18) but not separately for children. Therefore the intake of children above 5 years should follow the DRVs for adults. Up to the age of 5 years it is expected that the proportion of energy derived from dietary fats will fall from about 50%, as supplied by breast feeding or infant formula, to those recommended for adults. This change should not occur before 2 years old. In practice this means that the change from whole fat milk to semi-skimmed or even skimmed milk should be delayed until the age of 2. Below this age a high energy density of foods is important, and in addition if low-fat foods are given to toddlers there can be associated rapid gastric emptying and diarrhoea.

Saturated Fatty Acids

A diet low in saturated fat can lower total and low-density lipoprotein (LDL) cholesterol (28), which are strong predictors of coronary heart disease. In European adults with Type 1 diabetes, the saturated fatty acid intake represents 14–17% of total energy (29). In children without diabetes it is 14 (22) and although at the lower end of the adult range, it is above the 10–11% of dietary energy recommended (1,2,3,18). These figures support the view that children as well as adults require greater practical advice on reducing saturated fat intake.

Polyunsaturated Fatty Acids (PUFAs)

The DRV for PUFAs is 6.5% (18); WHO recommendations for the general population are 3–7% (18) and the ISPAD Consensus Guidelines 2000 (1) for children with diabetes are < 10% of total energy.

   Cis polyunsaturated fatty acids can be divided into two main groups, *cis n*-3 and *cis n*-6. These groups have different beneficial biological functions and are found in different foods. Fish oils are the richest source of *cis n*-3, with seed oils and margarines also providing alternative sources. *Cis n*-6 polyunsaturated fatty acids are found mainly in plant oils, including soya, corn and sunflower oils, and margarines manufactured from these oils.

   In the UK childhood population the average total intake of energy from *cis* polyunsaturated fatty acid is 6% (22). For infants, children and adults the DRV recommendations (18) are that linoleic acid (*cis n*-6) should provide at least 1% of total energy and α-linolenic acid (*cis n*-3) at least 0.2% of total energy. A report on nutritional aspects of cardiovascular disease (30) recommended that no further increase in average intakes in respect of *cis n*-6 was required but *cis n*-3 should increase from around 0.1 g a day to 0.2 g. Data are not available for individual fatty acids intakes for the general childhood population, however intakes of total *cis n*-3 and *cis n*-6 are above the DRVs set for individual fatty acids (22), suggesting that young people meet the DRV levels. Guidance with emphasis on a good balance of both *cis n*-3 and *cis n*-6 seems appropriate, as encouraging moderate intakes of these polyunsaturated fatty acids in a mixed diet will in consequence help to reduce overall saturated fat intake. Supplementation is not recommended as evidence of any benefit is conflicting on LDL cholesterol or glycaemic control.

Cis Monounsaturated Fatty Acids (MUFAs)

Ideally most dietary energy should be derived from a combination of *cis* MUFAs (13% of total energy) and high soluble-fibre carbohydrate. High MUFA intakes have several potential metabolic advantages including improving insulin sensitivity, glycaemic control and possibly reducing atheroma (28). A major benefit of a higher MUFA diet is palatability and aiding compliance to an otherwise low-fat diet. Donaghue *et al.* (31) have shown that even a modest increase in monounsaturated fat in adolescents with Type 1 diabetes seemed to improve insulin sensitivity.

The mean MUFA intake for the childhood population without diabetes is 11.8% of total energy (22). The intakes of children with diabetes are likely to be similar, however sources of MUFA in the UK are not as readily available as in other European countries, particularly some of the Mediterranean countries. Practical advice to increase MUFA intake should include promoting olive oil or rape seed oil and other rich sources such as specific margarines with a high monounsaturated fat content.

Trans-isomer Fatty Acids

Some *trans*-isomers of PUFAs occur naturally but most are formed during partial hydrogenation of vegetable oils to produce margarines and vegetable shortening found in baked goods and pastries. The *trans*-isomers of PUFAs have similar detrimental metabolic effects as saturated fatty acids and for practical purposes should be considered the same. The present mean intake of children without diabetes is 1.4% of total energy (22).

Lower Fat Snacks

The school snack, mid-morning, is often the most difficult one of the day, as it has to be taken or bought at school, carried in the school bag, and most importantly acceptable to peer group scrutiny. In the UK this often allows for few healthy alternatives as children do not want to eat fruit in front of their friends, in other European countries this is less of a problem as children usually choose much healthier snacks (32). Nevertheless dietary education should centre on lower fat snacks that are familiar to children. The fat content of snacks such as fruit or a bag of crisps can range from 0–12 g fat per portion, respectively, with similar carbohydrate values. The lower fat products such as corn chips, potato sticks, etc. should be encouraged and discussed with the child to help them in selection. Pictorial illustrations are often useful.

Vitamins and Antioxidant Micronutrients

Foods naturally rich in vitamins and dietary antioxidants (tocopherols, carotenoids, vitamin C and possibly flavonoids) should be strongly encouraged. Highly reactive oxygen free radicals are increasingly implicated in the pathogenesis of atherosclerosis and foods rich in antioxidants, such as fresh fruit and vegetables, may provide a means of protecting against long-term cardiovascular disease in populations at increased risk.

Unfortunately the intake of vitamins and dietary antioxidants in the UK is low among young children (22). Scientific evidence on their benefits is still evolving and further research is required in children before firm recommendations can be made. In the meantime it is appropriate to achieve at least the DRVs for vitamins and to promote foods that naturally contain significant quantities of dietary vitamins and antioxidants (33). Present evidence does not support the use of dietary supplementation with vitamins or minerals.

Non-starch Polysaccharide (Previously Known as Fibre)

Non-starch polysaccharides may be classified into two broad categories – *soluble* (including gums, gels, pectin) and *insoluble* (including cellulose and lignin). Intakes are recommended to the level suggested for the general population. However intakes may be low in European countries and meeting desired targets may involve considerable change for some children and their families (34). A reasonable first target would be 1 g/100 kcal/day (similar to non-diabetic children), rising to 2 g/100 kcal/day, with emphasis on soluble fibre (20). Soluble fibre can benefit both glycaemic control and lipid metabolism, reducing both fasting and post-prandial glucose values. An improvement in insulin sensitivity is postulated as the mechanism by which soluble fibre can improve fasting hyperglycaemia. The benefits of increasing soluble fibre are supported by studies in children (19). Fruit and vegetables are good sources of soluble fibre and emphasis should be placed on increasing intake, as most children with diabetes, like non-diabetic children in the UK, eat considerably less than the daily five portions of fruit and vegetables recommended (22).

Salt

Salt intake is in general too high and in Western countries difficult to decrease as it is added to many processed foods (only 20% of intake is added at the table and in cooking). Two-thirds of the children in the National Diet and Nutrition Survey had salt added to their cooking and salt was added to food at the table, either usually or occasionally, by about half of the young people (22). Dietary habits are learned in childhood and difficult to change. Therefore these practices should be discouraged for the whole family and practical advice to develop cooking skills to reduce the intake of processed foods would help to reduce salt consumption. Reduction is recommended to that of the general adult population. In most European countries this constitutes a reduction of 50%, to less than 6 g of salt daily.

Alcohol

Alcohol has no place in the normal nutrition of young people with or without diabetes, and in many countries alcohol ingestion in children and young teenagers is either illegal or culturally unacceptable. However, since most UK adolescents do experience and experiment with alcoholic drinks the effect of alcohol on their diabetes requires discussion. It is important to explain the risks of alcohol-induced hypoglycaemia and stress the dangers of nocturnal hypoglycaemia induced by inhibition of gluconeogenesis. The benefits of taking complex carbohydrates before, during and after drinking alcohol to reduce the risk of hypoglycaemia need to be explained.

Nutritive Sweeteners

These include glucose, sucrose, fructose and sugar alcohols such as sorbitol. All contain energy and should be considered if weight is a problem. The sugar alcohols have a lower glycaemic response than sucrose and have a slightly lower energy value. Large quantities may cause osmotic diarrhoea and some children are particularly sensitive.

Non-nutritive Sweeteners

These include saccharin, aspartame, acesulfame K, cyclamates, alitame and sucralase and may be used in low-sugar products to improve variety and compliance. Acceptable daily intakes have been established. Fears that these sweeteners may contribute to hyperactivity in children have not been substantiated.

'ACHIEVE AND MAINTAIN IDEAL BODY WEIGHT'

The diagnosis of Type 1 diabetes in a child is usually preceded by weight loss and initially extra energy is required to re-establish optimal weight. The appetite and food intake may double in the first 2–3 weeks after diagnosis and parents need to be reassured that this is a healthy physiological reaction that will settle. This increased appetite is a good opportunity to establish a regular carbohydrate intake and introduce new healthy foods that may become established in the future diet. This is a critical time to ensure that there is not an overshoot towards excessive weight gain.

Weight management during puberty is an important issue. Paradoxically (particularly in girls) energy requirements may actually decrease due to an unfortunate decline in the frequency and intensity of exercise, and when this occurs weight gain can become a problem. Puberty is also associated with insulin resistance and insulin doses need to increase to prevent hyperglycaemia but weight gain may accompany this increase in insulin administration. Regular monitoring of weight and height will help to identify potential weight problems in puberty, too much or too little, and allow insulin, food and weight management advice to be given promptly. Prevention of weight gain is a major priority because it is difficult to lose once gained and often the problem is transferred into adulthood. All aspects of diabetic control are compromised when the body mass index (BMI) rises; insulin sensitivity decreases, glycaemic control deteriorates and dyslipidaemias and hypertension can manifest themselves (35).

Intensive Insulin Management

Intensified insulin therapy to improve glycaemic control may have the negative effect of increasing weight, as demonstrated in the Diabetes Control and Complications Trial (17). Close nutritional supervision and weight management should accompany intensive therapy to prevent weight gain (17,36).

The intensive therapy group in the DCCT also experienced a threefold increase in hypoglycaemia (17). The need to carefully balance nutritional intake to insulin therapy was one of the important conclusions of the DCCT and stressed the importance of dietary re-education when intensified insulin management is introduced. Advice is difficult, as it needs to be directed simultaneously to reducing total energy and the fat/carbohydrate ratio, avoiding hypoglycaemia with regular carbohydrate while improving or maintaining good glycaemic control.

'ACHIEVE AND MAINTAIN OPTIMAL GLYCAEMIC CONTROL ON AN INDIVIDUAL BASIS, BALANCING FOOD INTAKE WITH METABOLIC REQUIREMENTS, PHYSICAL ACTIVITY AND INSULIN TREATMENT'

Initial Consultations

The newly diagnosed child and parent have an enormous volume of information to assimilate. This ranges from factual issues, such as what is diabetes, to technical issues, such as how to inject and adjust insulin and monitor blood sugars. In addition they are given information on what they can eat and how all these factors affect each other. This deluge of information is often overwhelming and frightening. Additional issues that health care professionals may feel important should be considered carefully and where possible delivered later. Initial consultations should be used to develop a trusting relationship with the child and parent establishing rapport, confidence and understanding. This time should be spent on how the child feels, and is coping with the initial tasks of diabetes. The focus should be on their immediate questions and real concerns. Usually the first question parents ask is 'What can we eat?' Useful prompts at these times include:

- *'How do you feel about the diabetes?'*
- *'What are your worries about food and diabetes?'*
- *'How will your eating habits at home affect diabetes?'*
- *'Do you think you will have to change the way you and the family eat?'*

It is particularly important to establish if other family members have diabetes and the influence this already has on the family eating pattern.

The interplay of insulin with food, eating habits, the timing of meals and snacks and even a wider discussion of insulin effects on metabolism in general should take place, if appropriate to the individual's level of understanding and perception of diabetes management.

A diet history should be taken to support any changes suggested, although this need not occur at the first appointment, if the parent or child has raised a number of emotional issues and concerns that need addressing. Completion of a food diary for review at a future appointment is often a more productive use of time. All information should be provided at a level appropriate to assist the child to achieve their immediate goals while addressing any concerns. Appropriate information at this stage may be very practical advice for the next supermarket shop or how to read food labels.

Events during the early days and weeks after diagnosis undoubtedly have a lasting impact on long-term control (see Chapter 3) and there is some evidence that if glycaemic control is good in the first 5 years long-term diabetic outcomes are improved (37–39). It is essential that the dietitian is perceived at this important time as being an ally and not prescriptive or dogmatic, taking little notice of immediate fears, crucial cultural and behavioural aspects of the family and their eating pattern. The DCCT showed conclusively that dietitians need to develop skills in communication, counselling and motivational interviewing to facilitate necessary effective changes (36).

Education Methods

The DCCT also showed that meticulous attention to both diet (36,40) and insulin management (17) produced better glycaemic control and reduced complication rates. Dietary education tools need to be selected carefully for each child and family to achieve maximum understanding and compliance.

Educational tools should be varied, appropriate to the needs of the family and staged at a pace with which the family is comfortable. As families become more confident with managing diabetes, education may become more complex and as children grow and take more responsibility, regular re-education is essential. The dietitian should have developed the skills to deliver any of the following methods and in this way the needs of the individual child and family can be met. The mode of transfer of the information should also be appropriate to the child's age and developmental level.

Food pyramids, Figure 5.1, and plate models, Figure 5.2, are useful in providing basic nutritional information and healthy eating concepts. They also illustrate visually carbohydrate in relation to the other food components and should be attractive visual aids for children.

Carbohydrate Management

Many methods of counting or estimating carbohydrate intake are used in paediatric practice, for example, intensive nutritional management with

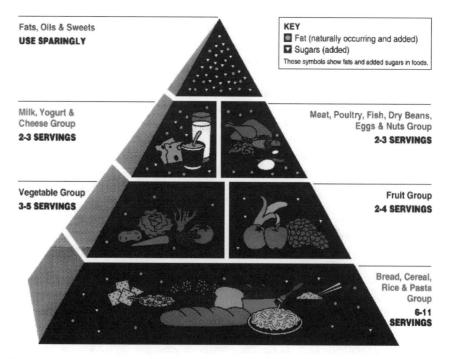

Figure 5.1 Food pyramid. Reproduced from US Department of Agriculture: Food and Nutrition Information Center, USA

estimation of carbohydrate effects, carbohydrate exchanges, portions/servings, low glycaemic index or a qualitative approach (41,42). There is no consensus in favour of one particular method and some methods are better suited to particular children and families. What is becoming clearer is that if we are aiming at really tight metabolic control to improve diabetes outcomes there seems to be a need for some form of carbohydrate estimation to counterbalance insulin doses (4).

The significant *diet behaviours* associated with improved HbA1c in the DCCT (40) were:

- Adherence to the agreed meal plan
- Adjusting food and insulin in response to hyperglycaemia
- Appropriate treatment of hypoglycaemia
- Consumption of agreed snacks within the meal plan

The DCCT also showed that intensive nutrition education, not necessarily carbohydrate assessment, with frequent blood glucose monitoring in conjunction

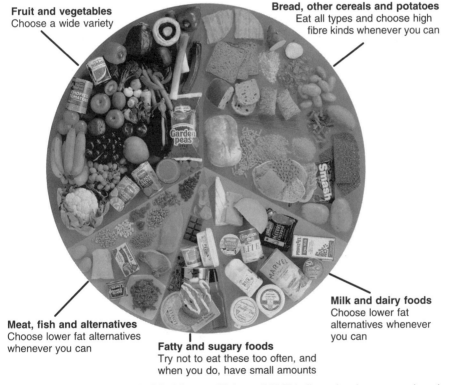

Fruit and vegetables
Choose a wide variety

Bread, other cereals and potatoes
Eat all types and choose high fibre kinds whenever you can

Milk and dairy foods
Choose lower fat alternatives whenever you can

Meat, fish and alternatives
Choose lower fat alternatives whenever you can

Fatty and sugary foods
Try not to eat these too often, and when you do, have small amounts

Figure 5.2 Plate model. Modified from: ©Diabetes UK. This figure has been reproduced with the kind permission of Diabetes UK. Adapted February 2001, from the Balance of Good Health: Food Standards Agency

with adjustment of insulin doses on a meal-to-meal and day-to-day basis, improved glycaemic control. This requires motivation, recording blood glucose results and altering insulin doses according to experience and often using an insulin adjustment algorithm. Moreover, the evaluation of intensified nutrition education programmes using carbohydrate assessment techniques in adults (43,44) has produced very good glycaemic outcomes.

Carbohydrate Assessment

The necessity and efficacy of using some form of carbohydrate assessment to achieve optimal glycaemic control is still hotly debated and questioned (4,45). In the past, exchange diets or carbohydrate portion systems were used rigidly, the person with diabetes was expected to eat the same amount of carbohydrate per meal or snack to balance their prescription of insulin and the patient was not encouraged to adjust their own insulin doses (46). Understandably, dietary adherence to such a system was poor (47–49) and made no allowances for diversity of energy expenditure (50) and growth. Also unless rigorously reviewed there was the danger that such dietary 'prescriptions' would lead to carbohydrate constraint as the child was growing, resulting in restricted growth and creating abnormal eating practices that are detrimental to normal family functioning (51). These dysfunctional approaches to eating may also contribute to disordered eating behaviours or eating disorders (52,53).

Most traditional teaching methods include some form of estimating or counting of carbohydrate. This may place misguided emphasis on quantifying carbohydrate and may alter the nutritional balance of the diet compared with non-diabetic peers. The subsequent suppression of carbohydrate then causes an increase in total fat (48,49,54,55) and potentially increases cardiovascular risk factors. Therefore whatever the educational method used there must also be a consideration of the balance of all the major nutrients.

The fundamental paradigm for carbohydrate education is the development of an understanding of the relationship between food and the post-prandial meal effect. This has to involve pre- and post-prandial blood glucose testing. The child and parents then need to be taught the skills to interpret the blood glucose tests and adjust insulin accordingly if optimal glycaemic control and a reduction in complications is to be achieved.

Optimal metabolic control as assessed by the level of glycated haemoglobin (HbA1c) is the gold standard of monitoring treatment of diabetes and the only evidence-based risk factor for future microvascular complications (17). However the DCCT (56) also suggests that post prandial glycaemic excursions play a significant role in increasing the risk of complications. This evidence supports a symbiotic link between the nutritional management of diabetes, blood glucose monitoring and insulin adjustment. Thus all three elements must be considered together.

Carbohydrate Assessment Methods

The following are descriptions of methods used to assess carbohydrate and their application will depend upon the preference of the child and family and their changing needs.

Carbohydrate Counting

Modern carbohydrate counting is a meal planning approach that focuses on improving glycaemic control and allowing maximum flexibility of food choices, so is especially suitable for children and young adults. Three levels of carbohydrate counting have been identified by the American Dietetic Association and can be considered as a stepwise approach (57,58).

- *Level 1* – basic, and introduces the concept of carbohydrate as the food component that raises blood glucose. A consistent intake of carbohydrate is encouraged using exchange or portion lists of measured quantities of food that contain all types of sugars and starches. Allowing a greater variety of carbohydrate foods (based on knowledge of the glycaemic index) than was previously accepted. With a regular carbohydrate intake and the results of blood glucose monitoring it is then possible for the dietitian, diabetes specialist nurse or doctor to advise on the appropriate insulin dose.
- *Level 2* – the intermediate step, in which the individual continues to eat regular carbohydrate and frequently monitors blood glucose levels, but learns to recognise patterns of blood glucose response to carbohydrate intake modified by insulin and exercise. They learn to make their own adjustments to insulin doses, or alter carbohydrate intake or timing of exercise to achieve blood glucose goals. Alterations of insulin should be made in response to a pattern of blood glucose results over a few days not based on a single high or low blood glucose.
- *Level 3* – for people on multiple injections or insulin pumps, requires a good understanding of the first two levels and motivation to closely monitor blood glucose levels. Once the appropriate insulin doses have been established on a regular intake of carbohydrate, an insulin/carbohydrate ratio can be calculated, e.g. 1.5 units rapid-acting insulin = 15 g carbohydrate exchange for additional carbohydrate. With this insulin/carbohydrate ratio the patient can begin to vary the amount of carbohydrate eaten at any particular meal and increase or decrease the insulin dose keeping the same ratio. This provides greater dietary flexibility than a traditional exchange diet and helps reduce the frequency of hypoglycaemia as well as high blood glucose levels after large meals.

The carbohydrate counting system at level 3 requires intensive education, extensive reassessment by an experienced dietitian and highly motivated patients. However levels 1 and 2 may assist in achieving better compliance and improved blood glucose control when not using multiple injection regimens (59).

Glycaemic Index (GI)

See Chapter 11.

Qualitative Advice

The evidence base behind using the exchange system has been questioned as above and some studies have recommended a less prescriptive qualitative approach (48,49). This dietary education method is distinctly different from the 'free' diet. It has all the qualities of healthy eating principles plus a clearly defined carbohydrate structure to the meal plan. Studies have shown that children who follow this type of advice have comparable glycaemic control to children who follow exchanges (48,49), although in these studies glycaemic control was far from optimal and the DCCT has shown the significant benefits of intensive management. A recent study also showed reasonable glycaemic control in a group of children that had received qualitative advice from diagnosis (23). Although it appears reasonable glycaemic control can be achieved using this method the negative aspect is there is no mechanism to prevent post-prandial blood glucose excursions.

Intensive Nutrition Education

A programme of intensive nutrition and insulin management has *not* been widely used in the UK up to the present time but it has been positively evaluated in some European centres in adults with Type 1 diabetes (43,44). It encourages self-management and is based upon changing insulin doses according to blood glucose monitoring and assessment of carbohydrate at each meal and snack. A recent pilot study has taken place in the UK in adults with Type 1 diabetes, called the DAFNE (Dose Adjustment For Normal Eating) Study (60). It involves a five-day outpatient skills-based training and treatment programme. The feasibility of this programme in children and adolescents with diabetes is being considered at the present time and the results will be crucial in finding out whether it is possible with this regimen to improve glycaemic control in children and adolescents with diabetes in the UK.

One of the concerns of this approach is the potential increase in hypoglycaemia as demonstrated by the DCCT where the intensive group had a threefold increase in the rate of hypoglycaemia (17). However, later paediatric studies have shown that good glycaemic control can be achieved without adversely affecting hypoglycaemia rates (59,61). The careful balancing of nutritional intake to insulin therapy was one of the important conclusions of the DCCT analysis and it seems clear that regular dietary re-education is essential when intensified management is introduced.

Insulin Types, Regimens and Action Profiles

General advice on balancing carbohydrate intake against the insulin action profile:

- Regular and frequent carbohydrate intake is advisable to prevent hypoglycaemia during inevitable periods of hyperinsulinaemia when the insulin regimen is twice daily mixtures of quick- and slower-acting insulins.
- A more flexible carbohydrate intake is possible when the insulin regimen is of multiple pre-prandial doses of quick or rapid-acting insulin.
- Carbohydrate intake is required before bedtime to prevent nocturnal hypoglycaemia in most insulin regimens.
- Extra carbohydrate is required before, during and after increased exercise and sport to balance increased energy needs and prevent hypoglycaemia.
- A 'grazing' or 'little and often' style of eating, often seen in younger children, may be suited to an insulin regimen consisting mainly of longer acting insulins.
- Flexible carbohydrate intake is possible when prandial boosts of insulin are given on multiple injection regimens or during continuous subcutaneous insulin infusions (CSSI 'pump treatment').

Insulin Analogues

Advice on balancing the insulin against an estimated carbohydrate intake has become more relevant and precise since the introduction of insulin analogues and CSSI management. The two rapid-acting insulin analogues currently available, lispro and aspart, have benefits over conventional soluble insulin:

- Very rapid onset of action within 10–15 min of subcutaneous injection
- A time action profile reducing the post-prandial blood glucose excursion
- Shorter duration of action reducing later hypoglycaemia several hours after insulin injection, including a reduction in nocturnal hypoglycaemia

However, it has become clear that to improve overall glycaemic control by the use of rapid-acting analogues, the slower-acting insulins also have to be carefully adjusted, and this may be made easier with the introduction of the newer longer acting analogue insulins.

In children the rapid-acting analogues are proving useful when:

- Injected *after a meal* when a young child's food intake is unpredictable
- Given as opportunistic extra doses when a child binges to satisfy hunger

- Injected as a calculated dose for particular levels of hyperglycaemia (it is useful to give specific guidelines on extra doses for particular levels of hyperglycaemia in relation to the age of the child – see below)
- Used in the evening instead of conventional soluble insulin to avoid nocturnal hypoglycaemia
- Used as a regular third injection after school to accommodate large volumes of food eaten at this time
- Used to reduce hyperglycaemia and ketosis in the management of intercurrent illnesses

Physical Activity

Physical activity in young people with or without diabetes is erratic and unpredictable: it is often spontaneous, usually unplanned and varies enormously in duration, type and intensity. Although regular physical activity and sports are highly recommended in all children and especially those with diabetes, the effects on glycaemic control are highly variable and difficult to manage. There are also great inter-individual differences with regard to physical activity and adjustments of both insulin and carbohydrate intake will be necessary to prevent hypoglycaemia which is a common complication (50,62). Intensive blood glucose testing is strongly advised at the beginning and after each new activity to develop some understanding of the relationship between the required insulin and the amount and type of food to sustain reasonable blood sugar levels.

The blood glucose-lowering effect of heavy exercise may occur several hours after the cessation of physical activity. The possibility of such late post-exercise hypoglycaemia should be remembered when planning meals and snacks. Insulin may need to be reduced and/or carbohydrate increased.

'PREVENT HYPO- AND/OR HYPERGLYCAEMIA DUE TO INSULIN, ILLNESS AND EXERCISE'

Hypoglycaemia

There seems little doubt from personal experience and studies such as the DCCT and others (59,61) that repeated expert dietetic advice as part of comprehensive diabetes management can reduce the incidence of hypoglycaemia. In contrast if diet is ignored as a major determinant of control and especially in extreme activity, hypoglycaemia rates can be worryingly high (50,64).

Guidelines (verbal and written) both for prevention and treatment of hypoglycaemia should be available soon after diagnosis with particular emphasis on regular carbohydrate intake. Hypoglycaemia should be discussed frequently at clinic appointments and investigated with respect to poor dietary management. Moreover if parents and other carers are given clear guidelines on how to treat with urgency episodes of severe hypoglycaemia, the frequency of hospital admissions may decrease to very low levels.

The dietitian should be able to supply useful information in relation to sport, exercise and travelling with diabetes, all of which require careful planning and organisation. Increased blood glucose monitoring (before and 2 h after) is advised for new activities. Nocturnal hypoglycaemia in relation to new activities, long duration and intense exercise should be discussed and changes in treatment may be necessary. The options for change may be either a reduction in insulin or increasing carbohydrate intake, and often both are necessary (50). Educational holidays (76,77) such as those organised by Diabetes UK are a rich source of education for dietitians with respect to planning outings, travel, preventing and treating hypoglycaemia, and arranging meal times to suit a variety of activities.

Hyperglycaemia

One of the most significant diet behaviours in the DCCT that reduced HbA1c was 'adjusting food and/or insulin in response to hyperglycaemia' (40). Dietetic advice should include an appraisal of the usual carbohydrate intake of the day in relation to blood glucose monitoring (BGM). Advice on timings of BGM will be necessary with the aim of developing the child's and parents' understanding of the glycaemic effect of different carbohydrates. The availability of rapid-acting insulin analogues has improved the management of isolated episodes of hyperglycaemia. Due to its short action profile parents feel confident about using these analogues, especially later in the evening. Also these insulins can be used prior to foods known to have a hyperglycaemic effect in the individual child.

Guidelines for extra rapid-acting insulin given for isolated high blood glucose levels or prior to extra carbohydrate loads are as follows:

Age	BG > 15 mmol/l	BG > 17 mmol/l	BG > 20 mmol/l
< 6 years	0.5–1.0 units	1–2 units	2–4 units
6–12 years	1–2 units	2–4 units	3–6 units
> 12 years	2–4 units	3–6 units	5–10 units

These doses may be repeated after 2 h if the BG shows no significant decrease.

Illness

The dietitian along with the diabetes care team should provide clear guidelines on managing diabetes during intercurrent illnesses. Normal food intake may be dramatically reduced and easily digested carbohydrate foods should be offered. It may be necessary to substitute food completely with sweet liquids during complete food refusal. Frequent BGM is essential during this period and adjustment of insulin may be necessary. Insulin should never be stopped but may be increased or decreased depending upon the type of illness and the results of BGM. It is important to recognise the childhood illness that is most likely to cause hypoglycaemia is gastroenteritis with vomiting and diarrhoea. Most other infections with fever cause hyperglycaemia. Written guidelines for 'sick days' are helpful and reassurance is often necessary during these troublesome episodes, especially when a young child will not eat. Adequate fluid intake is essential during hyperglycaemia and fever to prevent dehydration.

'REDUCE THE RISK OF LONG TERM MICRO- AND MACROVASCULAR COMPLICATIONS THROUGH OPTIMUM GLYCAEMIC CONTROL'

The most significant contribution to proving that a reduction in glycated haemoglobin is associated with a reduced risk of microvascular complications in adolescents with Type 1 diabetes was the DCCT (17). The DCCT enrolled 195 adolescents (13 to 17 years at entry) into the trial, 14% of the total participants: 125 with no retinopathy at baseline were recruited (primary prevention cohort) and 70 subjects with mild retinopathy (secondary intervention cohort). In the primary prevention cohort, intensive therapy decreased the risk of retinopathy by 53% in comparison with the conventional group. In the secondary intervention cohort, intensive therapy decreased the risk of retinopathy progression by 70% and the occurrence of microalbuminuria by 55%.

Dietary analysis of the DCCT confirmed the value of *regular* dietary advice and education (63).

'REDUCING THE RISK OF MACROVASCULAR COMPLICATIONS'

High Morbidity and Mortality in Young People with Diabetes

Young people with Type 1 diabetes diagnosed under the age of 30 years have an increased risk of cardiovascular disease. They suffer two to four times higher mortality compared with their peer group and cardiovascular disease is responsible for the majority of deaths above the age of 30 years (5). There is also increasing evidence that macrovascular changes may be present in young people with Type 1 diabetes (65,85). Promoting cardiovascular health is essential from the day of diagnosis.

Achieving Diabetes Nutritional Recommendations

The aetiology of cardiovascular disease is multi-factorial and nutritional intake is only one component. Dietary fats, especially saturated fats, play a key role and the importance of cardio-protective factors such as antioxidants is emerging. The combination and balance between other nutrients and all components of the dietary recommendations are important (1–3,31).

Although the total fat intake of children in the UK has decreased over the last decade (22) children with diabetes still appear to find it difficult to achieve diabetes recommendations (23) and total fat intake remains above recommendations. The indigenous diet of the UK and the unhealthy snack choices made by children may be responsible for this (32). Dorchy and Bourguet (66) also report the difficulty in reducing total fat even with intense dietary education. In comparison other countries report low fat intakes in children with diabetes, (67–72). However even with low fat intakes the fatty acid composition of the diet may not be ideal. Pinelli *et al.* (67) reported the ideal profile, saturated fat 8%, monounsaturated fat 21% and polyunsaturated fat 4% of total energy. The study by Donaghue *et al.* (31) shows how a diet rich in monounsaturates changes the lipid profile, and cell membrane characteristics would appear to be important. Children in the general population in the UK have a very poor profile with high saturated fat levels of 14% (22), and studies in children with diabetes also reflect this pattern (68,69,71,72,73). The importance of saturated fat in relation to cholesterol and LDL as cardiovascular risk factors suggests nutrition education should focus not only on total fat but also on the fatty acid profile. Due to the eating style of the average UK child this may be difficult to achieve. It is helpful therefore to give parents practical advice on identifying those foods with a high saturated fat content and to suggest lower fat (and palatable) alternatives.

Careful evaluation of the efficacy of education programmes along with prospective, randomised controlled trials in relation to dietary modification and cardiovascular risks are urgently needed.

PRESERVE SOCIAL AND PSYCHOLOGICAL WELL-BEING

Psychosocial Aspects of Meals and Food Intake

Food is often seen as the major issue for parents. The child has a great opportunity for aggravating and manipulating parents through food refusal. It is important that the family is encouraged to treat the child with diabetes and siblings the same from the first days after diagnosis. Virtanen *et al.* (74) have shown positive dietary changes can occur throughout the whole family due to the presence of a child with diabetes and therefore recommend that advice should be directed at the whole family from the beginning. Some parents will resist this because they do not want to deny siblings previous (often excessive) intake of sweets, chocolates and sweeter foods. This approach will cause feelings of isolation and stigmatisation. These feelings may also be acutely felt when with the child's peer group, especially in the school surroundings. The child is often embarrassed to eat snacks when other children are not allowed to, sometimes resulting in hypoglycaemia. The school timetable should be examined carefully and snacks placed within natural school breaks if possible. The teachers and lunch supervisors need instructions on the importance of regular carbohydrate and the individual child's signs and symptoms of hypoglycaemia and action to take if hypoglycaemia occurs. The 'School Pack' designed by Diabetes UK is useful in this context (75).

It is most unfortunate that the trend in the UK is not to eat meals at the family table with parents and siblings. Good eating habits are therefore not encouraged. It is important to counsel families, encouraging them back to more traditional eating patterns and to establish better supervision, communication and enjoyment at family meals.

Infants and Toddlers

Breast feeding is to be encouraged with infants diagnosed with Type 1 diabetes. Frequent small meals in infants and toddlers are compatible with good overall glycaemic control, especially when a long-acting insulin is the main insulin prescribed. In toddlers, eating as a family may help promote greater co-operation at meal times. Providing suitable foods with a variety of tastes, colours and textures can also improve a toddler's compliance with their diet. Of course this age group is renowned for food refusal and food fads, which is extremely anxiety provoking for the parent. This situation requires delicate handling because the child can hold the parent to ransom by refusing to eat and consequently parents 'give in' to the child and a poor dietary intake is established. Behaviour tactics are necessary; the parent should not get into conflict over these problems or give in to demands. Insulin analogues are extremely useful in this situation, especially given after the child has eaten.

School Children

Advice on prevention of disruptive, confidence-shattering hypoglycaemia is most important. School staff should be aware that children with diabetes need quick and easy access to food at all times, and this especially includes periods related to physical activity. Specific holiday and travel advice should be made available. Unfortunately, some schools continue to exclude children with diabetes from excursions and holidays and this needs to be assisted by health care professionals who can help by providing responsible advice to parents and teachers.

Young people with diabetes (and dietitians) may learn greatly from the experience of attending either local or nationally organised educational holidays (76,77). They are extremely useful educational events where skills can be developed in adjusting carbohydrate and insulin around different activities.

Adolescents

The normal physiological, psychological and metabolic changes of puberty are often associated with poor glycaemic control. Insulin requirements usually increase greatly with the physiological increase in insulin resistance and rapid growth. There is a tendency for excessive weight gain, particularly in girls. Careful review of insulin dosage, energy input and output is advisable throughout adolescence. Excessive weight gain may result from attempts to obtain excellent glycaemic control by matching insulin requirements with food intake. Weight monitoring is important for both the early recognition of excessive weight gain and also weight loss, as this can be the first sign of a potential eating disorder. Delayed puberty and poor linear growth may be an indication of insufficient energy intake, inappropriate insulin and/or poor glycaemic control. All children must have regular height as well as weight monitoring and be plotted on appropriate growth charts. While a degree of rebellious behaviour is usual in all adolescents it can be dangerous in diabetes when associated with failure to take insulin and erratic eating behaviour (7,79). Access to expert psychological support and counselling should be available. All adolescents should receive advice on the potential dangers of excessive alcohol intake.

Eating Disorders

The incidence of eating disorders in adolescent girls with diabetes is higher than that in the non-diabetic population and its incidence is increasing (79). This may be partly a consequence of intrusive dietetic management of diabetes at an earlier age. In association with eating disorders, the omission of insulin is a well-described tactic in attempts at weight loss in overweight insulin-treated patients (80,81). Individuals with eating disorders have higher HbA1c levels and an earlier age of onset of diabetic complications, one study reporting that eating disorders were associated with a threefold increase in risk of diabetic retinopathy (79).

It is not only teenage girls with eating disorders who require additional support but all teenagers are potentially vulnerable as there is some indication that binge eating and misuse of insulin is common among both teenage boys and girls. Evidence from the Young Diabetes Conference in 1987 indicated that

71% of young people with Type 1 diabetes admit to 'binge' eating which is often associated with feelings of extreme guilt (78).

The Acheson Report recommended 'policies which promote the adoption of healthier lifestyles, particularly in respect of factors which show a strong social gradient in prevalence or consequences' (82). Eating disorders have serious consequences for metabolic control and consequent acceleration of the onset of complications. They are also an indication of mental health problems requiring psychological support (82). There is a need to research effective methods of tackling these problems; to train health care professionals to deal with eating disorders. This will inevitably require sufficient resources. Indicators that could be used to show effective treatment are increased uptake of insulin usage, better glycaemic control and fewer admissions with diabetic ketoacidosis.

Parties, Festivities and Special Events

Children with diabetes should be encouraged to attend and participate in all family, social and religious events to which their non-diabetic siblings and friends are included and not to hide behind their diabetes. Special dispensation is usually given to children with diabetes during fasts such as Ramadan. Parents are recommended to advise other parents and care givers on their child's food preferences including low-sugar drinks. Occasional sugary food treats may not cause hyperglycaemia if physical activity levels are also high. To prevent or treat hyperglycaemia resulting from social events that include unusual amounts of eating, the use of additional short or rapid-acting insulins may be useful (see extra insulin guidelines above). As with all age groups, friends and other care givers should know how to recognise and treat hypoglycaemia.

DIABETES IN CHILDREN AND ADOLESCENTS NOT DUE TO TYPE 1 DIABETES

Type 2 Diabetes

Non-insulin-dependent, non-immune-mediated Type 2 diabetes has always been considered rare in children. However, in Japan it is more common than Type 1 diabetes and has increased greatly in incidence in the last two decades (83). Also in recent years in certain paediatric populations in the USA Type 2 diabetes has accounted for up to 45% of newly diagnosed diabetes (9,10) and there is evidence that this type of diabetes is now on the increase in the UK (11). The highest risk groups for Type 2 diabetes in youth are obese, physically inactive, female adolescents with a family history of diabetes, particularly from ethnic minority communities (12,13).

In adults, Type 2 diabetes is difficult to manage and there is a high reported incidence of serious vascular complications. Its emergence in adolescence is therefore a major public health concern, particularly as in this age group non-adherence in terms of clinic attendance and treatment regimens is common (7).

An essential component of nutritional management is a review of eating habits and lifestyle, and almost always there will need to be both a reduction of energy intake and an increase of physical activity to promote weight loss. Unfortunately these behavioural changes present major obstacles to effective education. Close surveillance will be necessary and if weight loss does not occur with simple healthy eating advice more detailed advice should be given on energy reduction. Nutritional advice will depend on the type of treatment prescribed and advice given on hypoglycaemia if necessary.

Carefully organised multicentre trials of lifestyle management and interventions amongst young people are required (84).

DIABETES SECONDARY TO CHRONIC DISEASES OF CHILDHOOD

Cystic Fibrosis (CF)-related Diabetes

As life expectancy in CF improves, slowly evolving, non-ketotic, glucose intolerance and diabetes is becoming more frequent (14). The diabetes is predominantly due to insulin deficiency but there are elements of insulin resistance and, because of co-existing pancreatic exocrine deficiency, there is a need for high-energy, complex carbohydrate and high-fat foods which conflicts with the usual advice for diabetes in terms of cardiovascular risk.

Moreover it is common practice in CF to use overnight gastrostomy feeds to improve nutrition and steroid therapy is often prescribed. Both of these increase glucose intolerance (and may initially precipitate diabetes). Alterations of food intake and absorption and constantly changing treatments demand flexibility in both nutrition education and insulin regimens, especially as the diagnosis of diabetes in addition to CF is particularly demoralising.

Haemoglobinopathies

Treated β-thalassaemia with chronic iron overload is associated with decreasing tissue sensitivity to insulin, pancreatic insulin deficiency and diabetes (15). Insulin doses may be high and the diabetes difficult to manage as in CF because of the double diagnosis. Chronic glycosuria may be associated with poor weight gain and effective nutritional management becomes important in trying to persuade patients to increase energy intake in association with escalating insulin doses.

Genetic Defects of β-cell Function

This group of rare disorders was formerly known as maturity-onset diabetes in the young (MODY) and comprises at least six subtypes of genetically inherited disorders of insulin secretion usually presenting under the age of 25 years and also present in several other family members in different generations (16). It is important to recognise the small number of this unusual and 'mild' type of diabetes in a paediatric clinic (confirmed by special tests in a molecular genetic laboratory) because of the treatment implications.

The two commonest types are:

- *Glucokinase deficiency* (25% total) – a defect in the glucose-sensing gene resulting in mild persistent hyperglycaemia from birth, but with a very low risk of long-term complications. The only treatment required is healthy eating advice to improve levels of glycaemia.
- *HNF-1α deficiency* (55% total) – involves progressive β cell failure from puberty, managed initially by healthy eating advice like Type 2 diabetes but subsequently treated with low dose sulphonylurea tablets and later insulin so that nutritional advice on hypoglycaemia as described elsewhere is required.

SUMMARY

The care of children with diabetes is complex. It involves not only the child but also the family and multiple carers. It requires a deep understanding of the relationship between treatment regimens and constantly changing physiological requirements, including growth, fluctuations in appetite associated with changes in growth velocity, varying nutritional requirements and sporadic episodes of physical activity. In addition diabetes management is set within the current context of frequently dysfunctional family dynamics, deteriorating national dietary characteristics, issues of non-compliance, peer pressure, emerging independence and the ultimate aim of maintaining quality of life. However evidence suggests it is possible to improve diabetes outcomes through meticulous attention to nutritional management. This requires a clear focus of the dietetic targets in relation to glycaemic control and the reduction in cardiovascular risk.

The fundamental premise of success for the paediatric diabetes specialist dietitian is the development of a trusting relationship between the child and family, which will facilitate behaviour change during the challenges and turbulence of childhood and adolescent development.

LOOKING TO THE FUTURE

The management of childhood diabetes will continue to present special challenges to all members of the paediatric diabetes team. These challenges are perhaps greatest for the dietitian whose success depends so much on trying to promote significant changes of behaviour related to food, eating and weight control. All of these areas of human behaviour are notoriously resistant to change, particularly in adolescents and family groups.

Despite these difficulties there will be developments in management that should improve the prospects for the dietitian. Specialist paediatric diabetes dietitians will have more specific and extensive training and will become a more effective member of the multi-disciplinary diabetes team. With better training the knowledge base in both paediatrics and diabetes will increase and be more practical. Also the skills to effect behaviour change, which include counselling, motivational interviewing and the ability to be flexible by using various education tools to suit different families, will be far more extensive than at present. Better communication between team members will be seen as essential in providing comprehensive, co-ordinated professional support and optimal care of the child and family.

Nutritional management will have targets more clearly linked to the two major diabetes outcomes of maintaining much tighter glycaemic control associated with a substantial reduction in microvascular complications and far better prevention of cardiovascular disease.

The highly trained and experienced dietitian will have an extended role in the team and will be confident not only to advise on food changes but also to help adjust insulins to reduce post-prandial blood glucose excursions. These adjustments will become more flexible and appropriate because of more frequent use of rapid-acting insulin analogues, continuous insulin infusions and perhaps other modes of insulin delivery such as inhaled insulin.

Methods of continuous monitoring of blood glucose will become easier and more sophisticated so that the glycaemic effects of certain types of carbohydrate intake will become more readily apparent to the child and family.

Thus the devolution back towards carbohydrate assessment or measurement in some form will continue so that a more precise balance between food and insulin can be achieved.

It has become clear that the specialist paediatric diabetes dietitian must also focus attention on reducing cardiovascular risk factors. Evidence is accumulating that increases in anti-oxidants and modifications in fatty acid intake may induce beneficial changes in cell membranes and these changes must be initiated in childhood to minimise the progression of atherosclerosis.

These are exciting innovations but unfortunately they are set against a nutritional environment in the UK which encourages unhealthy eating practices with increasing reliance on high-fat, high-salt fast foods, disorganised family eating patterns and even a reluctance by many influential agencies to promote healthier eating along the lines of those in some other areas and countries such as around the Mediterranean and Scandinavia.

To counterbalance this the dietetic community must improve the scientific evaluation of dietary practices by more extensive and better research. In paediatric practice where numbers are relatively small this can only be achieved by well-structured, multi-centre projects similar to DCCT and DAFNE (see above).

To enable all these exciting changes in practice to come to fruition there will need to be a recognition by health authorities that specialist paediatric diabetes dietitians are an important investment in the future of children with diabetes. It is then essential that there is more adequate resourcing for paediatric centres of excellence to be established as specialist training centres.

REFERENCES

1. International Society for Pediatric and Adolescent Diabetes (ISPAD). *Consensus Guidelines 2000*. Medforum, Ziest, Netherlands. Ed. PGF Swift.
2. The Diabetes Nutrition Study Group of the European Association for the Study of Diabetes (EASD). Recommendations for the nutritional management of patients with diabetes mellitus. *Eur J Clin Nutr* 2000; 54: 353–355.
3. American Diabetes Association. Evidence-Based Nutrition Principles and Recommendations for the Treatment and Prevention of Diabetes and Related Complications. *Diabetes Care* 2002; 25: S50–S60.
4. Scott A, Donnelly R. Improving outcomes for young people with diabetes: use of new technology and a skill-based training approach is urgently needed. *Diabet Med* 2001; 18: 861–863.
5. Laing SP, Swerdlow AJ, Slater SD, Botha JL, Burden AC, Waugh NR, Smith AWM, Hill RD, Bingley PJ, Patterson CC, Qiao Z, Keen H. The British Diabetic Association Cohort Study, 11: cause specific mortality in patients with insulin treated diabetes mellitus. *Diabet Med* 1999; 16: 466–471.
6. Betts P, Buckley M, Davies R, McEvilly E, Swift P. The care of young people with diabetes. *Diabet Med* 1996; 13: S54–S59.
7. Morris AD, Boyle DIR, McMahon AD, Greene SAG, MacDonald TM, Newton RW. Adherence to insulin treatment, glycaemic control, and ketoacidosis in insulin-dependent diabetes mellitus. *Lancet* 1997; 350: 1505–1510.
8. American Diabetes Association. Type 2 diabetes in children and adolescents. *Diabetes Care* 2000; 23: 381–389.
9. Rosenbloom A, Roe J, Young RS, Winter WE. Emerging epidemic of type 2 diabetes in youth. *Diabetes Care* 1999; 22: 345–354.
10. Fagot-Campagna A. Emergence of type 2 diabetes mellitus in children: epidemiological evidence. *J Pediatr Endo Metab* 2000; 13 (Suppl 6): 1395–1402.
11. Ehtisham S, Barrett TG, Shaw NJ. Type 2 diabetes mellitus in UK children – an emerging problem. *Diabet Med* 2000; 17: 867–871.
12. Fagot-Campagna A, Venkat-Narayan KM, Imperatore G. Type 2 diabetes in children. *Br Med J* 2001; 322: 377–378.

13. Fagot-Campagna A, Pettitt DJ, Engelgau MM, Rios Burrows N, Geiss LS, Valdes R *et al.* Type 2 diabetes among North American children and adolescents: an epidemiological review and public health perspective. *J Pediatr* 2000; 136: 664–672.
14. Moran A, Hardin D, Rodman D, Allen HF, Beall RJ *et al.* Diagnosis, screening and management of cystic fibrosis related diabetes – Consensus report. *Diab Res and Clin Pract* 1999; 45: 61–73.
15. De Sanctis V, Zurlo M, Senesi E *et al.* Insulin dependent diabetes in thalassemia. *Arch Dis Child* 1988; 63: 58–62.
16. Hattersley AT. Maturity-onset diabetes of the young: clinical heterogeneity explained by genetic heterogeneity. *Diabet Med* 1998; 15: 15–24.
17. Diabetes Control and Complications Trial Research Group. Effect of intensive diabetes treatment on the development and progression of long-term complication in adolescents with IDDM: DCCT. *J Pediatr* 1994; 125: 177–188.
18. Department of Health. *Dietary Reference Values for Food Energy and Nutrients for the United Kingdom.* Report on Health and Social Subjects, 41. London: HMSO, 1991.
19. British Diabetic Association. Dietary recommendations for children and adolescents with diabetes. *Diabet Med* 1993; 6: 537–547.
20. Kinmonth AL. Studies on diet and diabetic control in childhood. MD Thesis, Cambridge University, 1983.
21. Cohen D, Dodds R, Viberti G. Effect of protein restriction in insulin dependent diabetics at risk of nephropathy. *Br Med J* 1987; 294: 795–798.
22. National Diet and Nutrition Survey: young people aged 4 to 18 years. Food Standards Agency, 2000 (ISBN 0 11 621265 9).
23. Waldron S, Swift PGF. Can children in the UK achieve the ISPAD Nutritional Guidelines? *J Pediatr Endo Metab* 2000; 13 (Suppl 4): 1222.
24. Wolever TMS. The glycaemic index. *World Rev Nutr Diet* 1990; 62: 120–185.
25. Bantle JP, Swanson JE, Thomas W, Laine DC. Metabolic effects of sucrose in Type 2 diabetic subjects. *Diabetes Care* 1993; 16: 1301–1305.
26. Loghmani E, Richard K, Washburne I *et al.* Glycaemic response to sucrose-containing mixed meals in diets of children with insulin-dependent diabetes mellitus. *J. Paediatr* 1991; 119: 531–537.
27. Shimakwa T, Warram JH, Herrera-Acena MG, Krolewski AS. Usual dietary intake and haemoglobin A1 level in patients with insulin dependent diabetes. *J Am Diet Assoc* 1993; 93: 1409–1412.
28. Ha TKK, Lean MEJ. Technical review recommendations for the nutritional management of patients with diabetes mellitus. *Eur J Clin Nutr* 1998; 52: 467–481.
29. Toeller M, Klischan A, Heitkamp G, Schumacher W. Nutritional intakes of 2868 IDDM patients from 30 centres in Europe. *Diabetologia* 1996; 39: 929–939.
30. Department of Health. *Nutritional Aspects of Cardiovascular Disease.* Report on Health and Social Subjects: 46. London: HMSO, 1994.
31. Donaghue KC, Pena MM, Chan AKF, Blades BL, King J, Storlien LH, Silink M. Beneficial effects of increasing monounsaturated fat intake in adolescents with Type 1 diabetes. *Diabetes Res Clin Prac* 2000; 48: 193–199.
32. Alexander V, Howells L, Wilson A, Waldron S, Swift PGF, Greene S. Type 1 diabetes in children under 5: a multi-centre survey of dietary habits and parental attitudes. *Diabetes Res Clin Prac* 1991; 44: (S1-48 PS16): 18.
33. World Health Organisation. *Diet, Nutrition and the Prevention of Chronic Diseases.* Technical Report Series, 797. Geneva: WHO, 1990.

34. Kinmonth A-L, Angus RM, Jenkins PA, Smith MA, Baum JD. Whole foods and increased dietary fibre improved blood glucose control in diabetic children. *Arch Dis Child* 1982; 57: 187–194.
35. Goldstein DJ. Beneficial health effects of modest weight loss. *Int J Obes* 1992; 16: 397–415.
36. DCCT Research Group. Expanded role of the dietitian in the Diabetes Control and Complications Trial: implications for clinical practice. *J Am Diet Assoc* 1993; 93: 7.
37. Palta Mari Shen G, Allen C, Klrin R, D'Alessio D. Longitudinal patterns of glycaemic control and diabetes care from diagnosis in a population-based cohort with type 1 diabetes. *Am J Epidemiol* 1996; 144: 954–961.
38. Danne T, Mortensen HB, Hougaard P *et al.* Persistent differences among centers over 3 years in glycemic control and hypoglycemia in a study of 3805 children and adolescents with type 1 diabetes from the Hvidore Study Group. *Diabetes Care* 2001; 24: 1342–1347.
39. Jorde R, Sundsfjord J. Intra-individual variability and longitudinal changes in glycaemic control in patients with type1 diabetes. *Diabet Med* 2000; 17: 451–456.
40. Delahanty LM, Halford BN. The role of diet behaviours in achieving improved glycaemic control in intensively treated patients in the Diabetes Control and Complications Trial. *Diabetes Care* 1993; 16 (11): 1453–1458.
41. *Insulin-Dependent Diabetes in Children, Adolescents and Adults*, ed. R Hanas. Uddevalla, Sweden: Piara HB, 1998.
42. Waldron S, Swift PGF, Raymond NT, Botha JL. A survey of the dietary management of children's diabetes. *Diabet Med* 1997; 14: 698–702.
43. Pieber TR, Brunner GA, Schnedl WJ, Schattenberg S, Kaufman P, Krejs GJ. Evaluation of a structured outpatient group education program for intensive insulin therapy. *Diabetes Care* 1995; 18: 625–630.
44. Muhlhauser I, Berger M. Implementation of intensive insulin therapy: a European perspective. *Diabet Med* 1995; 12: 201–208.
45. Waldron S. Current controversies in the dietary management of diabetes in childhood and adolescence. *Br J Hosp Med* 1996; 56 (9): 450–455.
46. Lawrence RD. *The Diabetic Life. Its Control by Diet and Insulin.* Churchill, 1925.
47. Lorenz RA, Nedra K, Christensen RD, Pickert JW. Diet related knowledge, skill and adherence among children with insulin dependent diabetes mellitus. *Paediatrics* 1985; 75: 872–876.
48. Price KJ, Lang JD, Eiser C, Tripp SK. Prescribed versus unrestricted carbohydrate diets in children with type 1 diabetes. *Diabet Med* 1993; 10: 962–967.
49. Hackett AF, Court S, McCowen C, Parkin JM. Dietary survey of diabetics. *Arch Dis Child* 1986; 61: 67–71.
50. Swift PGF. Flexible carbohydrate *Diabet Med* 1997; 14: 187–188.
51. Swift PGF, Waldron S, Glass C. A child with diabetes: distress, discrepancies and dietetic debate. *Pract Diabetes Int* 1995; 12 (2): 59–62.
52. Steel JM, Young RJ, Lloyd GG, MacIntyre CCA. Abnormal eating attitudes in young insulin dependent diabetics. *Br J Psychiatry* 1989; 155: 515–521.
53. Rodin GM, Daneman D. IDDM and eating disorders are common conditions in young women. *Diabetes Care* 1992; 15 (10): 1402–1412.
54. Kalk WJ, Kruger, Slabbert A, Osler C, Raal FJ. Fat, protein and carbohydrate content of diets of white insulin-dependent diabetic adolescents and young adults. *S Afr Med J* 1992; 81: 399–402.
55. Schmidt LE, Klover R, Arfken C, Delamater AM, Hobson D. Compliance with dietary prescriptions in children and adolescents with insulin-dependent diabetes mellitus. *J Am Diet Assoc* 1992; 92: 567–570.

56. DCCT Research Group. Relationship between glycaemic exposure (HbA1c) to the risk of development and progression of retinopathy in the DCCT. *Diabetes* 1995; 44: 968–983.
57. Gillespie SJ, Kulkarni KD, Daly AE. Using carbohydrate counting in diabetes clinical practice. *J Am Diet Assoc* 1998; 98: 897–905.
58. Rabasa-Lhoret R, Garon J, Langelier H, Poisson D, Chiasson JL. Effects of meal carbohydrate content on insulin requirements in Type 1 diabetic patients treated with the basal-bolus (Ultralente-Regular) insulin regimen. *Diabetes Care* 1999; 22: 667–673.
59. Dorchy H. Glycated hemoglobin and related factors in diabetic children and adolescents under 18 years of age: a Belgian experience. *Diabetes Care* 1997; 20 (1).
60. DAFNE Study Group. Training in flexible, intensive insulin management to enable dietary freedom in people with type 1 diabetes: dose adjustment for normal eating (DAFNE) randomised controlled trial. *Br Med J* 2002; 325: 746–752.
61. Nordfeld S, Ludvigsson J. Severe hypoglycaemia in children with IDDM – a prospective population study 1992–1994. *Diabetes Care* 1997; 20: 497–502.
62. Frost GF, Hodges S, Swift PGF. Dietary carbohydrate deficits and hypoglycaemia in the young diabetic on holiday. *Diabet Med* 1986; 3: 250–252.
63. Delahanty LM. Clinical significance of medical nutrition therapy in achieving diabetes outcomes and the importance of process. *J Am Diet Assoc* 1998; 98: 28–30.
64. Braatvedt GD, Mildenhall L, Patten C, Harris G. Insulin requirements and metabolic control in children with diabetes mellitus attending a summer camp. *Diabet Med* 1996; 14: 258–261.
65. Valsania P. Severity of Coronary Artery Disease in young patients with insulin-dependent diabetes. *Am Heart J* 1991; 122: 693–700.
66. Dorchy H, Bourguet K. Nutritional intake of Belgian diabetic children. *Diabetes Care* 1997; 20: 1046–1047.
67. Pinelli L, Mormile R, Gonfiantini E, Busato A, Kaufmann P, Piccoli R, Chiarelli F. Recommended Dietary Allowances (RDA) in the dietary management of children and adolescents with IDDM: an unfeasible target or an achievable cornerstone? *J Pediatr Endo Metab* 1998; 11: 335–346.
68. Randecker GA, Smiciklas-Wright H, McKenzie JM, Shannon BM, Mitchell DC, Becker DJ, Kieselhorst K. The dietary intake of children with IDDM. *Diabetes Care* 1996; 19: 1370–1374.
69. Forsander G. Clinical management of children with type 1 diabetes mellitus. MD thesis. Stockholm 2000.
70. Schober E, Langergraber B, Rupprecht G, Rami B. Dietary intake of Austrian diabetic children 10–14 years of age. *J Pediatr Gastroenterol Nutr* 1999; 29(2): 144–147.
71. Virtanen S, Ylönen K, Räsänen L, Ala-Venna E, Mäenpää J, Åkerblom H. Two year prospective dietary survey of newly diagnosed children with diabetes aged less than 6 years. *Arch Dis Child* 2000; 82: 21–26.
72. Pietiläinen KH, Virtanen SM, Rissanen A, Rita H, Mäenpää J. Diet, obesity, and metabolic control in girls with insulin dependent diabetes mellitus. *Arch Dis Child* 1995; 73: 398-402.
73. Virtanen SM, Räsänen L, Tumme R, Laitinen S, Mäenpää J, Virtanen M, Åkerblom H. A follow-up study of the diet of Finnish diabetic adolescents. *Acta Paediatr* 1992; 81: 153–157.
74. Virtanen SM, Virta-Autio P, Räsänen L, Åkerblom H. Changes in food habits in families with a newly diagnosed child with type 1 diabetes mellitus. *J Pediatr Endo Metab* 2001; 14: 627–636.

75. Diabetes UK, London, Ref. 6001.
76. Newton RW, Isles T, Farquhar JW. The Firbush project – sharing a way of life. *Diabet Med* 1985; 2: 217–224.
77. Thompson C, Greene SA, Newton RW. Camps for diabetic children and teenagers. In: *Childhood and Adolescent Diabetes*. London: Chapman and Hall, 1995.
78. Newton RW, Connacher A, Morris AD, Thompson CJ, Greene SA, Davies R. Dilemmas and directions in the care of the diabetic teenager: the Arnold Bloom Lecture. *Pract Diabetes Int* 2000; 17: 15–20.
79. Jones JM, Lawson ML, Daneman D, Olmsted MP, Rodin G. Eating disorders in adolescent females with and without type 1 diabetes: cross sectional study. *Br Med J* 2000; 320: 1563–1566.
80. Takii M, Komaki G, Uchigata Y, Maeda M, Omori Y, Kubo C. Differences between bulimia nervosa and binge-eating disorder in females with type 1 diabetes: the important role of insulin omission. *J Psychosom Res* 1999; 47: 221–231.
81. Bryden KS, Neil A, Mayou RA, Peveler RC, Fairburn CG, Dunger DB. Eating habits, body weight, and insulin misuse. A longitudinal study of teenagers and young adults with type 1 diabetes. *Diabetes Care* 1999; 22: 1956–1960.
82. Acheson D. *Independent Inquiry into Inequalities in Health*. London: HMSO, 1998.
83. Kitigawa T, Owada M, Urakami T, Yamauchi IC. Increased incidence of non-insulin-dependent diabetes mellitus among Japanese school children correlates with an increased intake of animal protein and fat. *Clin Pediatr* 1998; 37: 111–115.
84. Dabelea D, Pettitt DJ, Jones KL, Arslanian SA. Type 2 diabetes in minority children and adolescents. *Endo Metab Clin N Am* 1999; 28 (4): 709–729.
85. Larsen J, Brekke M, Sandvik L, Arnesen H, Hanssen KF, Dahl-Jorgensen K. Silent coronary atheromatosis in type 1 diabetic patients and its relation to long-term glycemic control. *Diabetes* 2002; 51: 2637–2641.

6

An Introduction to Type 2 Diabetes

GARY FROST

Imperial School of Medicine, London, UK

Type 2 diabetes should not be viewed as a less severe version of type 1 as it is a highly malignant condition with 50% of affected individuals dying within 10 years of the diagnosis. This chapter however is specifically short as the treatment of type 2 diabetes is extensively covered in other chapters in this book, specifically chapters 2, 3 and 8, which cover obesity management, counselling and exercise.

A major contributing factor to the development of Type 2 diabetes is body weight and the incidence of type 2 diabetes begins to rise at a BMI of 23 kg/m². Type 2 diabetes is increasing worldwide in parallel with the increase in the numbers of people who are overweight or obese. Those populations with the greatest genetic predisposition for Type 2 diabetes are the populations most vulnerable to the environmental and behavioural changes that cause obesity and physical inactivity.

The UK Prospective Diabetic Study (UKPDS) demonstrated that Type 2 diabetes is a progressive disease characterised by a progressive loss of b-cell function. With time there is an inevitable loss of glycaemic control. Different treatment modalities are required at different times in the natural history of type 2 diabetes with insulin treatment frequently required after ten years. The UKPDS demonstrated that with good glycaemic control the microvascular complications of Type 2 diabetes could be reduced (1).

DIETARY GOALS

Reflecting the aims in chapter 1 dietary recommendations for type 2 can be simply broken down as follows

Nutritional Management of Diabetes Mellitus. Edited by G. Frost, A. Dornhorst and R. Moses
© 2003 John Wiley & Sons, Ltd. ISBN 0 471 49751 7

- A regular meal pattern
- Starchy carbohydrate in each meal/snack, especially low glycaemic index carbohydrate
- A reduction in total fat intakes, replacing saturated fat with monounsaturated rich fats and oils
- Five portions of fruit and vegetables each day
- A reduction in sugar intake and replacing with sweeteners
- Two-three portions of oily fish each week
- A reduction in salt intake, a 'no added salt diet'
- Moderate alcohol consumption, a maximum of 1–2 drinks per day (unless medically contraindicated)
- A reduction in daily energy intake by 500 kcal, where appropriate

DIETARY TREATMENT SHOULD HAVE STANDARDS OF PRACTICE

On diagnosis with diabetes or when seen for an initial consultation any background information that influences diabetic/dietetic management should be collected. This will include:

- Reason for referral
- Diagnosis
- Past medical history and any co-existing morbidity
- Medication
- Home monitoring data from urine or blood testing
- Relevant social/cultural circumstances
- Special needs

Anthropometric measurements recorded:

- Height (m)
- Weight (kg)
- BMI (kg/m^2)
- Waist circumference (cm)

Also any clinical parameters pertinent to the treatment of diabetes which might include:

- Blood pressure
- Fasting/random blood glucose (mmol/l)
- HbA1c (%)
- Total, HDL and LDL cholesterol levels (mmol/l)
- Triglycerides (mmol/l)

and where appropriate indicators of renal function (and liver function).

A diet history/24-hour recall is used as the basis for giving dietary advice. This should take the form of open questions about his/her diet over a typical 24-hour period. The time-frame to discuss should commence when the patient wakes up and finish 24 hours later. Due to differences in employment circumstances this time-frame may not be morning to night. Times of eating and drinking should be noted and portion sizes estimated. The checklist on the back of the dietetic record card can be used to determine more detailed information.

A three-day food diary is useful when further dietary information is required.

DIETARY MANAGEMENT

On the basis of the patient's dietary assessment, a dietary treatment plan needs to be agreed on to improve or maintain the patient's nutritional status, glycaemic control and cardiovascular risk factors, such as hyperlipidaemia and hypertension. This treatment plan must take into account the patient's medical, social and cultural requirements and dietary advice tailored to the individual's specific needs. A number of dietary targets may be agreed depending on the patient's understanding and their ability to make informed changes. It is important that the patient is aware that for maximum benefit life long compliance is usually required and therefore all changes should be realistically maintainable over the long term.

If the patient is overweight or obese a target weight should be agreed. The target weight should represent a maximum weight loss of 10%. This target will not necessarily be an ideal weight for the patient's height, but will bring about an improvement in BMI and a reduction in risk factors.

Follow up appointments need to be arranged, to continue dietary education, as and when the dietitian feels it is necessary, but under the St Vincent Declaration it is stated that 'every person with diabetes should be able to see a dietitian at diagnosis and annually for a dietary review' [2].

OBESITY (see chapter 8)

Obesity is a risk factor for the development of Type 2 diabetes. Weight gain (particularly centrally distributed) is associated with metabolic processes that increase the risk of cardiovascular disease. These metabolic disturbances include an atherogenic lipid profile, hyperinsulinaemia, hypertension and thrombogenesis.

Diabetes UK estimate 75–90% of people with diabetes have Type 2 diabetes, of these 80% are overweight or obese. The risks of hypertension, dyslipidaemia, atherogenesis and premature death from cardiovascular disease are all increased with increasing obesity in Type 2 DM. This is illustrated by the ten-fold increased risk of premature death when Type 2 DM is associated with a BMI above $36 \, \text{kg/m}^2$. By contrast, intentional weight loss of between 8–13 kg can reduce mortality by 33% in obese diabetic subjects.

For overweight Type 2 diabetic patients, the most important dietary objective is to achieve and maintain a desirable weight and BMI. However, the weight loss required to achieve this is often not realistic, even in the long term and weight loss of 5% can result in some clinical improvement. Whereas 10% weight loss can produce major benefits improving glycaemic control by reducing insulin resistance; improving lipid profile and reducing hypertension [3].

Weight loss can only be accomplished by reduction of total energy intake below the level of energy expenditure. It is important that the weight loss targets and diet are realistic. Each individual's requirements will vary and are hard to determine accurately. It is usual to determine normal intake from a diet history. From this, modification of the diet is suggested to reduce energy intake usually involving a reduction of energy dense foods, those high in fat and sugar. If this is unsuccessful a more prescriptive diet can be given based on a calculation of energy expenditure using Lean and James formula which is reduced by 500 kcal to give a more precise dietary target [4].

DIET AND ORAL HYPOGLYCAEMIC DRUGS

Anti-diabetic drugs should be taken as prescribed at the appropriate time interval in relation to food intakes. In order to prevent hypoglycaemia, in patients taking insulin secretagogues, and to maintain good glycaemic control in all subjects, an even distribution of food intakes, including some carbohydrate is essential. Foods with a low glycaemic index should be encouraged. Patients treated by diet alone can be more flexible about their food intakes, but the basic/good dietary principles still apply.

As Type 2 diabetes is a progressive disease, worsening glycaemic control should not be seen as necessarily being due to non-compliance with drug therapy or diet. Large prospective type 2 diabetic studies have clearly demonstrated that to maintain good glycaemic control most diabetic patients progress from diet alone, to monotherapy and then to combination therapy with oral agents before finally requiring insulin. Polypharmacy is difficult to avoid in the majority of Type 2 diabetic patients, as hypertensive medication, antithrombolytic therapy and lipid lowering drugs are also frequently required [1] [5] [7].

INSULIN THERAPY

As a consequence of the relentless deterioration in beta cell function in Type 2 diabetic patients with little, if any, improvement in insulin resistance with time exogenous insulin therapy is required to achieve adequate glycaemic control. During the UKPDS approximately 30% of obese and 22% of non-obese Type 2 DM patients required insulin within six years of diagnosis [1]. The introduction of insulin in Type 2 DM patients is however associated with weight gain which itself is likely to be detrimental to the underlying metabolic syndrome, glycaemic control and cardiac risk.

Although the UKPDS study showed the benefit of insulin therapy on glycaemic control, there is little data on whether the introduction of insulin therapy favourably influences insulin resistance syndrome, lipid profiles or blood pressure. There is a need for planned obesity management and weight maintenance as outlined in chapter 1 for any patients starting insulin.

SALT RESTRICTION

There is evidence that salt reduction will lower blood pressure in the general population and Type 2 diabetics. The importance of achieving good blood pressure control was again demonstrated in the UKPDS [6]. Advice should therefore be given to reduce the amount of salt added in cooking and at the table and to reduce intakes of salty foods especially for hypertensive diabetic patients.

All other aspects on management are reflected in the recommendation section of this book

SUMMARY

Management of type 2 diabetes remains a nutritional challenge with the main focus on management of obesity and coronary risk factors.

REFERENCES

1. UK Prospective Diabetes Study Group. UK Prospective Diabetes Study (UKDPS) 16: Overview of 6 years' of therapy of Type II diabetes: a progressive disease. *Diabetes* 1995; 44: 1258–1258.
2. St Vincent Declaration. Diabetic care and research in Europe. *Diabet Med* 1990; 7: 360.
3. Goldstein DJ. Beneficial health effects of modest weight loss. *J Obesity* 1992; 16: 397–415.

4. Lean MEJ, Brenchley S, Connor H, Elkeles RS, Govindji A, Hartland BV. Dietary recommendations for people with diabetes: An update for the 1990s. Nutrition subcommittee of the British Diabetic Association's Professional Advisory Committee. *Diabet Med* 1992; 9: 189–202.
5. Gaede P, Vedel P, Parving HH, Pedersen O. Intensified multifactorial intervention in patients with type 2 diabetes mellitus and microalbuminuria: the Steno type 2 randomised study. *Lancet* 1999; 353: 617–622.
6. UK Prospective Diabetes Study Group. Tight blood pressure control and risk of macrovascular and microvascular complications in type 2 diabetes: UKPDS 38. *BMJ* 1998; 317: 703–713.
7. Gaede P, Vedel P, Larsen N *et al*. Multifactorial intervention and cardiovascular disease in patients with Type 2 diabetes. *N Engl J Med* 2003; 343: 383–393.

7

The Dietary Management of Diabetic Pregnancies

ANNE DORNHORST AND GARY FROST

Imperial School of Medicine, London, UK

INTRODUCTION

There are general nutritional principles that apply to all pregnancies and there are specific nutritional issues that surround the management of pregnant women with diabetes. The nutritional needs of women with pre-existing Type 1 diabetes and Type 2 diabetes differ, as do those for women who become glucose-intolerant in pregnancy. Ideally nutritional advice should start before pregnancy and continue throughout the pregnancy, being modified as necessary at each antenatal visit. The dietitian is an integral part of the multidisciplinary diabetic–obstetric team and should be involved in all aspects of the patient's care plan. The prescribed diet has to accommodate the metabolic and physiological changes associated with a diabetic pregnancy and the dietitian must be familiar with these changes.

Over the last few decades the Western antenatal population has become older, more obese, less physically active and more ethnically diverse. These demographic changes explain the rise in the numbers of pregnant women with pre-existing Type 2 diabetes and gestational diabetes (1). Although the actual number of pregnant women with pre-existing Type 1 diabetes has remained relatively constant, the duration of diabetes prior to pregnancy has increased, due to women delaying childbirth for personal reasons and the earlier onset of Type 1 diabetes that has occurred over recent years. Both the age of the mother and the duration of her diabetes contribute to the clinical

Nutritional Management of Diabetes Mellitus. Edited by G. Frost, A. Dornhorst and R. Moses
© 2003 John Wiley & Sons, Ltd. ISBN 0 471 49751 7

complications encountered in a Type 1 diabetic pregnancy. Although pregnancy outcomes continue to improve in women with Type 1 diabetes, perinatal morbidity and mortality remain fourfold higher than for the non-diabetic population (2,3).

Active dietary management for all types of diabetic pregnancies can lessen complications during pregnancy and improve pregnancy outcome for the mother and her child.

CONSEQUENCES OF A DIABETIC PREGNANCY

Maternal hyperglycaemia results in an excess maternal–foetal transfer of glucose. The placental glucose transporter protein, GLUT1, is increased in diabetic pregnancies, and maternal hyperglycaemia quickly results in foetal hyperglycaemia and foetal hyperinsulinaemia (4). Maternal hyperglycaemia is not only a critical factor in glucose-mediated congenital malformations, but also in many aspects of foetal development, neonatal well-being and future health, see Table 7.1.

An accelerated foetal growth pattern and a large-for-gestational-age (LGA) infant at birth is the hallmark of a poorly controlled diabetic pregnancy. Foetal insulin is the main foetal anabolic hormone and hyperinsulinaemia can cause excess fat accumulation, organomegaly, especially of the heart and liver, and high birthweight. An LGA infant is a potential cause for birth trauma and a high Caesarean rate. Foetal hyperinsulinaemia is also believed to contribute to adverse foetal metabolic complications in late pregnancy including a tendency to high lactate levels and an increased risk of stillbirth. Foetal hyperinsulinaemia at delivery can cause transient hypoglycaemia and hypocalcaemia. There is increasing and tantalising evidence that by optimising maternal glycaemia and avoiding foetal hyperinsulinaemia one can reduce the long-term risk of the child becoming obese and insulin-resistant in adult life (5).

Table 7.1 The intrauterine influence of maternal hyperglycaemia on foetal and childhood development

Period of influence	Consequence of maternal hyperglycaemia
First trimester	Congenital malformations
Second trimester	Foetal cell programming, foetal hyperinsulinaemia
Third trimester	Accelerated foetal growth and stillbirth
Neonatal period	Transient hypoglycaemia; hypocalcaemia and cardiomyopathy
Adolescence	Obesity, impaired glucose tolerance and insulin resistance
Adulthood	Insulin resistance, obesity and Type 2 diabetes

THE THERAPEUTIC AIM IN THE MANAGEMENT OF DIABETIC PREGNANCIES

The aim in the management of all diabetic pregnancies is to achieve normoglycaemia while avoiding maternal hypoglycaemia. This approach will optimise foetal growth and minimise short- and long-term complications. As the immediate post-prandial period is when maternal glucose levels are at their highest, dietary and insulin therapies need to specifically target this time (6). The glycaemic targets for all types of diabetic pregnancies should be the same, namely a fasting glucose of < 5 mmol/l and a 1 h post-prandial glucose < 7.8 mmol/l. While these goals will inevitably require insulin in women with pre-pregnancy diabetes, many women with gestational diabetes (GDM) will be able to achieve them with dietary intervention alone, with insulin being reserved for women who, after a trial of dietary therapy, are above these glycaemic target values. The use of oral agents that do not cross the placenta, such as glibenclamide, in the management of GDM, although probably safe, are best suited for women with Type 2 diabetes and GDM in areas of the world where insulin availability is limited (7).

Due to the lack of adequate controlled dietary studies in diabetic pregnancies, conflicting dietary advice is often advocated. Debate still surrounds the total energy content of the diet and the optimal proportions and type of dietary carbohydrate and fat to be prescribed. The benefits, if any, of whether the dietary advice given during pregnancy actually leads to behavioural changes that reduce the future recurrence of GDM or the development of diabetes in the mother are unknown. Also the influence of maternal diets on foetal programming and the future risk of childhood and adult obesity and diabetes are not fully understood.

PRECONCEPTION NUTRITIONAL COUNSELLING IN DIABETIC PREGNANCIES

All women attempting pregnancy should take a minimum of 400 µg folic acid supplements a day to prevent neural tube defects (8). The higher dose of 5 mg folic acid a day is frequently recommended for diabetic women, despite any actual trial evidence for this, the rationale being that neural tube defects are commoner in this group. In Britain, where the dietary folate intakes are relatively low despite numerous public health campaigns, less than 10% of women actually take folate supplements in early pregnancy (9).

The preconception period is a time when women with diabetes are encouraged to achieve the best glycaemic control possible. Congenital malformations account for approximately 40% of all diabetic perinatal mortality, and can be significantly reduced when HbA_{1c} levels are within the normal range. To achieve this insulin regimens usually need to be intensified and many women with Type 2 diabetes will be started on insulin for the first time. Dietetic input is required to build confidence, reduce hypoglycaemia and limit unnecessary weight gain (10).

Achieving near-normal glycaemic control is possible in most women with Type 2 and Type 1 diabetes. However, in women with a long duration of Type 1 diabetes and significant autonomic neuropathy the risk of severe hypoglycaemia is high. Poor hypoglycaemia awareness and impaired counter-regulatory hormonal responses increase with the duration of Type 1 diabetes. Dietary advice is essential to ensure adequate carbohydrate is being taken with each meal and that suitable low glycaemic carbohydrate snacks are being consumed between meals.

The preconception period is a good time to encourage weight loss and exercise in obese women with pre-existing Type 2 diabetes or a previous history of gestational diabetes. Maternal obesity is independently associated with increased perinatal morbidity and mortality rates (11). Epidemiological studies suggest that when obesity and diabetes coexist an adverse synergistic effect on pregnancy outcome occurs, including an unexplained increase in congenital malformation rates (12–14). Potentially a weight-reducing diet in obese women prior to conception will improve both glycaemic control and pregnancy outcome.

GENERAL DIETETIC ADVICE FOR PREGNANCY

Once pregnancy has been confirmed the diet should be reviewed to ensure the recommended vitamin and mineral intakes, including folate and iron, for pregnancy are met. Ensuring adequate amounts of antioxidants in the diet may help to lessen the risk of pre-eclampsia and congenital malformation. Recently dietary supplementation with the antioxidant vitamins C and E have been shown to reduce the incidence of pre-eclampsia in high-risk women (15). Animal, but so far not human, studies have shown that these vitamins also protect embryos from the teratogenic effects of hyperglycaemia (16).

Calcium and vitamin D supplements during both pregnancy and lactation should be considered for Indian/Asian women and others with poor sunlight exposure or low calcium intakes (17,18). Observational studies have linked low vitamin D levels with insulin resistance and diabetes (19,20) and, given the high incidence of diabetes among Asian women, ensuring adequate vitamin D in the diet seems prudent.

All women should be reminded of the dangers of excess alcohol (21), and the potentially harmful effects of uncooked meats and soft cheese.

RECOMMENDED MATERNAL WEIGHT GAINS IN NON-DIABETIC PREGNANCIES

Optimal weight gain for pregnancy needs to reflect the woman's pre-pregnancy weight (22). The guidelines on recommended maternal weight gains are based on large obstetric surveys in non-diabetic women in the United States (23). The maternal weight gain required to minimise the frequency of small-for-gestational-age (SGA) infants is higher for underweight (BMI < 19.8 kg/m^2) than overweight or obese women, see Table 7.2. As the majority of women with pre-existing Type 2 and GDM are already obese it is important that the dietary advice given does not result in higher post-partum than pre-pregnancy weights.

When the pre-pregnancy BMI is > 35 kg/m^2, the risk of a SGA infant is low and even when little or no maternal weight gain occurs the risk of a SGA infant does not appear to increase (11). Overweight (BMI 26.1–29 kg/m^2) and obese (BMI > 29 kg/m^2) women are more likely to give birth to a LGA infant than normal weight women and this risk increases with increasing maternal weight gain. The US obstetric recommendation for a minimum 7 kg weight gain for all obese women (23,24) may not be universally appropriate (11,25). Nutritional advice given in pregnancy should include appropriate weight gain targets set in early pregnancy and based on pre-pregnancy weight.

ENERGY REQUIREMENTS IN PREGNANCY

Pregnancy is an anabolic state requiring energy for the products of conception, the foetal–placental unit and the increase in maternal tissues. Newly synthesised maternal tissues account for a 15–26% increase in metabolic rate in pregnancy (26). The total calculated energy cost for pregnancy is around 355 640 kJ (85 000 kcal) and this translates into an extra 1191.3 kJ (285 kcal) a day (27,28). These theoretical energy costs, originally derived in the 1960s by Hytten and Leitch, have been confirmed by more recent physiological measurements (29).

Maternal physiology is highly adaptable and pregnancy can progress during times of extreme food deprivation and/or physical activity (30). Under adverse

Table 7.2 The 1990 guidelines of the United States Institute of Medicine on maternal weight gain targets according to pre-pregnancy BMI

	Underweight < 19.8 kg/m^2	Normal weight 19.8–26 kg/m^2	Overweight > 26 kg/m^2
Weight gain term target	12.5–18 kg	11.5–16 kg	7.0–11.5 kg

environmental conditions maternal adipose deposition is limited, and diet-induced thermogenesis can fall which, when combined with a small decrease in physical activity, can conserve sufficient energy for foetal development (29,31,32). With extreme calorie restriction in the first half of pregnancy, maternal basal metabolic rate can also fall (30).

The energy requirements of pregnancy are seldom, if ever, met by increased dietary intake as shown by cross-sectional and longitudinal nutritional studies (30). Well-nourished women only obtain 20% of their pregnancy energy requirement from increased dietary intake (29). In fact no increase in maternal energy intake is required providing maternal physical activity falls by 20% during pregnancy (27). In women with high physical energy expenditures before pregnancy decreases in physical activity contribute significantly to the overall energy costs of the pregnancy (29,33). Despite these observational studies many of the dietary recommendations for pregnancy are based on providing the total energy costs of pregnancy from increased energy intake (34).

METABOLIC CHANGES IN NON-DIABETIC PREGNANCY

Metabolic changes occur throughout pregnancy to ensure optimal foetal growth. Maternal glucose is the primary foetal oxidative substrate (35) and by late pregnancy 17–26 g glucose is metabolised per day (36). The maternal respiratory quotient rises during pregnancy as foetal carbohydrate metabolism increases (29). Metabolic changes occur to maximise the maternal–foetal transfer of glucose. Several placental hormones are lipolytic and increase maternal circulating free fatty acids that increase maternal peripheral insulin resistance (37). This increase in maternal insulin resistance diverts glucose away from maternal peripheral tissues to the foetus (35,38,39,40). Post-prandial glucose and insulin concentrations rise during pregnancy in women consuming a typical Western diet. The ability to remain glucose-tolerant while pregnant requires a trebling of insulin secretion by the end of pregnancy to counter this increase in insulin resistance (41). Observational studies suggest that habitual diet and lifestyle factors can influence maternal glucose tolerance and insulin sensitivity in pregnancy (42). Active women consuming low glycaemic index diets have significantly lower post-prandial glucose and insulin levels in pregnancy than women consuming high glycaemic index diets (43,44).

The higher post-prandial insulin levels encountered in pregnancy facilitate maternal fat deposition (45,46), which in well-nourished women approximates to a minimum of 4 kg of adipose tissue (46) and in undernourished women to 2 kg (32). A fall in fatty acid oxidation in late pregnancy also contributes to adipose deposition (29).

Other maternal metabolic changes occur to ensure a steady supply of glucose to the foetus. Lipolytic placental hormones increase maternal lipolysis during the post-absorbative periods, generating sufficient gluconeogenic substrates in the form of ketone bodies and glycerol to provide the necessary glucose for foetal use (45). An increase in maternal hepatic glucose output ensures a necessary glucose supply to the foetus during fasting (48,49). Although ketone bodies can cross the placenta and be used as foetal fuels, non-esterified acids cannot.

SPECIFIC METABOLIC CHANGES ASSOCIATED WITH TYPE 1 DIABETES

Dietary factors, insulin adjustments and blood glucose values are so interdependent in women with Type 1 diabetes that one should not consider any one in isolation. Women with Type 1 diabetes have an absolute deficiency of insulin and their glycaemic control is totally dependent on exogenous insulin and dietary intake. The metabolic and physiological changes occurring in early pregnancy make these women especially vulnerable to hypoglycaemia, and this is further compounded if food intake falls due to pregnancy-induced nausea or vomiting. In later pregnancy, due to the increase in maternal lipolysis during the post-absorbative and fasting periods, ketoacidosis may develop rapidly. To minimise metabolic complications one needs to continually match and adjust the insulin doses to the carbohydrate intake. Maternal ketosis, as assessed by urine strips, is usually an indication for an increase in both dietary carbohydrate and insulin treatment.

Diets need to be individual and flexible enough to adjust to any of the numerous co-morbidities encountered in pregnancy, such as hyperemesis gravidarum or gastroparesis. If nausea is a problem in early pregnancy the use of liquid meals should be considered, as these are often better tolerated than solids. Going without regular food and insulin in this group is not an option.

SPECIFIC METABOLIC CHANGES ASSOCIATED WITH TYPE 2 DIABETES

Women with Type 2 diabetes have a relative rather than an absolute deficiency of insulin. These women are already insulin-resistant and with the physiological increase in insulin resistance that occurs in pregnancy their insulin deficiency is further compromised. Very large doses of exogenous insulin are often required to obtain the necessary blood glucose target values. Avoiding excessive weight gain in these obese women being treated with large insulin doses requires considerable dietary education and intervention early in pregnancy. The use of low-calorie foods and snacks should be encouraged. Appropriate weight targets should be set and a degree of energy restriction considered, see below.

SPECIFIC METABOLIC CHANGES ASSOCIATED WITH GESTATIONAL DIABETES

A degree of β-cell dysfunction is universal in women with GDM, both during and following pregnancy (50–52). Women who develop GDM not only have insufficient β-cell reserve to remain glucose-tolerant in pregnancy, but higher peripheral and hepatic insulin resistance than glucose-tolerant women (53). The β-cell defect is more apparent in the non-obese than obese GDM women in whom insulin resistance is often a greater contributing factor (54). These metabolic defects result in abnormalities of post-prandial lipoprotein metabolism (55) that can further reduce insulin sensitivity and compromise β-cell function (37,56). The diet should be aimed at lessening these metabolic abnormalities. As with the Type 2 diabetic women, most of the women who develop GDM are obese and weight gain targets should be set and a degree of energy restriction considered, see below. However, unlike the Type 2 diabetic women most can achieve adequate glycaemic control with diet alone. For this reason the dietary recommendations for GDM will be considered in further detail below.

GENERAL DIETARY RECOMMENDATIONS FOR GDM

A dogmatic approach to the dietary advice for GDM should be avoided as only four randomised trials of primary dietary management of GDM against no treatment were considered to be of sufficient standard to include in a recent Cochrane systematic review (57). This pooled data analysis of 612 women failed to show any benefit of dietary intervention on final birthweight, risk of LGA infants and/or Caesarean deliveries (57). However, ignoring all clinical and observational nutritional studies that have no non-intervention arm is probably unwise, and until definitively controlled studies are done each available study should be considered on its own merit.

The objectives in the dietary management of GDM include glycaemic control, balancing adequate nourishment for the mother and foetus, while limiting excessive weight gain, and establishing healthy eating habits that will continue beyond the pregnancy. Lifestyle changes encompassing diet and exercise should be started during the pregnancy itself, when access to a qualified dietitian is likely to be greater than at any future time.

It is important that women with gestational diabetes understand why dietary intervention during the pregnancy is so important to obstetric care. It is worth stressing that adherence to a diet in pregnancy can in most women improve glycaemic control. Understanding that a diet will reduce her risk of having a very large baby and the need for insulin therapy in pregnancy will help compliance. The importance of avoiding unnecessary weight gain needs to be emphasised, and women need to know that too much weight gain increases the risk of delivering an LGA infant and increased obesity post partum (58). Unnecessary weight gain will also increase the future risk of developing GDM in a subsequent pregnancy (59), and diabetes in later life (60).

CALCULATING TOTAL ENERGY FOR THE DIET AND SETTING SAFE WEIGHT GAIN TARGETS

In our practice we calculate an individual's energy requirement using the pre-pregnancy weight to calculate resting energy expenditure, using Schofield's formula (61), and a physical activity ratio of 1.6. To this we add 200 kcal for the energy requirements for the third trimester. If we wish to induce a mild degree of negative energy balance we subtract 500 kcal from this calculated daily energy requirement to provide the total energy for the diet.

The American Diabetic Association (ADA) have endorsed dietary guidelines for diabetes in pregnancy (62) that are based on pre-pregnancy weights, see Table 7.3.

As previously mentioned, current American guidelines recommend a minimum weight gain of 7.0 kg for all obese (BMI > 29 kg/m^2) women, both diabetic (63) and non-diabetic (24). No equivalent weight or daily calorie guidelines exist for the UK. Our own unit limits weight gains in diabetic pregnancies to the bottom rather than the top of those recommended for average, overweight and obese women. For Type 2 diabetic women and those with GDM if the BMI is > 34 kg/m^2 we set no minimum weight gain. Ideally we like to achieve no overall weight gain in the overweight woman post partum and weight loss in the morbidly obese woman.

Table 7.3

Pre-pregnancy weight (% ideal body weight)	Daily calorie intake (kcal/kg)
< 90%	36–40
90–120%	30
121–150%	24
> 150%	12–18

CALORIE RESTRICTION IN THE OBESE WOMAN WITH GDM

The safety of calorie restriction in pregnancy is not known and genuine concerns exist around infant psychological or physical development. Long-term follow-up of children born to mothers exposed to famine suggests that future health is compromised. Infants born to previously well-nourished Dutch women restricted to 800 kcal/day in late pregnancy during the five months of famine in 1944/5 developed normally, although thinner at birth and at 18 years (64). However, when middle-aged these children had a higher incidence of glucose intolerance and diabetes (65).

Maternal ketosis, induced by calorie restriction, has been implicated to impaired foetal neuro-physiological and cognitive development (66,67). While there is a general reluctance to recommend severe calorie restriction in pregnancy even in obese women, modest calorie constraint for those with GDM may be safe as these women are relatively protected against ketosis by their high hepatic glucose outputs (54,68,69). Theoretically maternal ketosis can be lessened during modest calorie restriction when small frequent meals containing slowly absorbed carbohydrates are taken, as such diets are associated with an attenuated insulin response that delays lipolysis and ketogenesis (70).

We have previously reported that when the daily energy is restricted to 20–25 kcal/kg/day for obese women with GDM (pre-pregnancy BMI > 28 kg/m^2) from the 24th week of gestation, weight gain is half that of women with a similar pre-pregnancy weight who receive no dietary intervention, and their risk of delivering an LGA infant is similarly reduced (71). This degree of modest calorie restraint has also been shown to improve glycaemic control (69). Frequent small meals containing slowly absorbed carbohydrates help to prevent ketosis.

All women receiving a diet that is calorie restricted should have regular foetal ultrasound examinations to ensure that foetal growth is not compromised.

THE OPTIMAL MIX OF DIETARY CARBOHYDRATE AND FAT FOR GDM

The diet for the diabetic mother needs to limit excess maternal–foetal transfer of glucose. As post-prandial hyperglycaemia is the time of maximal maternal–foetal glucose transfer, treatment interventions need to target this period (6). Controversy exists on how best to achieve this. Some authorities recommend limiting carbohydrate at the expense of increasing dietary fat, while others favour high-carbohydrate diets with a low glycaemic response. It is the authors' belief that promoting diets that actively limit carbohydrate over fat sends out the wrong lifetime educational message. Clinical studies suggest that it is the type of carbohydrate and fat rather than the absolute amount that dictates the glycaemic and metabolic responses to a meal. As a degree of gastric stasis is common in pregnancy, the glycaemic response of many carbohydrates is blunted.

The American Diabetic Association (62) recommend limiting carbohydrate to 40% of the total energy content by increasing dietary fat to 40%. This advice is based on clinical studies showing women with GDM have better glycaemic control when consuming less than 45%, rather than more than 45%, of their calorie intake as carbohydrate (72,73). The American approach gives no acknowledgement to the fact that different ingested carbohydrates have different glycaemic responses as measured by their glycaemic index (74).

British advice on the diabetic diet in pregnancy does not recommend limiting carbohydrate to 40% of the total energy and indeed suggests this figure should be nearer 55%, with the majority of carbohydrate having a low glycaemic index (75). Low glycaemic index diets can in fact increase insulin sensitivity in both pregnant and non-pregnant individuals (42–44,76). In pregnancy glycaemic control deteriorates when refined carbohydrate contributes more than 45% of the total energy (72). By contrast when refined carbohydrates are exchanged for low glycaemic index carbohydrates, 60% of the total dietary energy can be consumed in this form without any change in glucose tolerance (42–44). As the glycaemic response to rapidly absorbed refined sugars is greatest in the early morning, advice on suitable commercial breakfast cereals should be given (77).

DIETARY FAT

The short-term dietary studies that demonstrated a benefit of high-fat versus high-carbohydrate diets on post-prandial blood glucose values (72,77) may, as discussed above, have been accounted for by the use of high glycaemic index carbohydrates in these studies. Jovanovic's group (78) have also stated that the addition of dietary saturated fat to a test meal produces a significantly lower glycaemic and insulin response than when the test meal contains the equivalent proportion of monounsaturated fat. The differences may be explained by slower gastric emptying when the meal contains a high saturated fat content. However, we believe that even if the glycaemic response mid-morning can be lowered by increasing the saturated fat content of the breakfast, advocating such a diet to women at future risk of diabetes and cardiovascular disease remains highly questionable, when epidemiological and clinical studies show that high-fat diets are associated with insulin resistance, β-cell dysfunction, and recurrent GDM pregnancy and future diabetes (56,59). Also the long-term effects of a high maternal saturated fat diet on cardiovascular health is unknown. Animal studies certainly suggest caution as high-fat diets in pregnant rodents can promote cardiovascular disease in the next generation (79,80). Increasing the saturation content of the diet in pregnant rats leads both to unfavourable changes in fatty acid compositions and function of the major arterial vessels. High-fat diets in pregnancy have also been associated with severe hyperemesis gravidarum, with a 5.4-fold increased risk reported for every additional 15 g/day of dietary saturated fat (81).

Increasing the polyunsaturated fat (PUFA) content of the diet while restricting the saturated fat may provide an alternative approach to safely reducing the overall dietary carbohydrate content. A large epidemiological study in China reported that a high habitual intake of dietary PUFA with a correspondingly raised low dietary polyunsaturated to saturated fat ratio protected against gestational diabetes (57). It remains to be proven whether Western women would achieve a similar benefit, as their PUFA intake is highly correlated with saturated fat intake.

The potential benefits of increasing monounsaturated fat (MUFA) intake in pregnancy still need to be shown. A recent small Danish study failed to show any improvement in insulin sensitivity in late pregnancy when women with GDM eat diets high in MUFA rather than high in carbohydrates, although a favourable effect on blood pressure was reported (82). Outside pregnancy improved insulin resistance and lipid profiles have been reported when either a high-carbohydrate diet or a monosaturated-enriched diet replaces dietary saturated fat, with reductions in plasma LDL cholesterol observed (83,84). If high-MUFA diets are to be promoted over a high-carbohydrate diet, one needs to ensure that overall calorie intake leading to unnecessary weight gain does not occur (85).

A large Swedish epidemiological study has suggested that increasing dietary long-chain n-3 fatty acids (omega-3 fatty acids) by increasing fish and fish oils may provide some protection against low birth weights and pre-term deliveries (86). Similar diets in Type 2 diabetic subjects have been shown to have some favourable metabolic effects on serum triglycerides but not plasma LDL cholesterol (87,88). Other food sources of n-3 polyunsaturated fatty acids include flaxseed and flaxseed oil, canola oil, soybean oil and nuts. Population studies suggest that foods containing n-3 fatty acids, specifically eicosapentaenoic acid and docosahexaenoic acid, may provide long-term cardio-protection (89,90). There are therefore potential theoretical benefits for increasing dietary long-chain n-3 fatty acids in diabetic women both in and out of pregnancy.

In the face of no real clinical-based studies on the optimal ratio between saturated, poly, mono and fish oils for pregnancy, it is our policy to aim for a ratio of sat:poly:mono of 1:1:1, with the specific advice to eat oily fish three times a week (91). These recommendations are similar to those for people with diabetes and coronary heart disease.

DIET AND INSULIN THERAPY FOR GDM

Once diet alone can no longer consistently ensure fasting glucose values below 5.5 mmol/l and a 1 h post-prandial value below 7 mmol/l, the introduction of insulin should be considered (63). It is important to recognise that a small proportion of women will require insulin early in pregnancy and not to assume dietary non-compliance (92). Those requiring insulin are the most metabolically compromised and tend to have both the highest perinatal complications and the fastest deterioration to diabetes after pregnancy (93). Insulin is also occasionally introduced in later pregnancy for obstetric rather than glycaemic reasons; this might occur for accelerated foetal growth or unexplained polyhydramnios (94).

It is important to stress that once insulin is introduced for the management of GDM the dietary management remains equally important. The need to limit weight gain remains for obese women who now need to balance this with having sufficient carbohydrate snacks throughout the day to prevent hypoglycaemia. Although short periods of hypoglycaemia are not detrimental to the foetus they are unpleasant for the woman and frequently result in sudden rises of blood sugar due to the action of counter-regulatory hormones and the consumption of sugary drinks. Frequent episodes of hypoglycaemia often result in women chasing these high-rebound glucose levels by increasing their insulin dosage, which can result in further hypoglycaemic attacks and unnecessary weight gain.

When starting on insulin women should be advised to take low glycaemic index carbohydrates at meal times and for snacks between meals and before bed. Fruit is ideal for snacks as it is low in fat and calories. Fruit, by being slowly absorbed, reduces the risk of hypoglycaemia while allowing post-prandial glucose levels to be lowered without having to increase the insulin dose.

LONG-TERM DIETARY ADVICE FOR THE MOTHER AND HER CHILD

As most women with GDM are obese and all have at least one child at increased risk of adolescent obesity and diabetes, providing dietary education and advice that extends beyond the pregnancy is extremely important. Lifestyle changes encompassing diet and exercise have been shown to reduce the risk of GDM in subsequent pregnancies as well as delaying the progression to Type 2 diabetes (59,95,96). Women with a history of GDM are an ideal group to target, not only because of their own heightened risk of future diabetes (97,98) but to ensure a healthy lifestyle within the family unit, hence reducing the risk of obesity and future diabetes in the children also.

Ideally all women with GDM should receive lifestyle advice and education in pregnancy that is relevant to after pregnancy. It will be an important challenge to find methods of delivering dietetic education and advice both effectively and cheaply to enable all women with GDM to receive the necessary ongoing support and care they require after pregnancy in the community.

THE NEED AND FEASIBILITY OF FUTURE DIETARY STUDIES IN PREGNANCY

There remains a lack of good randomised studies on the dietary management of diabetic pregnancies. Such studies are required for both short-term pregnancy outcomes and long-term outcomes for the mother and her child. One of the main difficulties in conducting such studies is the control arm; even when no dietary advice is given, women once diagnosed with GDM make lifestyle changes based on family beliefs or information gathered from a variety of sources. Also if the health care providers are aware of the diagnosis they too unintentionally are likely to influence lifestyle factors. The need to blind both the women and the health care staff to the diagnosis is difficult and often considered unethical, as GDM if ignored can carry a risk to the pregnancy (99). It is hoped that the HAPO Study (Hyperglycaemia Adverse Pregnancy Outcome Study) currently underway, looking at pregnancy outcomes in 25 000 pregnant women in whom lesser degrees of glucose intolerance will go untreated, will help to answer some of these questions.

SUMMARY

Diabetes is a common complication of pregnancy. Nutritional advice, intervention and education are a central part of the management of all women with diabetes in pregnancy. Dietary intervention, either alone or with insulin, can improve pregnancy outcomes. Appropriate advice to obese women with Type 2 diabetes and GDM should aim to avoid excessive maternal weight gain and worsening glucose tolerance after pregnancy. For women with GDM dietary advice in pregnancy should extend beyond the pregnancy itself, aimed at reducing the lifetime risk of future diabetes for both the mother and her child.

REFERENCES

1. Brydon P, Smith T, Proffitt M, Gee H, Holder R, Dunne F. Pregnancy outcome in women with Type 2 diabetes mellitus needs to be addressed. *Int J Clin Prac* 2000; 54: 418–419.
2. Casson IF, Clarke CA, Howard CV et al. Outcomes of pregnancy in insulin dependent diabetic women: results of a five year population cohort study. *Br Med J* 1997; 315: 275–278.
3. Hawthorne G, Robson S, Ryall E, Sen D, Roberts SH, Ward Platt MP. Prospective population based survey of outcome of pregnancy in diabetic women: results of the Northern Diabetic Pregnancy Audit. *Br Med J* 1997; 315: 279–281.
4. Hahn T, Hahn D, Blaschitz A, Korgun ET, Desoye G, Dohr G. Hyperglycaemia-induced subcellular redistribution of GLUT1 glucose transporters in cultured human term placental trophoblast cells. *Diabetologia* 2000; 43: 173–80.
5. Weiss PA, Scholz HS, Haas J, Tamussino KF, Seissler J, Borkenstein MH, Long-term follow-up of infants of mothers with Type 1 diabetes: evidence for hereditary and nonhereditary transmission of diabetes and precursors. *Diabetes Care* 2000; 23: 905–911.
6. DeVeciana M, Major CA, Morgan MA. Postprandial versus preprandial glucose monitoring in women with gestational diabetes mellitus requiring insulin therapy. *N Engl J Med* 1995; 333: 1237–1241.
7. Langer O, Conway DL, Berkus MD, Xenakis EM-J, Gonzales O. A Comparison of glyburide and insulin in women with gestational diabetes mellitus. *N Engl J Med* 2000; 343: 1134–1138.
8. The MRC Vitamin Research Study Group. Prevention of neural tube defects: the results of the Medical Research Council Vitamin Study, 1991. London: MRC.
9. Rogers I, Emmett P. England ALSPAC Study Team. Avon Longitudinal Study of Pregnancy and Childhood. *Eur J Clin Nutr* 1998; 52: 246–250.
10. Dickinson PJ, Dornhorst A, Frost GS. A retrospective case control study of initiating insulin therapy in type 2 diabetes. *Pract Diabetes Int* 2002; 19: 67–70.
11. Bianco A, Smilen S, Davis Y, Lopez S, Lapinski R, Lockwood C. Pregnancy outcome and weight gain recommendations for the morbidly obese woman. *Obstet Gynecol* 1998; 91: 97–102.
12. Watkins ML, Botto L. Maternal prepregnancy weight and congenital heart defects in the offspring. *Epidemiology* 2001; 12: 439–446.
13. Moore L, Singer M, Bradlee ML, Rothman K, Milunsky A. A prospective study of the risk of congenital defects associated with maternal obesity and diabetes mellitus. *Epidemiology* 2000; 11: 689–694.
14. Baeten J, Bukusi E, Lambe M. Pregnancy complications and outcomes among overweight and obese nulliparous women. *Am J Public Health* 2001; 91: 436–440.
15. Chappell LC, Seed PT, Briley AL et al. Effects on antioxidants on the occurrence of pre-eclampsia in women at increased risk: a randomised trial. *Lancet* 1999; 354: 810–816.
16. Siman C, Eriksson U. Vitamin E decreases the occurrence of malformations in the offspring of diabetic rats. *Diabetes* 1997; 46: 1054–1061.
17. Daaboul J, Sanderson S. Vitamin D deficiency in pregnant and breast-feeding women and their infants. *J Perinatol* 1997; 17: 10–14.
18. Waiters B, Godel JC, Basu TK. Perinatal vitamin D and calcium status of northern Canadian mothers and their newborn infants. *J Am Coll Nutr* 1999; 18: 122–126.
19. Boucher BJ. Inadequate vitamin D status: does it contribute to the disorders comprising syndrome 'X'? *Br J Nutr* 1998; 79: 315–327.

20. Hitman GA, Mannan N, McDermott MF *et al.* Vitamin D receptor gene polymorphisms influence insulin secretion in Bangladeshi Asians. *Diabetes* 1998; 47: 688–690.
21. Janerich DT. Alcohol and pregnancy. An epidemiologic perspective. *Ann Epidemiol* 1990; 1: 179–185.
22. Pitkin RM. Energy in pregnancy. *Am J Clin Nutr* 1999; 69: 583.
23. Institute of Medicine. *Nutrition during Pregnancy: Weight Gain and Nutritional Supplements.* Washington DC: National Academy Press, 1990.
24. American College of Obstetricians and Gynaecologists. Nutrition during pregnancy. *ACOG Tech Bull* 1993: 1–7.
25. Feig D, Naylor CD. Eating for two: are guidelines for weight gain during pregnancy too liberal? *Lancet* 1998; 351: 1054–1055.
26. Butte NF, Hopkinson JM, Mehta N, Moon JK, Smith EO. Adjustments in energy expenditure and substrate utilisation during late pregnancy and lactation. *Am J Clin Nutr* 1999; 69: 299–307.
27. Hytten F, Leitch I. *The Physiology of Human Pregnancy.* Oxford: Blackwell Scientific, 1964.
28. Hytten FF. Nutrition. In: *Clinical Physiology in Obstetrics*, eds E Hytten and G Chamberlain. Oxford: Blackwell Scientific, 1980: 163–192.
29. Kopp-Hoolihan LE, van Loan MD, Wong WW, King JC. Longitudinal assessment of energy balance in well nourished, pregnant women. *Am J Clin Nutr* 1999; 69: 697–704.
30. Durnin J. Energy requirements of pregnancy: an integrated study in five countries. Background and methods. *Lancet* 1987; II: 895–897.
31. Illingsworth PJ, Jung RT, Howie PW. Reduction in post-prandial energy expenditure during pregnancy. *Br Med J* 1987; 294: 1573–1576.
32. Poppitt SD, Prentice AM, Jequier E, Schutz Y, Whitehead RG. Evidence of energy sparing in Gambian women during pregnancy: a longitudinal study using whole-body calorimetry. *Am J Clin Nutr* 1993; 57: 353–364.
33. Lawrence M, Whitehead RG. Physical activity and total energy expenditure of child-bearing Gambian village women. *Eur J Clin Nutr* 1987; 42: 145–160.
34. National Research Council. *Recommended Dietary Allowance.* Washington, DC: National Academic Press, 1989.
35. Hay WWJ. The role of placental–fetal interaction in fetal nutrition. *Semin Perinatol* 1991; 15: 424–433.
36. Hay WWJ. Placental supply of energy and protein substrate to the fetus. *Acta Paediatr* 1994; 405 (Suppl): 13–19.
37. Sivan E, Homko CJ, Chen X, Reece EA, Boden G. Free fatty acids and insulin resistance during pregnancy. *J Clin Endocrin Metab* 1998; 83: 2338–2342.
38. Kalkhoff RK, Richardson BL, Beck P. Relative effects of pregnancy human placental lactogen and prednisolone on carbohydrate tolerance in normal and subclinical diabetic subjects. *Diabetes* 1969; 18: 153–175.
39. Langhoff-Roos J, Wibell L, Gebre-Medhin M, Lindmark G. Placental hormones and maternal glucose tolerance: a study of fetal growth in normal pregnancy. *Br J Obstet Gynaecol* 1989; 96: 320–326.
40. Leturque A, Hauguel S, Sutter-Dub MT, Girard J. Effects of placental lactogen and progesterone on insulin stimulated glucose metabolism in rat muscles in vitro. *Diabetes Metab* 1989; 15: 176–181.
41. Spellacy WN, Goetz FC. Plasma insulin in normal late pregnancy. *N Engl J Med* 1963; 268: 988–991.

42. Clapp J. Effect of dietary carbohydrate on the glucose and insulin response to mixed caloric intake and exercise in both nonpregnant and pregnant women. *Diabetes Care* 1998; 21 (Suppl 2): B107–112.
43. Fraser RB. The normal range of OGTT in the African female: pregnant and non-pregnant. *East Afr Med J* 1981; 58: 90–94.
44. Fraser R, Ford F, Lawrence G. Insulin sensitivity in third trimester pregnancy. A randomized study of dietary effects. *Br J Obstet Gynaecol* 1988; 95: 223–229.
45. Freinkel N. Banting Lecture 1980: of pregnancy and progeny. *Diabetes* 1980; 29: 1023–1035.
46. Freinkel N, Metzger BE, Phelps RL *et al.* Gestational diabetes mellitus: heterogeneity of maternal age, weight, insulin secretion, HLA antigens, and islet cell antibodies and the impact of maternal metabolism on pancreatic β-cell function and somatic growth in the offspring. *Diabetes* 1985; 34 (Suppl 2): 1–7.
47. Highman TJ, Friedman JE, Huston L, Wong WW, Catalano PM. Longitudinal studies in maternal leptin concentrations, body composition, and resting metabolic rate in pregnancy. *Am J Obstet Gynecol* 1998; 178: 1010–1015.
48. Kalhan SC, D'Angelo LJ, Savin SM, Adam PAJ. Glucose production in pregnant women at term gestation. *J Clin Invest* 1979; 63: 388–394.
49. Kalhan S, Rossi K, Gruca L, Burkett E, O'Brien A. Glucose turnover and gluconeogenesis in human pregnancy. *J Clin Invest* 1997; 100: 1775–1781.
50. Kühl C, Hornnes P. Aetiological factors in gestational diabetes. In: *Carbohydrate Metabolism in Pregnancy and the Newborn*, ed. HWSaKM Stowers. Edinburgh: Churchill Livingstone, 1984; 12–22.
51. Kühl C. Insulin secretion and insulin resistance in pregnancy and GDM. Implications for diagnosis and management. *Diabetes* 1991; 40 (Suppl 2): 18–24.
52. Kautzky-Willer A, Prager R, Waldhäusl W *et al.* Pronounced insulin resistance and inadequate β-cell secretion characterizes lean gestational diabetes during and after pregnancy. *Diabetes Care* 1997; 20: 1717–1723.
53. Catalano PM, Tyzbir ED, Wolfe RR *et al.* Carbohydrate metabolism during pregnancy in control subjects and women with gestational diabetes. *Am J Physiol* 1993; 264: E60–E67.
54. Catalano PM, Huston L, Amini SB, Kalhan SC. Longitudinal changes in glucose metabolism during pregnancy in obese women with normal glucose tolerance and gestational diabetes mellitus. *Am J Obstet Gynecol* 1999; 180: 903–916.
55. Cowett RM, Carr SR, Ogburn PL. Lipid tolerance testing in pregnancy. *Diabetes Care* 1993; 16: 5–56.
56. Boden G, Chen X. Effects of fatty acids and ketone bodies on basal insulin secretion in type 2 diabetes. *Diabetes* 1999; 48: 577–583.
57. Wang Y, Storlien L, Jenkins A *et al.* Dietary variables and glucose tolerance in pregnancy. *Diabetes Care* 2000; 23: 460–464.
58. Scholl TO, Hediger ML, Schall JI, Ances IG, Smith WK. Gestational weight gain, pregnancy outcome, and postpartum weight retention. *Obstet Gynecol* 1995; 86: 423–427.
59. Moses RG, Shand JL, Tapsell LC. The recurrence of gestational diabetes: could dietary differences in fat intake be an explanation? *Diabetes Care* 1997; 20: 1647–1650.
60. O'Sullivan JB. Body weight and subsequent diabetes mellitus. *J Am Med Assoc* 1982; 248: 949–952.
61. Schofield WN, Schofield C, James WPT. Basal metabolic rate review and prediction, together with annotated source material. *Human Nutr Appl Nutr* 1985; 39C: 5–96.

62. American Diabetes Association. Nutritional management. In: *Medical Management of Pregnancy Complicated by Diabetes*. Virginia: American Diabetes Association, 1995: 47–56.

63. Metzger BE. Summary and recommendations of the Fourth International Workshop – Conference on Gestational Diabetes Mellitus. *Diabetes Care* 1998; 21 (Suppl 2): B1–B167.

64. Ravelli GP, Stein ZA, Susser MW. Obesity in young men after famine exposure in utero and early infancy. *N Engl J Med* 1976; 295: 349–353.

65. Ravelli ACJ, van der Meulen JHP, Michels RP *et al*. Glucose tolerance in adults after prenatal exposure to famine. *Lancet* 1998; 351: 173–177.

66. Churchill JA, Berendez HW, Nemore J. Neuropsychological deficits in children of diabetic mothers. *Am J Obstet Gynecol* 1966; 105: 257–268.

67. Rizzo T, Metzger BE, Burns WJ, Burns K. Correlation between antepartum maternal metabolism and intelligence of offspring. *N Engl J Med* 1991; 325: 408–413.

68. Buchanan TA, Metzger BE, Freinkel N. Accelerated starvation in late pregnancy: a comparison between obese normal pregnant women and women with gestational diabetes. *Am J Obstet Gynecol* 1990; 162: 1015–1020.

69. Knopp RH, Magee MS, Raisys V, Benedetti T. Metabolic effects of hypocaloric diets in management of gestational diabetes. *Diabetes* 1991; 40 (Suppl 2): 165–171.

70. Wolever TM, Bentum-Williams A, Jenkins DJ. Physiological modulation of plasma free fatty acid concentrations by diet. Metabolic implications in nondiabetic subjects. *Diabetes Care* 1995; 18: 962–970.

71. Dornhorst A, Nicholls JSD, Probst F *et al*. Calorie restriction for the treatment of gestational diabetes. *Diabetes* 1991; 40 (Suppl 2): 161–164.

72. Major C, Henry M, De Veciana M, Morgan M. The effects of carbohydrate restriction in patients with diet-controlled gestational diabetes. *Obstet Gynecol* 1998; 91: 600–604.

73. Jovanovic L. American Diabetes Association, Fourth International Workshop – Conference on Gestational Diabetes Mellitus. Summary and Discussion: therapeutic interventions. *Diabetes Care* 1998; 21 (Suppl 2): 131–137.

74. Wolever TM. The glycemic index. *World Rev Nutr Diet* 1990; 62: 120–185.

75. Dornhorst A, Frost GS. The principles of dietary management of gestational diabetes: reflection on current evidence. *Br J Human Nutr Diet* 2002; 15: 145–156.

76. Frost G, Leeds TA, Dornhorst A. Insulin sensitivity in women at risk of coronary heart disease and the effect of a low glycaemic diet. *Metabolism* 1998; 47: 1245–1251.

77. Peterson CM, Jovanovic-Peterson L. Percentage of carbohydrate and glycaemic response to breakfast, lunch and dinner in women with gestational diabetes. *Diabetes* 1991; 40 (Suppl 2): 172–174.

78. Ilic S, Jovanovic L, Pettitt D. Comparison of the effect of saturated and monounsaturated fat on postprandial plasma glucose and insulin concentration in women with gestational diabetes mellitus. *Am J Perinatol* 1999; 16: 489–495.

79. Ghosh P, Bitsanis D, Ghebremeskel K, Crawford M, Poston L. Abnormal aortic fatty acid composition and small artery function in offspring of rats fed a high fat diet in pregnancy. *J Physiol* 2001; 533 (3): 815–822.

80. Kucera J. Rate and type of congenital anomalies among offspring in diabetic women. *J Reproduct Med* 1971; 7: 61–70.

81. Signorello L, Harlow B, Wang S, Erick M. Saturated fat intake and the risk of severe hyperemesis gravidarum. *Epidemiology* 1998; 9: 636–640.

82. Lauszus FF, Klebe JG, Flyvbjerg A. Macrosomia associated with maternal serum insulin-like growth factor-I and -II in diabetic pregnancy. *Obstet Gynecol* 2001; 97: 734–741.

83. Georgopoulous A, Bantle JP, Noutsou M, Swaim WR, Parker SJ. Differences in the metabolism of postprandial lipoproteins after a high-monounsaturated-fat versus a high-carbohydrate diet in patients with type 1 diabetes mellitus. *Arterioscler Thromb Vasc Biol* 1998; 18: 773–782.

84. Garg A, Bantle JP, Henry RR *et al*. Effects of varying carbohydrate content of diet in patients with non-insulin dependent diabetes mellitus. *J Am Med Assoc* 1994; 271: 1421–1428.

85. Yu-Poth S, Zhao G, Etherton T, Naglak M, Jonnalagadda S, Kris-Etherton PM. Effect of National Cholesterol Education Program's Step I and Step II dietary interventon programs of cardiovascular disease risk factors; a meta-analysis. *Am J Clin Nutr* 1999; 69: 632–646.

86. Olsen SF, Secher NJ. Low consumption of seafood in early pregnancy as a risk factor for preterm delivery: prospective cohort study. *Br Med J* 2002: 447–450.

87. Glauber H, Wallace P, Griver K, Brechtel G. Adverse metabolic effect of omega-3 fatty acids in non-insulin-dependent diabetes mellitus. *Ann Intern Med* 1988; 108: 663–668.

88. Westerveld HT, deGraaf JC, van Breugel HH *et al*. Effects of low-dose EPA-E on glycemic control, lipid profile, lipoprotein (a), platelet aggregation, viscosity, and platelet and vessel wall interaction in NIDDM. *Diabetes Care* 1993; 16: 683–688.

89. de Lorgeril M, Salen P, Martin JL, Monjaud I, Delaye J, Mamelle N. Mediterranean diet, traditional risk factors, and the rate of cardiovascular complications after myocardial infarction: final of the Lyon Diet Heart Study. *Circulation* 1999; 99: 733–735.

90. Daviglus ML, Stamler J, Orencia AJ *et al*. Fish consumption and the 30-year risk of fatal myocardial infarction. *N Engl J Med* 1997; 336: 1046–1053.

91. Lean MEJ, Brenchley S, Connor H, Elkeles RS, Govindji A, Hartland BV. Dietary recommendations for people with diabetes: an update for the 1990s. Nutrition Subcommittee of the British Diabetic Association's Professional Advisory Committee. *Diabet Med* 1992; 9: 189–202.

92. McFarland MB, Langer O, Conway DL, Berkus MD. Dietary therapy for gestational diabetes: how long is long enough? *Obstet Gynecol* 1999; 93: 978–982.

93. Metzger BE, Cho NH, Roston SM, Radvany R. Prepregnancy weight and antepartum insulin secretion predict glucose tolerance five years after gestational diabetes mellitus. *Diabetes Care* 1993; 16: 1598–1605.

94. Buchanan TA, Kjos SL, Montoro MN *et al*. Use of fetal ultrasound to select metabolic therapy for pregnancies complicated by mild gestational diabetes. *Diabetes Care* 1994; 17: 275–283.

95. Diabetes Prevention Program Research Group. Reduction in the incidence of type 2 diabetes with lifestyle intervention or metformin. *N Engl J Med* 2002; 346: 393–403.

96. Tuomilehto J, Lindström J, Eriksson JG *et al*. Prevention of type 2 diabetes mellitus by changes in lifestyle among subjects with impaired glucose tolerance. *N Engl J Med* 2001; 344: 1343–1350.

97. Damm PD, Molsted-Pedersen LMP, Kühl CK. High incidence of diabetes mellitus and impaired glucose tolerance in women with previous gestational diabetes (Abstract). *Diabetologia* 1989; 32: 479A.

98. Dornhorst A, Bailey PC, Anyaoku V, Elkeles RS, Johnston DG, Beard RW. Abnormalities of glucose tolerance following gestational diabetes. *Q J Med* 1990; 284 (New Series 77): 1219–1228.

99. Adams KM, Li H, Nelson RL, Ogburn PLJ, Danilenko-Dixon DR. Sequelae of unrecognised gestational diabetes. *Am J Obstet Gynecol* 1998; 178: 1321–1332.

8

Obesity and Diabetes

KAREN SLEVIN, JACQUELINE CLEATOR AND JOHN WILDING

University Hospital Aintree, Liverpool, UK

INTRODUCTION

Obesity has recently been highlighted as having a substantial human cost, by contributing to the onset of disease and premature mortality, as well as having serious financial consequences for the health service and the economy (1). There is a strong relationship between diabetes and obesity, and excess body fat has been shown to affect both the development and progression of this chronic endocrine condition. Obesity is most closely associated with Type 2 diabetes and evidence suggests that a substantial number of the cases of Type 2 diabetes could be avoided if individuals were to stay within a healthy weight range (2). The mean body mass index (BMI) at diagnosis of Type 2 diabetes is $29\,kg/m^2$ (3), with the risk of developing the disease increasing exponentially with an increase in BMI. For example, the risk is 80-fold greater in an individual with morbid obesity $(BMI > 40\,kg/m^2)$ compared with an individual with a $BMI \leqslant 22\,kg/m^2$ (4). Several studies have also shown that even modest degrees of overweight in early age are predictive of diabetes risk in middle age (4,5).

The prevalence of obesity in the UK has almost tripled since 1980, and this trend shows no sign of reversing (1). It follows, therefore, that there has been an increase in the incidence of Type 2 diabetes, with 180 million cases predicted world-wide by the year 2010 (6). Alarmingly, as the levels of obesity have increased, a greater number of cases of Type 2 diabetes have emerged in both children and young adults. No longer can Type 2 diabetes be considered as a 'late-onset' condition. The management costs of diabetes are already exceptionally high (7) and this shift in the age of onset of Type 2 diabetes will have

---

Nutritional Management of Diabetes Mellitus. Edited by G. Frost, A. Dornhorst and R. Moses
© 2003 John Wiley & Sons, Ltd. ISBN 0 471 49751 7

devastating implications for both the medical and social costs of diabetes. While such statistics are alarming, it is important to recognise that obesity is also the most modifiable risk factor for Type 2 diabetes. It must be remembered, however, that correlation does not prove causation and that obesity is not obligatory for the development of diabetes. Obesity must interact to a variable degree with other environmental and genetic factors that determine insulin resistance and β-cell dysfunction, in order to lead to Type 2 diabetes in an individual (8).

There is a substantial disease burden associated with obesity and overweight. However, in the presence of diabetes, the devastating metabolic consequences of insulin resistance further expose the obese individual to cardiogenic risk factors such as dyslipidaemia and hypertension. Atherosclerosis and ischaemic heart disease are more likely to develop, and the risk of premature death is 10-fold greater in a diabetic person with a $BMI > 36 \, kg/m^2$ compared with a similarly obese non-diabetic patient (9). While many of the complications associated with diabetes are linked to the metabolic consequences of increased adipose tissue mass, it is important to remember that other sequelae in the guise of obesity-related co-morbidities are common in diabetic patients. Most notable are: musculoskeletal disease, sleep apnoea, cancer, gall bladder disease, impaired mobility, respiratory problems, foot ulcers and perhaps most significantly for the individual, low self-esteem and poor quality of life. In addition, obese persons suffer from marked discrimination in society and often face prejudice from both the public and health professionals (10,11).

It is clear that weight management should form an integral part of the management of diabetes, with a strong emphasis on the prevention of obesity. It should be recognised however that obesity is a complex condition, the treatment of which is far from simple and requires the support of skilled helpers. Obesity treatment should be regarded as a long-term procedure, which is threaded into the management of diabetes. The primary focus of this chapter is to consider the mechanisms which link obesity and diabetes, the benefits of weight loss in diabetes, and how to manage obesity within a model of life-long diabetes care.

DEFINING OBESITY

Obesity is a condition in which there is excessive reserves of body fat. Clinically, obesity is classified in terms of the BMI (kg/m^2). The different classifications of

Table 8.1 Categories of BMI [weight (kg)/height (m^2)]

Normal weight	Overweight	Pre-obese	Obese Class 1	Obese Class 2	Obese Class 3
18.5–24.9	$\geqslant 25$	25.0–29.9	30.0–34.9	35.0–39.9	$\geqslant 40$

BMI are outlined in Table 8.1, with obesity defined as a BMI $> 30\,kg/m^2$ and morbid obesity as a BMI $> 40\,kg/m^2$.

OBESITY AND TYPE 1 DIABETES

The strong association between obesity and Type 2 diabetes has generally overshadowed obesity in relation to Type 1 diabetes. Obesity is relevant, however, as increases in body fat stores generally dictate an increase in insulin requirements, mainly as a result of a further decline in insulin sensitivity. Conversely, excessive dosages of insulin can lead to weight gain, presumably through the lipogenic effects of hyperinsulinaeima and possibly compounded by overeating during the hypoglycaemic episodes, which become more frequent as insulin therapy is intensified. Weight gain, following intensive treatment of those with Type 1 diabetes, has been shown to induce unfavourable changes in lipid levels and blood pressure, similar to those observed in the insulin resistance syndrome (12). However, if intensive therapy results in improvements in glycaemic control, this can reduce the impact of weight gain on such cardiovascular risk factors (13).

Of concern also is that obesity, or the fear of it, can have detrimental effects, particularly in young (predominantly female) patients with Type 1 diabetes. The desire to remain thin can lead these patients to reduce or omit insulin dosages and/ or to engage in purging and laxative abuse (14–16). This particular form of 'eating disorder' is probably one of the prevailing causes of 'brittle' or unstable diabetes, and often leads to recurrent episodes of diabetic ketoacidosis with an increased risk of developing chronic diabetic complications and of premature death (17). Consideration should therefore be given to the management of those with Type 1 diabetes who are obese or at risk of becoming obese, and to vulnerable individuals who are in danger of adversely controlling their own treatment for fear of becoming obese. It remains true, however, that the prevalence of being overweight in Type 1 diabetes is lower than that in the general population (13).

THE ASSOCIATION BETWEEN OBESITY AND TYPE 2 DIABETES

The link between obesity and Type 2 diabetes has long been established and a visit to any diabetes clinic will confirm the alarming statistic that 90% of those with Type 2 diabetes are also estimated to be obese (18). It is not currently known whether insulin resistance is the cause of obesity, the result of obesity, or whether the two conditions arise independently from each other (19). It is known that the prevalence of insulin resistance is greater among the obese, however, there are normal weight individuals who are equally insulin resistant

(20). Without question, reduction in weight is associated with improvements in insulin sensitivity (21,22). It is also clear that regular physical activity improves insulin action, although the exact mechanisms involved are not clear.

Several mechanisms have been proposed to explain how excessive body weight is associated with Type 2 diabetes. In general, the accumulation of fat mass is associated with a decline in whole body insulin sensitivity. The distribution of obesity is important, with resistance to the action of insulin and glucose intolerance most closely associated with excess abdominal adipose tissue. As visceral adipose tissue increases plasma triglyceride (TG) concentrations are elevated, high-density lipoprotein (HDL) cholesterol decreases and low-density lipoprotein (LDL) cholesterol increases with a greater proportion of the more atherogenic small dense LDL particles (LDL subclass III). Other associated characteristics include an elevated plasma non-esterified fatty acid (NEFA) concentration, an increased plasminogen activator inhibitor 1 (PAI-1) concentration, hyperuricaemia and hypertension. Abdominal obesity is also associated with specific changes in skeletal muscle morphology, namely a reduction in capillary density and an increase in the proportion of 'white' or 'glycolytic' fibres which are less insulin sensitive than the red (oxidative) fibres (23). Within the adipocyte an increase in the expression of products such as tumour necrosis factor-α (TNF-α) and leptin may also contribute to the deterioration in insulin sensitivity. More recently a novel protein known as resistin has been reported as providing the missing link in explaining the molecular link between diabetes and obesity. Resistin is secreted by adipocytes. Its circulating levels correlate with obesity and it has been shown to cause insulin resistance in target tissues (24).

BENEFITS OF WEIGHT LOSS

Despite the expectations of the individual, the likelihood that an obese person will achieve sufficient weight loss to reach an 'ideal' body weight is remote (25). However, this does not imply that treating obesity is fruitless, as there is evidence that even a modest weight loss of 5–10% in obese diabetic subjects can produce clinical benefits. Improvements have been noted in all modifiable risk factors such as HbA$_{1c}$ levels, hypertension, dyslipidaemia, self-esteem and overall quality of life. Moreover, improvements in these risk factors have a favourable effect on mortality. A retrospective study of Type 2 diabetic patients receiving standard dietetic advice showed a mean weight loss of 2.6 kg for those with a BMI 25–30 kg/m^2 and a loss of 6.8 kg for those with a BMI > 30 kg/m^2 after 1 year. For the average patient each kilogram of weight loss was associated with a three- to four-month prolonged survival and a 10 kg weight loss predicted the restoration of about 35% in life expectancy (26).

GLYCAEMIC CONTROL

A reduction in body weight has a direct influence on glycaemic control by improving both hepatic and peripheral insulin sensitivity and decreasing insulin resistance (27). HbA_{1c} is the accepted measure of longer-term glycaemic control with a level $<7\%$ as the desired target (28). While several studies of Type 2 diabetic subjects have demonstrated improvements in fasting blood glucose, HbA_{1c} and plasma insulin after weight loss, it has been observed that the benefits are proportional to the amount of weight lost. A study by Wing *et al.* (29) showed that a weight loss of 10% of total body weight reduced HbA_{1c} levels by 1.6%. Correspondingly, there was a reduction in the need for oral diabetic agents. In fact, those losing 15% of their body weight were able to discontinue medication for diabetes altogether.

HYPERTENSION

Hypertension is a feature of Type 2 diabetes and is thought to result from a failure of insulin-induced vasodilation to counteract both renal sodium reabsorption and activation of the sympathetic nervous system (30). Indeed the UKPDS emphasised the importance of tight blood pressure (BP) control in Type 2 diabetes to reduce the risk of cardiovascular and macrovascular complications, with a recommended target BP of 140/85 mmHg (31). For the obese Type 2 diabetic patient, weight loss is pivotal to achieving this target as a weight loss of more than 10 kg has been shown to reduce the risk of hypertension by 26% (32). A more realistic intervention may be to prevent further weight gain, as it is estimated that a 1 kg increase in weight is associated with a 5% increase in risk of hypertension (32).

DYSLIPIDAEMIA

Adverse lipoprotein concentrations are commonly observed in those with Type 2 diabetes, with 40–50% of subjects having an abnormal profile (33). The most characteristic lipid pattern in diabetes is a high serum triglyceride level and a low HDL cholesterol level. Raised serum triglyceride levels lead to the synthesis of TG-enriched VLDL from the liver, promoting an unfavourable lipid exchange between lipoproteins. This results in an increased clearance of the more protective HDL cholesterol from the circulation and an increase in the more atherogenic LDL cholesterol. Weight loss can help to reverse this TG-driven atherogenic process and promote a more favourable shift in the LDL cholesterol profile of an individual, through the generation of larger and less dense LDL particles, which are less of an atherogenic threat (34). Lean *et al.* (26) investigated the effects of weight loss in newly diagnosed diabetic subjects. Their results support the benefit of modest amounts of weight loss and at 6 years they found that an initial and sustained weight loss of 9 kg had associated improvements in lipid and lipoprotein levels.

QUALITY OF LIFE

Although the evidence of the physical benefits of weight loss is sustained and unequivocal, arguably, it is improvements in the quality of life that are more significant for the obese individual with Type 2 diabetes. Diabetes itself is a chronic condition, which severely affects daily living. It is estimated that the average person with diabetes is willing to trade away 12% of his remaining life in return for a diabetes-free health state (35). For many with Type 2 diabetes, this is further compounded by the burden of obesity. Compared to the general population, obese subjects report significantly worse physical, social and role functioning and worse perceived general health, with the morbidly obese experiencing greater distress than the moderately to severely obese. In addition, the obese also report significantly greater disability due to bodily pain than patients with other chronic medical conditions (36). Encouragingly, a trial of 13 weeks weight loss treatment resulting in a mean weight loss of 8.6 ± 2.8 kg showed significant improvements in all of these domains.

APPROACHES TO WEIGHT MANAGEMENT

In theory, the management of the obese diabetic patient should not differ from that of the obese non-diabetic patient. However, it has been reported that weight loss is much more difficult for Type 2 diabetic subjects than obese non-diabetic subjects. For example, 12 overweight diabetic patients treated in a behavioural weight loss programme for 20 weeks lost significantly less weight than their non-diabetic spouses on the same programme (29). Although it appears that dietary adherence alone may account for the difference, a small sample size and family dynamics may be confounding factors in these results. Indeed a more recent study using larger numbers and unrelated subjects showed that, on the contrary, Type 2 diabetic subjects can lose as much weight as their non-diabetic peers during active treatment but that the diabetic subjects regain significantly more weight at 1 year follow-up (37). This suggests that weight loss maintenance rather than initial weight loss is the main problem for these individuals. Both studies demonstrate the complex interplay between obesity and diabetes. Indeed the many physical, social and psychological burdens of these two chronic conditions make it important from the outset to build a trusting and non-judgemental relationship with the patient. The aim of the initial assessment should be to gather information needed to make a decision about the direction of future treatment (38). The general goals of weight management can be considered as follows:

1. To prevent further weight gain
2. To reduce body weight
3. To promote long-term maintenance of weight loss

ASSESSMENT OF OBESITY

Measurement of height and weight, in order to determine the BMI, is the initial step in the clinical assessment of obesity. Waist and hip circumference measurements provide information as to the distribution of weight, with a waist circumference measure of > 102 cm in men and > 88 cm in women associated with increased risk of CHD (39). More sophisticated measures of body fat can be made using other techniques such as bioelectrical impedance, dual energy X-ray absorptiometry, densitometry and isotope dilution, although these techniques tend to be expensive, complex and are generally confined to a research setting.

RISK FACTORS FOR OBESITY

The patient's age is important in determining risk from obesity and generally there is greater risk from obesity in those under 40 years of age. Taking a weight history can ascertain the onset and duration of obesity as well as the pattern of weight gain and weight loss throughout the individual's life. Longitudinal studies have shown that weight gain confers a greater risk of cardiovascular disease than an unchanging level of obesity (40). In addition, the longer the duration of obesity the more difficult treatment may be. Gender is another variable that impacts on the development of obesity, with women generally having a higher prevalence of obesity compared to men, especially in middle age (41). Reproductive function can be affected in younger women, with menstrual disorders including irregular bleeding and amenorrhea being more common among obese females.

Various medical/genetic causes of obesity must also be considered. Endocrine conditions associated with weight gain include hypothyroidism, Cushing's syndrome, hypogonadism in the male, polycystic ovary syndrome (PCOS) in the female and growth hormone deficiency (42). Rare genetic causes of obesity include Prader–Willi syndrome, Bardet–Biedl syndrome and Cohen's syndrome. Diabetes can be an obvious consequence of the severe obesity associated with such syndromes.

FAMILY HISTORY

It is important also to establish a family weight history. Estimates of the heritability of obesity vary, with some early estimates as high as 70% (43) to more recent estimates of 30–40% (44,45). The children of those with diabetes are at an increased risk of developing the condition and the involvement of the whole family in treating and preventing obesity should be encouraged.

ASSESSMENT OF CO-MORBIDITY

It is important to determine the presence of any cardiac risk factors such as hypertension, hyperlipidaemia and cigarette smoking and to provide appropriate advice and therapy. The physical symptoms of obesity include reduced mobility, joint pain, chest pain, breathing difficulties and sleeping difficulties, and these should also be assessed. Conditions such as osteoarthritis and gastrointestinal disorders such as gastric reflux can also be exacerbated by excess weight. As well as measures of glycaemic control, measurements of biochemical indices such as lipid levels and thyroid levels are advisable.

DIETARY HISTORY

A history of eating behaviour and if appropriate a current diet history can provide information as to the eating patterns and food preferences of the individual and can be used to begin to identify the changes needed. Encouraging patients to monitor their own food intake and activity patterns can be helpful in providing feedback to the patient on how to improve the nutritional quality of the diet and how to identify and overcome barriers that lead to overeating. Consideration should also be given to socio-economic and cultural factors that influence the eating patterns of an individual, particularly since diabetes is strongly associated with the Asian and African–Caribbean populations in the UK.

Eating disorders and in particular binge eating are common among the obese, with prevalence estimates of 23–46% in those seeking treatment (46). Binge eating disorder has also been reported to be associated with Type 2 diabetes, but would appear to precede Type 2 diabetes in most patients. The prevalence of binge eating disorder in those with Type 2 diabetes was recently estimated as 10% among a sample of 322 German patients (47). Other forms of disordered eating, including night eating syndrome, should also be considered when assessing an obese individual.

ASSESSING MOTIVATION TO LOSE WEIGHT

When conducting an assessment of obesity, it is important to establish the ability and motivation of the individual to make lifestyle changes at that time. The style of the therapist can be crucial in facilitating behaviour change (48) and enhancing the confidence of the individual to be able to sustain changes. Key skills include the core counselling skills of listening and reflecting, motivational interviewing techniques, as well as strategies such as cognitive behavioural therapy (CBT).

OBESITY TREATMENT

It is a basic fact that excess body fat results from an imbalance between energy input and energy output. Any obesity treatment will therefore have to attempt to reverse this imbalance so that energy intake is less than energy expenditure. However, obesity is a complex condition that involves the integration of social, behavioural, cultural, physiological, psychological, metabolic and genetic factors. It follows therefore that no single treatment option is likely to address all components. Treatments need to be interwoven so that dietary counselling, physical activity, behavioural therapy, pharmacotherapy and even surgical treatment are provided in tandem. A multidisciplinary approach to weight management is generally advocated, although where resources are limited this may not always be achievable.

DIETARY MANAGEMENT

The dietary management of diabetes is focused on measures that will improve glycaemic control. The high-fibre, high-carbohydrate and low-fat advice advocated is a type of dietary regimen which should also encourage weight loss. Increasingly, attention has also been given to the glycaemic index (GI) within the dietary management of diabetes. It is interesting to note that diets based on low glycaemic foods have been shown not only to improve blood glucose control but also to cause greater weight loss than diets based on high GI meals (49).

Ultimately, in order to lose weight, a reduction in overall energy intake is required. A useful first step, therefore, is to calculate the energy requirements of an individual based on their current body weight, age, gender and activity levels using prediction equations such as those recommended by Lean and James (50). Aiming for a weight loss of 0.5–1 kg/week involves reducing energy intake by 500–1000 kcal/day. In conjunction with the individual, it is possible to devise an eating plan which will provide a modest reduction in energy intake and be more achievable than standard prescribed energy diets. Blanket energy prescription, usually 1200 kcal for women and 1500 kcal for men, has been shown to produce significant weight loss in several studies (51–53). For those most overweight, however, a standard energy prescription can be several thousand calories below their requirements. Frost *et al.* (54) compared a 1200 kcal dietary prescription to a daily energy deficit of 500 kcal in a group of patients attending a dietetic weight management clinic. Their results showed that those in the daily deficit group achieved a greater weight loss than those in the standard prescribed diet group, suggesting a greater compliance to a more modest energy reduction. As well as aiming for a realistic reduction in energy intake, the nutritional quality of the diet is important and it should provide all of the essential nutrients in order to maintain health.

Several studies have looked at the effect of very low calorie diets (VLCDs) in the treatment of diabetes (55,56). VLCDs are 'nutrient-enriched' regimens, usually in the form of liquid drinks, which aim to provide less than 3300 kJ/ 800 kcal of dietary energy per day. Mean weight losses with a VLCD range from 1.5–2.5 kg/week, so that use over 12–16 weeks should produce close to a 20 kg weight loss. In practice, however, such weight loss is not always observed, indicating that as with other dietary regimes, this change is difficult to sustain. Maintenance of weight loss may be of particular concern with a VLCD regimen, due to the significant calorie reduction from actual energy requirements and the sharp divergence from normal eating patterns (57). Following the termination of severe energy restriction, subsequent overeating could be a compensatory response to the physiological or psychological effects of food deprivation (58). VLCD regimens have been used in many short-term studies with considerably fewer examining their long-term use. Often improvements in glycaemic control in the obese diabetic patient are seen within days of caloric restriction, suggesting that calorie restriction as well as actual weight loss is responsible for improvements in blood glucose control. The mechanisms for improved glycaemic control through calorie restriction are unclear, but are thought to relate to a reduction in hepatic glucose output. Wing et al. (59) studied a group of 93 obese Type 2 diabetic patients who were randomised to receive two different degrees of calorie restriction, i.e. 400 or 1000 kcal/day. The study showed that the degree of calorie restriction, independent of differences in the magnitude of weight loss, affected fasting glucose levels and insulin sensitivity. It is recommended that VLCDs are carried out under medical supervision only, with consideration given to long-term maintenance of weight loss.

Whichever type of dietary regimen is adopted it is important to remember that dissemination of information and direct persuasion alone are unlikely to bring about sustained dietary change (60). Adopting a counselling approach and developing skills in communication that facilitate behaviour change are recommended to help people through the process of change necessary in obesity treatment (61).

BENEFITS OF ACTIVITY

Regular physical activity has been shown to confer a protective effect against the development of diabetes, particularly in those individuals who are at greatest risk of developing the condition (62–65). For the obese individual who has already developed diabetes, regular physical exercise also has several clinical benefits. In any weight management programme, therefore, it is essential that consideration be given to increasing physical activity. Treatment strategies that combine physical activity with dietary changes are generally much more effective than treatments which are exclusive to one or other strategy (66). In general, any measure that increases modest daily activity, such as avoiding lifts, or getting off the bus one stop earlier, is beneficial in increasing energy expenditure. A sedentary obese individual performing 3 h of any activity standing up rather than sitting down will increase his 24-h energy output from 40% to more than 75% above the BMR (67). However, for the obese individual with Type 2 diabetes, increasing daily activity patterns may not be enough, and more intensive degrees of exercise need to be considered on an individual basis.

Physical activity has a positive effect on insulin action, thus improving glucose control and insulin sensitivity (68). In addition, exercise improves lipid profiles by reducing serum TG and VLDL and raising HDL concentrations. Improvements in blood pressure have also been observed, independent of weight loss. Cardiac fitness is improved, with the risk of myocardial infarction reduced by 35–50% (69). Evidence suggests that these benefits are not uniform and that, in general, younger (40–54 years) individuals with Type 2 diabetes, in the early stage of disease, are more likely to benefit from the effects of exercise (70). In addition, the greatest benefits from physical activity may be in the weight maintenance phase of obesity management (71).

The psychological benefits of exercise are equally important for the obese individual with Type 2 diabetes. Reductions in anxiety levels, improved body image and higher self-esteem promote greater self-efficacy and help the individual to cope with stressful situations which often result in overeating and relapses (71,72).

While exercise improves insulin action, the effects of physical training disappear within days when discontinued, so consideration must be given to the nature and duration of the activity. Programme activities need to be regular and of at least moderate intensity (73). Aerobic activities, e.g. walking, swimming, cycling, for 20–60 min at moderate or greater intensity for 3–4 days/ week will benefit glycaemic control and at least 5 days a week will assist weight loss (74,75). The value of walking as an exercise strategy for those with Type 2 diabetes should not be overlooked. Those asked to walk 10 000 steps a day, and maintain a 1000 kcal deficit diet, lost more weight and had greater improvements in insulin sensitivity than those on diet alone (76).

Unfortunately, obese persons with Type 2 diabetes identify more barriers to exercise than to any other aspect of the diabetes self-care regimen, with specific complaints of physical discomfort, fear of hypoglycaemia, being too overweight to exercise and lack of family support (77). Physical discomfort as a limiting factor has to be considered from the perspective of both obesity and diabetes. Obese women report higher degrees of perceived pain and exertion when walking than non-obese, suggesting that this moderate intensity activity is actually more intense for the obese due to the greater relative oxygen cost of walking (78). In addition, the myriad of macrovascular and microvascular complications associated with diabetes may increase discomfort during activity and limit endurance and flexibility (71). Patients with proliferative retinopathy or hypertension, for example, should avoid resistance training and high-intensity exercises and those with peripheral neuropathy are advised to pursue activities such as swimming, where the ankle and foot are not under stress. Advice regarding appropriate footwear, foot inspection and adequate hydration should be given and those at risk of hypoglycaemia should take care to adjust insulin doses and consume sufficient carbohydrates (79). The emergence of exercise referral schemes may be an important development for the treatment of obesity in Type 2 diabetes (1).

BEHAVIOURAL THERAPY

Behavioural treatments for obesity originated in the 1960s and were founded on the concept that altering behaviours associated with eating and activity could be central to weight loss. Specific strategies include self-monitoring of both eating habits and physical activity, stress management, stimulus control, problem solving, contingency management, cognitive restructuring and social support. Treatments employing cognitive behavioural therapy (CBT) generally achieve levels of between 5–10% weight loss. A notable fact with regard to studies which have investigated CBT as a treatment strategy is that drop-out rates are very low. Over 80% of subjects who enter behavioural treatments complete the programme and are available for follow-up (80). It is recognised that CBT may produce the best results when combined with other treatments (81).

PHARMACOLOGICAL MANAGEMENT

There is incontrovertible evidence to show that early pharmaceutical intervention achieves better glycaemic control and reduces macrovascular and microvascular outcomes for Type 2 diabetic subjects (82). However, the conflict for obese diabetic patients between the need to achieve glycaemic control whilst minimising weight gain poses a challenging dilemma, as weight gain is an unfortunate consequence of several diabetic medications, a summary of which is provided in Table 8.2 (83).

Despite the undoubted ability of insulin to influence glycaemic control and microvascular outcomes, the mean weight gain by insulin-treated Type 2 obese subjects after 6 years is 10.4 kg. Sulphonylureas have a similar, but less pronounced effect, with a mean gain of 4.9 kg (84). For this reason, there is a general reluctance to use insulin in particular with the obese, although there is

Table 8.2 Anti-diabetic agents and their impact on body weight

Anti-diabetic agent	Effect on body weight
Sulphonylureas (e.g. gliclazide)	+
Biguanides (e.g. metformin)	−
α-Glucosidase inhibitors (e.g. acarbose)	−
Thiazolidinediones (e.g. pioglitazone, rosiglitazone)	+
Insulin	+ +

Source: Adapted from Hauner (83).

some evidence that the use of basal insulin as opposed to meal-time insulin will lessen the weight gain effect (85). Newer agents such as the thiozolidinedione insulin sensitisers remain controversial, as the impact of undesirable subcutaneous weight gain, despite reductions in the more harmful visceral fat, continues to be debated (8).

α-Glucosidase inhibitors such as acarbose, although generally less effective hypoglycaemic agents, may have some value in the management of the obese Type 2 diabetic patient. Although they generally have a neutral effect on weight, some studies suggest they cause modest weight loss and are thought to act by reducing the energy available from carbohydrates by delaying fermentation in the gut (86).

Biguanides such as metformin, on the other hand, have a weak anorectic action, and were shown by the UKPDS to be the treatment of choice for the obese Type 2 diabetic patient, causing no weight gain relative to conventional policy and demonstrating a cardio-protective effect by reducing the rates of mortality and myocardial infarction (87).

Furthermore, there is some evidence that the combination of metformin with intensive insulin therapy can negate the weight gain caused by insulin (88). However the effects of metformin on microvascular outcomes are less favourable than insulin, and for many patients its side-effects and contra-indications mean that it is not a viable option.

Clearly there is no easy way for an individual with diabetes who is obese to improve glycaemic control, reduce microvascular and macrovascular complications and lose weight at the same time. A more rational approach may be to address the problem of obesity first, using agents that cause weight loss as a primary effect and achieve reductions in hyperglycaemia as a desirable consequence. One such agent is orlistat, an intestinal lipase inhibitor, which acts enterically to inhibit the absorption of approximately 30% of dietary fat (89). Orlistat is recommended for use in those aged 18–75 years with a BMI 28–30 kg/m^2, in the presence of significant co-morbidities and in those with a BMI > 30 kg/m^2 with no associated co-morbidities. Patients are required to demonstrate a weight loss of at least 2.5 kg in the month prior to the drug being prescribed. The NICE (90) guidelines in the UK have also recently recommended that continuation of this therapy beyond three months should be supported by evidence of a loss of at least a further 5% of body weight, and beyond six months by evidence of at least 10% weight loss. Several clinical trials have been conducted to examine the efficacy of this drug treatment in obese diabetic and non-diabetic patients (89,91). While over a one-year period, Type 2 diabetic subjects taking sulphonylureas and orlistat lost less weight than non-diabetic subjects taking orlistat (mean 6.2 kg vs 9.5 kg), the subsequent improvements in HbA_{1c} reduced the need for diabetic medication and had favourable effects on lipid profiles and hypertension. In addition, improvements in the insulin resistance index of obese non-diabetic subjects, proportional to the degree of weight lost, suggest that orlistat may have a valuable role in the delay of onset or perhaps the prevention of Type 2 diabetes in the obese (92).

Sibutramine is a selective serotonin and noradrenaline reuptake inhibitor, which promotes weight loss. The blocking of serotonin reuptake has a satiety enhancing effect and inhibition of noradrenaline uptake promotes thermogenesis. Sibutramine has only recently been licensed in the UK, the drug having been available on prescription in the USA for considerably longer. The results of the clinical trials show that obese non-diabetic patients are more able to achieve a 5–10% weight loss with sibutramine than with placebo, although the positive effects are dose-related. A 10 mg dose results in a mean weight loss of 5.5% and a 15 mg dose a loss of 7.2% (93). For the Type 2 diabetic patient who loses weight with sibutramine, the ensuing improvements in all modifiable risk factors are proportional to the degree of weight lost, with significant improvements, specifically a reduction in HbA_{1c} of 0.4%, seen in those who lost > 5% of body weight (94). As a word of caution, slight increases in pulse and blood pressure (2–3 mmHg) are associated with sibutramine, but in the long term, weight loss results in a net decrease in blood pressure.

SURGICAL INTERVENTION

Surgery is a treatment option which is usually only advised for patients with severe obesity (BMI > 40 kg/m²), although some centres are now opting to use this in patients with a BMI > 35 kg/m² if significant co-morbidity is present. There are two types of obesity surgery: (1) restrictive procedures and (2) combined restrictive and malabsorptive procedures. Restrictive surgery uses bands or staples to create a stomach pouch, thereby producing a restriction in food intake. Examples of restrictive procedures include the vertical banded gastroplasty (VBG) and the laprascopic banding procedure. Combined restrictive and malabsorptive surgery involves a combination of restrictive surgery with bypass or malabsorptive surgery, in which the stomach is connected to the jejunum or ileum of the small intestine, bypassing the duodenum. Roux-en-Y gastric bypass is the most commonly performed gastric bypass procedure.

In terms of the percentage of excess weight loss, results range from 50% for restrictive procedures to 60–70% for malabsorptive procedures.

Results from the surgical treatment of obesity provide the most convincing evidence of the benefit of weight loss in Type 2 diabetes. The Swedish obese subjects (SOS) study is a recent prospective trial, which has demonstrated the effect of surgically induced weight loss on the incidence of diabetes mellitus (95). The intervention consists of a surgically treated group of severely obese individuals and a matched group of weight-stable obese controls. This study provides overwhelming evidence that weight loss not only helps reduce, treat and eliminate diabetes, but also that losing weight can prevent the onset of diabetes. The surgically treated patients lost an average of about 60% of their body weight, with the incidence of hyperinsulinaemia and high blood glucose significantly decreased compared with the medically treated group. For the 8 years these patients have been followed, one consistent factor has held up – weight loss maintains improvements in insulin sensitivity, helps decrease the incidence of diabetes, and effectively treats Type 2 diabetes. Pories *et al.* (96) followed 608 patients who had undergone gastric bypass surgery for up to 14 years. At 1 year, there was an average weight loss of 100 lb, which was maintained by the majority of patients at 5 years. About 83% of the 146 patients with diabetes experienced a return to normal levels of plasma glucose, glycosylated haemoglobin and insulin. In 152 patients with impaired glucose tolerance, more than 98% achieved normal glucose tolerance post-surgery. It is interesting to note however that even before a large weight loss was obtained, post-surgery glycaemic control improved.

Surgical intervention requires long-term follow up to help patients adjust to the surgery and change their eating habits. Vitamin supplementation, particularly vitamin B_{12}, will be necessary in patients who have undergone malabsorptive surgery.

While the results from the studies of obesity surgery are impressive, as pointed out by Pinkney *et al.* (97), it should be remembered that no trials have been designed with diabetes as the central focus and moreover few patients on oral agents or insulin have been reported on. There is a need therefore for more large-scale, long-term prospective studies specific to diabetes before firm conclusions can be drawn as to the role of obesity surgery in diabetes management.

CONSIDERATIONS IN MANAGING OBESITY WITHIN DIABETES CARE

It would be unusual to find the overweight patient with diabetes who has not at one time or another been advised to 'lose some weight'. For the patient faced with the prospect of attempting to achieve this it can be helpful first of all to quantify the amount of weight loss which we now know can bring clinically significant benefit, i.e. 5–10% of current body weight. Although the results of obesity surgery provide compelling evidence that an even greater amount of weight loss can significantly reduce the need for medication and in some cases eliminate the need for any further treatment, obesity surgery will not be appropriate for or accessible to many people with diabetes. It is important therefore that an achievable degree of weight loss is promoted and that a greater understanding of the benefits of a more modest amount of weight loss in the treatment of those with Type 2 diabetes is gained. In addition, with many studies demonstrating weight regain following a period of weight loss, the importance of weight maintenance needs to be more strongly emphasised.

Also in advising patients to 'lose some weight' it is to be questioned whether current services are designed to help patients to achieve this. Obesity, like no other condition, is considered to be solely under the control of the individual, and as such can lead to the view that there is little that can be done by the health professional to alter this. This belief could easily impact upon the priority given to weight management within the realm of diabetes care. It could be argued however that the 'medical' treatment of obesity is in effect still in its infancy, with only 50% of the health authorities surveyed in the National Audit Office report of England and Wales (1) indicating that they had a dedicated obesity strategy in place. Weight loss achieved through changes in lifestyle is not impossible and perhaps before we dismiss weight loss as an unattainable ideal we need to consider whether we offer adequately funded, comprehensive and effective weight management programmes.

In the pharmacological management of diabetes it has already been highlighted that finding a regimen which complements both glycaemic control and weight loss is a challenge. With a greater number of anti-obesity drugs emerging there is a need to investigate more fully their potential as front-line treatments in the management of the obese Type 2 diabetic patient. While it is not questioned that treating hyperglycaemia reduces complications in diabetes, the long-term benefit of reacting to what is in effect the consequence of obesity rather than reacting to the obesity itself is controversial. At a certain level of obesity, or if weight continues to increase, there will inevitably be a finite limit to the effectiveness of anti-diabetic agents and we need to consider whether a 'reactive' approach is the most effective in the long term.

Finally, more and more evidence is emerging to suggest that prevention strategies are extremely important, particularly since the escalation in the levels of obesity has seen a corresponding increase in the incidence of diabetes. Indeed in Europe alone, the number of diabetic patients is predicted to increase from 16 million in 1994 to 24 million in 2010 and indicates that the 21st century will herald an astounding increase in both the financial and social costs of diabetes (98). Impaired glucose tolerance is in effect the first stage of Type 2 diabetes and consideration must be given to (a) how such individuals can best be identified and (b) whether more rigorous intervention at this stage would be a more cost-effective method of tackling the impending diabetes epidemic in the long term. Modest weight loss, for example in high-risk subjects, could help to prevent a substantial number of cases of diabetes from ever developing (64, 65). The studies which have highlighted the benefits of weight loss in preventing progression to diabetes from IGT involved reductions in body weight of on average < 5 kg. These findings again lend credence to the message that weight loss does not have to be extensive in order to modify the risk of diabetes.

SUMMARY

- Obesity is a chronic condition that impacts greatly upon the development, the progression and the consequences of diabetes.
- Weight management should form an integral part of the management of diabetes, with a strong emphasis on the prevention of obesity.
- The traditional emphasis on achieving pharmacologically driven glycaemic control can make weight loss difficult. Consideration should be given to the provision of a multi-skilled weight management service as part of the front-line therapy in diabetes treatment.

REFERENCES

1. National Audit Office. *Tackling Obesity in England.* London: National Audit Office, 2001.
2. Tuomilehto J, Lindstrom J, Eriksson JG, Valle TT, Hamalainen H, Ilanne-Parikka P, Keinanen-Kiukaanniemi S, Laakso M, Louheranta A, Rastas M, Salminen V, Uusitupa M. Prevention of type 2 diabetes mellitus by changes in lifestyle among subjects with impaired glucose tolerance. *New Engl J Med* 2001; 344 (18): 1343–1350.
3. United Kingdom Prospective Diabetes Study group (UKPDS). Plasma lipids and lipoproteins at diagnosis of NIDDM by age and sex. UKPDS 27. *Diabetes Care* 1997; 20: 1683–1687.
4. Colditz GA, Willett WC, Rotnitzky A, Manson JF. Weight gain as a risk factor for clinical diabetes in women. *Ann Intern Med* 1995; 122: 481–486.
5. Brancati FL, Wang N-Y, Mead LA, Liang K-Y, Klag MJ. Body weight patterns from 20 to 49 years of age and subsequent risk for diabetes mellitus. *Arch Int Med* 1999; 159: 957–963.
6. WHO study group. Defining the problem of overweight and obesity. In: *Report of a WHO Consultation on Obesity. Obesity: Preventing and Managing the Global Epidemic.* Geneva: WHO, 1997: 7–16.
7. Jönsson B. The economic impact of diabetes. *Diabetes Care* 1998; 21: 7–10.
8. Wilding JPH. Is diabetes realistically treatable in type 2 diabetes? In: *Difficult Diabetes,* eds G Gill, J Pickup and G Williams. Oxford: Blackwell Science, 2001.
9. Williams G. Obesity and type 2 diabetes: conflict of interests? *Int J Obes* 1999; 23: S2–S4.
10. Anderson DA, Wadden TA. Treating the obese patient. *Arch Fam Med* 1998; 8: 156–167.

11. Kirk SF. Treatment of obesity: theory into practice. *Proc Nutr Soc* 1999; 58: 53–58.
12. Purnell JQ, Hokanson JE, Marcovina SM, Steffes MW, Cleary PA, Brunzell JD. Effects of excessive weight gain with intensive therapy of type I diabetes on lipid levels and blood pressure. *J Am Med Assoc* 1998; 280: 140–146.
13. Williams KV, Erbey JR, Becker D, Orchard TJ. Improved glycaemic control reduces the impact of weight gain on cardiovascular risk factors in type 1 diabetes. *Diabetes Care* 1999; 22: 1084–1091.
14. Rodin GM, Johnson LE, Garfinkel PE, Daneman D, Kenshole, AB. Eating disorders in female adolescents with insulin dependent diabetes mellitus. *Int J Psychiat Med* 1986; 16: 49–57.
15. Steel JM, Young RJ, Lloyd GG, MacIntyre CCA. Abnormal eating attitudes in young insulin dependent diabetes. *Br J Psychiatry* 1989; 155: 515–521.
16. Bryden KS, Neil A, Mayou RA, Peveler RC, Fairburn CG, Dunger DB. Eating habits, body weight and insulin misuse. A longitudinal study of teenagers and young adults with type 1 diabetes. *Diabetes Care* 1999: 22: 1956–1960.
17. Kent LA, Gill GV, Williams G. Mortality and outcome of patients with brittle diabetes and recurrent ketoacidosis. *Lancet* 1994: 778–781.
18. Albu J, Pi-Sunyer FX. Obesity and diabetes. In: *Handbook of Obesity*, eds GA Bray, C Bouchard and WPT James. New York: Marcel Dekker, 1998: 697–707.
19. Bessesen DH. Obesity as a factor. *Nutr Rev* 2000; 58: S12–S15.
20. Ruderman N, Chisholm D, Pi-Sunyer X, Schneider S. The metabolically obese, normal-weight individual revisited. *Diabetes* 1998; 47: 699–713.
21. Torjesen PA, Birkeland KI, Anderssen SA, Hjermann I, Holme I, Urdal P. Lifestyle changes may reverse development of the insulin resistance syndrome. The Oslo diet and exercise study: a randomized trial. *Diabetes Care* 1997; 20: 26–31.
22. Markovic TP, Campbell LV, Balasubramanian S, Jenkins AB, Fleury AC, Simons LA, Chisholm DJ. Beneficial effect on average lipid levels from energy restriction and fat loss in obese individuals with or without type 2 diabetes. *Diabetes Care* 1998: 21: 695–700.
23. Jung RT. Obesity and nutritional factors in the pathogenesis of non-insulin-dependent diabetes mellitus. In: *Textbook of Diabetes*, Vol. 1, eds J Pickup and G Williams. London: Blackwell Science, 1997: 19.1–19.22.
24. Steppan CM, Bailey ST, Bhat S, Brown EJ, Banerjee RR, Wright CM, Patel HR, Ahima RS, Mitchell AL. The hormone resistin links obesity to diabetes. *Nature* 2001; 409: 307–312.
25. Brownwell KD, Wadden TA. The heterogeneity of obesity: fitting treatments to individuals. *Behav Ther* 1991: 153–177.
26. Lean MEJ, Powrie JK, Anderson AS, Garthwaite PH. Obesity, weight loss and prognosis in type 2 diabetes. *Diabet Med* 1990; 7: 228–233.
27. Klein S. Outcome success in obesity. *Obes Res* 2001 (4): 354S–358S.
28. United Kingdom Prospective Diabetes Study group (UKPDS). Tight blood pressure control and risk of macrovascular and microvascular complications in type 2 diabetes. UKPDS 38. *Br Med J* 1998; 317: 720–726.
29. Wing RR, Koeske R, Epstein LH, Norwark MP, Gooding W, Becker D. Long term effects of modest weight loss in type 2 diabetics. *Arch Int Med* 1987; 147: 1749–1753.
30. Baron AD. Haemodynamic actions of insulin. *Am J Physiol* 1994; 267: E187–E202.
31. Ramsey LE, Williams B, Johnston JD, MacGregor GA, Poston L, Potter JF. British hypertension management. *Br Med J* 1999; 319: 630–635.
32. Huang Z, Willett WC, Manson JE *et al*. Body weight, weight change and risk for hypertension in women. *Ann Intern Med* 1998; 128: 81–88.

33. Tuck M. Macrovascular disease in type 2 diabetes. *Pract Diabetes Int* 2000; 17: S1–S4.
34. Griffin BA. Liporotein atherogenicity: an overview of current mechanisms. *Proc Nutr Soc* 1999; 58: 163–169.
35. Brown GC, Brown MM, Sharma S, Brown H, Gogin M, Denton P. Quality of life associated with diabetes mellitus in an adult population. *J Diabetes Comp* 2000; 14: 18–24.
36. Fontaine KR, Cheskin LJ, Barofsky I. Health-related quality of life in obese persons seeking treatment. *J Fam Prac* 1996; 43: 265–270.
37. Guare JC, Wing RR, Grant A. Comparison of obese NIDDM and non-diabetic women. *Obes Res* 1995; 3: 329–335.
38. British Dietetic Association Position Paper. Obesity treatment: future directions for the contribution of dietitians. *J Human Nutr Diet* 1997; 10: 95–101.
39. Lean MEJ, Hans TS, Morrison CE. Waist circumference indicates the need for weight management. *Br Med J* 1995; 311: 158–161.
40. National Research Council, Committee on Diet and Health. *Diet and Health: Implications for Reducing Chronic Disease.* The National Academies, 1989; 768 pp.
41. Seidell JC, Flegal KM. Assessing obesity: classification and epidemiology. *Br Med Bull* 1997; 53: 238–252.
42. McNulty SJ, Williams G. Obesity, an overview. *Proc R Coll Physicians Edinb* 1999; 29: 220–227.
43. Stunkard AJ, Harris JR, Pedersen NL, McClearn GE. The body mass index of twins who have been reared apart. *New Engl J Med* 1990; 322: 1483–1487.
44. Bouchard C (ed.) *The Genetics of Obesity.* London: CRC Press, 1994: 135–145.
45. Vogler G, Sorensen T, Stunkard A, Srinivasan M, Rao D. Influences of genes and shared family environment on adult body mass index assessed in an adoption study by a comprehensive path model. *Int J Obes* 1995; 19: 40–45.
46. Kolotkin RL, Revis ES, Kirkley BG, Janick L. Binge eating in obesity: associated MMPI characteristics. *J Consult Clin Psychol* 1987; 55: 872–876.
47. Herpertz S, Albus C, Wagener R, Kocnar M, Wagner R, Henning A, Best F, Foerster H, Schulze Schleppinghoff B, Thomas W, Köhle K, Mann K, Senf W. Comorbidity of diabetes and eating disorders. Does diabetes control reflect disturbed eating behaviour? *Diabetes Care* 1998; 21: 1110–1116.
48. Miller WR, Rollnick S. *Motivational Interviewing: Preparing People to Change Addictive Behaviour.* New York: Guilford Press, 1991.
49. Brand Miller JC, Foster-Powell K, Colagiuri S. *The G.I. Factor – The Glycaemic Index Solution.* Rydalmere: Hodder and Stoughton, 1996.
50. Lean MEJ, James WPT. Prescription of diabetic diets in the 1980s. *Lancet* 1986; 1: 723–725.
51. Sweeney ME, Hill JO, Heller PA, Baney R, DiGirolamo M. Severe vs moderate energy restriction with and without exercise in the treatment of obesity: efficiency of weight loss. *Am J Clin Nutr* 1993; 57: 127–134.
52. Svedsen OL, Hassager C, Christiansen C. Six months' follow up on exercise added to a short term diet in overweight postmenopausal women – effects on body composition, resting metabolic rate, cardiovascular risk factors and bone. *Int J Obes* 1994; 18: 692–698.
53. Jeffery JW, Hellerstedt WI, French SA, Baxter JE. A randomised trial of counselling for fat restriction versus calorie restriction in the treatment of obesity. *Int J Obes Rel Metab Disord* 1995; 19: 132–137.
54. Frost G, Masters K, King C et al. A new method of energy prescription to improve weight loss. *J Human Nutr Diet* 1991: 4: 369–373.

55. Wing RR. Use of very-low-calorie diets in the treatment of obese persons with non-insulin dependent diabetes mellitus. *J Am Diet Assoc* 1995; 95: 569–572.
56. Paisey RB, Harvey P, Rice S, Belka I, Bower L, Dunn M, Taylor P, Paisey RM, Frost J, Ash I. An intensive weight loss programme in established type 2 diabetes and controls: effects on weight and atherosclerosis risk factors at 1 year. *Diabet Med* 1998; 15: 73–79.
57. Flynn TJ, Walsh MF. Thirty-month evaluation of a popular very-low-calorie diet program. *Fam Med* 1993; 2: 1042–1048.
58. Wadden TA. Treatment of obesity by moderate and severe caloric restriction. Results of clinical research trials. *Ann Intern Med* 1993; 119: 688–693.
59. Wing R, Blair E, Bononi P, Marcus M, Watanabe R, Bergman R. Caloric restriction per se is a significant factor in improvements in glycaemic control and insulin sensitivity during weight loss in obese NIDDM patients. *Diabetes Care* 1994; 17: 30–36.
60. Rapoport L. Integrating cognitive behavioural therapy into dietetic practice: a challenge for dietitians. *J Human Nutr Diet* 1998; 11: 227–237.
61. Rapoport L, Nicholson Perry K. Do dietitians feel that that they have had adequate training in behaviour change methods. *J Hum Nutr Diet* 2000; 13: 287–298.
62. Helmrich SP, Ragland DR, Leung RW, Paffenbarger RS Jr. Physical activity and reduced occurrence of non-insulin-dependent diabetes mellitus. *New Engl J Med* 1991; 325: 147–152.
63. Manson JE, Rimm EB, Stampfer MJ *et al.* Physical activity and incidence of non-independent diabetes mellitus in women. *Lancet* 1991; 338: 774–778.
64. Eriksson J, Lindstrom J, Valle T, Aunola S *et al.* Prevention of type 2 diabetes in subjects with impaired glucose tolerance: the Diabetes Prevention Study (DPS) in Finland. *Diabetologia* 1999; 42: 793–801.
65. Uusitupa M, Louheranta A, Lindstrom J, Valle T, Sundvall J, Eriksson J, Tuomilehto J. The Finnish Diabetes Prevention Study. *Br J Nutr* 2000; 83: S137–S142.
66. Skender ML, Goodrick GK, Del-Junco DJ, Reeves RS, Darnell L, Gotto AM *et al.* Comparison of 2-year weight loss trends in behavioural treatments for obesity: diet, exercise, and combination interventions. *J Am Diet Assoc* 1996; 4: 342–346.
67. James WPT, Schofield EC. *Human Energy Requirements. A Manual for Planners and Nutritionalists.* FAO and Oxford University Press, 1990.
68. Bouchard C, Despres JP. Physical activity and health: atherosclerotic, metabolic and hypertensive diseases. *Res Q Ex Sport* 1996; 66: 268–275.
69. Lehmann R, Vokac A, Niedermann K, Agosti K, Spinas GA. Loss of abdominal fat and improvement of the cardiovascular risk profile by regular moderate exercise training in patients with NIDDM. *Diabetologia* 1995; 38: 1313–1319.
70. Barnard RJ, Jung T, Inkeles SB. Diet and exercise in the treatment of NIDDM. The need for early emphasis. *Diabetes Care* 1994; 17: 1469–1472.
71. Foreyt JP, Carlos Poston II WS. The challenge of diet, exercise and lifestyle modification in the management of the obese diabetic patient. *Int J Obes* 1999; 23 (Suppl 7): S5–S11.
72. Fox KR. The influences of physical activity on mental well being. *Public Health Nutr* 1999; 2: 18.
73. Wallberg-Henriksson H, Rincon J, Zierath JR. Exercise in the management of non-insulin dependent diabetes mellitus. *Sports Med* 1998; 25: 25–35.
74. Young JC. Exercise prescription for individuals with metabolic disorders: practical considerations. *Sports Med* 1995; 19: 43–54.

75. Eriksson J, Taimela S, Koivisto VA. Exercise and the metabolic syndrome. *Diabetologia* 1997; 40: 125–135.
76. Yamanouchi K, Shinozaki T, Chikada K, Nishikawa T *et al*. Daily walking combined with diet therapy is a useful means for obese NIDDM patients not only to reduce body weight but also to improve insulin sensitivity. *Diabetes Care* 1995; 18: 775–778.
77. Swift CS, Armstrong JE, Beerman KA, Campbell RK, Pond-Smith D. Attitudes and beliefs about exercise among persons with non-insulin dependent diabetes. *Diabetes Educ* 1995; 21: 533–540.
78. Mattsson E, Evers Larson U, Rossner S. Is walking for exercise too exhausting for obese women? *Int J Obes* 1997; 21: 380–386.
79. Zierath JR, Wallberg-Henriksson H. Exercise training in obese diabetic patients; special considerations. *Sports Med* 1992; 14: 171–189.
80. Wing RR. Behavioral treatment of severe obesity. *Am J Clin Nutr* 1992; 55: 545S–551S.
81. Wadden TA, Stunkard AJ. Controlled trial of very low calorie diet, behaviour therapy, and their combination in the treatment of obesity. *J Consult Clin Psychol* 1986; 54: 482–488.
82. United Kingdom Prospective Diabetes Study (UKPDS). Intensive blood glucose control with sulphonylureas or insulin compared with conventional treatment of risk of complications in patients with type 2 diabetes. UKPDS 33. *Lancet* 1998; 352: 837–853.
83. Hauner H. The impact of pharmacotherapy on weight management in type 2 diabetes. *Int J Obes* 1999; 23: S12–S17.
84. United Kingdom Prospective Diabetes Study group (UKPDS). A six year, randomised, controlled trial comparing sulfonylurea, insulin and metformin therapy in patients with newly diagnosed type 2 diabetes that could not be controlled with diet therapy. UKPDS 24. *Ann Intern Med* 1998; 128: 165–175.
85. Riddle MC. Should obese type 2 diabetic patients be treated with insulin? In: *Difficult Diabetes*, eds G Gill, J Pickup and G Williams. Oxford: Blackwell Science, 2001.
86. Coniff RF, Shapiro JA, Seaton TB, Bray GA. Multicenter, placebo-controlled trial comparing acarbose (Bay g 5421) with placebo, tolbutamide, and tolbutamide-plus-acarbose in non-insulin-dependent diabetes mellitus. *Am J Med* 1995; 98: 443–451.
87. United Kingdom Prospective Diabetes Study group (UKPDS). Effect of intensive blood glucose control with metformin on complications in overweight patients with type 2 diabetes. UKPDS 34. *Lancet* 1998; 352: 854–865.
88. Bergenstal R, Johnson M, Whipple D *et al*. Advantages of adding metformin to multiple dose insulin therapy in type 2 diabetes. *Diabetes* 1999; 47 (Suppl 1): A47.
89. Hollander PA, Elbein SC, Hirsh IB *et al*. Role of orlistat in the treatment of obese patients with type 2 diabetes – a 1 year randomised double-blind study. *Diabetes Care* 1998; 21: 1288–1294.
90. NICE guidelines. Orlistat for treatment of obesity in adults. National Institute for Clinical Excellence, 2001.
91. Sjöström L, Rissanen A, Andersen T, Boldrin M, Golay A, Koppeschaar HP, Krempf N. Randomised placebo-controlled trial of orlistat for weight loss and prevention of weight regain in obese patients. *Lancet* 1998; 352: 167–172.
92. Wilding JPH. Orlistat-induced weight loss improves insulin resistance in obese patients. *Diabetologia* 1999; 42 (Suppl 1): 807.

93. Apfelbaum M, Vague P, Ziegler O, Hantin C, Thomas F, Leutenegger E. Long term maintenance of weight loss after a very-low-calorie-diet: a randomised blinded trial of the efficacy and tolerability of sibutramine. *Am J Med* 1999; 106: 179–184.
94. Finer N, Bloom SR, Frost GS, Banks LM, Griffiths J. Sibutramine is effective for weight loss and diabetic control in obesity with type 2 diabetes: a randomised, double-blind, placebo controlled study. *Diab Obes Metab* 2000; 2: 105–112.
95. Sjöström CD, Lissner L, Wedel H, Sjöström L. Reduction in incidence of diabetes, hypertension and lipid disturbances after intentional weight loss induced by bariatric surgery: the SOS I intervention study. *Obes Res* 1999; 7: 477–484.
96. Pories WJ, Swanson MS, Macdonald KS, Long SB, Morris PG. Who would have thought it? An operation proves to be the most effective therapy for adult-onset diabetes mellitus. *Ann Surg* 1995; 222: 339–352.
97. Pinkney JH, Sjöström CD, Edwin AMG. Should surgeons treat diabetes in severely obese people? *Lancet* 2001; 357: 1357–1359.
98. Amos AF, McCarthy DJ, Zimmet P. The rising global burden of obesity and its complications: estimates and projections to the year 2010. *Diabet Med* 1997; 14: S7–S85.

9

Nutritional Management of Cardiac Risk Factors in Type 2 Diabetes

AUDREY BRYNES

Hammersmith Hospital, London, UK

INTRODUCTION

In people with diabetes three out of four deaths are caused by cardiovascular disease (1). There is a three- to fivefold increase in myocardial infarction (MI), with an increase up to 10–15-fold once diabetic neuropathy develops. Angina and left ventricular failure are common, while interventions such as angioplasty and coronary artery bypass grafting have worse outcomes in people with diabetes compared with non-diabetic people (2). Thus the management of Type 2 diabetes is largely about addressing cardiovascular risk factors.

The vast majority of people with Type 2 diabetes have associated insulin resistance which is now recognised as the key pathophysiological defect.

INSULIN RESISTANCE SYNDROME

Reaven, at his Banting Lecture in 1988 (3), first proposed a widespread role for insulin resistance in common diseases such as coronary heart disease, Type 2 diabetes, obesity and hypertension. He proposed an insulin resistance syndrome (IRS) (or Syndrome X) as a unifying theory for a cluster of adverse metabolic changes (Table 9.1). Each of these changes have been independently shown to be related to a risk of cardiovascular disease. Insulin resistance is also a strong marker for the risk of developing Type 2 diabetes and therefore a

Nutritional Management of Diabetes Mellitus. Edited by G. Frost, A. Dornhorst and R. Moses
© 2003 John Wiley & Sons, Ltd. ISBN 0 471 49751 7

Table 9.1 Metabolic and related disorders associated with the insulin resistance syndrome

Glucose metabolism	Hyperinsulinaemia
	Glucose intolerance
Lipid metabolism	Hypertriacylglycerolaemia (particularly elevation of VLDL-TG and VLDL-apolipoprotein B)
	Exaggerated postprandial lipaemia
	Decreased HDL-cholesterol concentrations (particularly HDL$_2$-cholesterol)
	Preponderance of small dense LDL-cholesterol particles
Other	Hypertension
	Increased coagulation (PAI-1)
	Central obesity
	Increased body flux of non-esterified fatty acids (particularly impaired postprandial suppression)
Clinical correlates	Cardiovascular disease
	Type 2 diabetes
	Gout
	Breast cancer

Source: Adapted from Reaven (4).

reduction in insulin resistance is a key goal which may delay the onset of Type 2 diabetes. Thus dietary advice to reduce insulin resistance (or increase insulin sensitivity) is essential.

IRS affects lipid metabolism as well as carbohydrate metabolism. Alterations in the lipid profile, as described in Table 9.1, are at the centre of the insulin resistance syndrome (4).

This cluster of risk factors is commonly seen in the presence of obesity, which is thought to contribute to the development of both Type 2 diabetes and increased cardiovascular risk.

In Europe, modest improvements in CHD mortality have occurred during the last two decades (5). It is likely that some of this reduction in CHD mortality is a result of health strategies first introduced in the 1960s that targeted modifiable CHD risk factors. These included discouraging smoking, treating hypertension and lowering cholesterol concentrations. Despite modest falls in the non-diabetic population, no improvement in CHD has occurred within the diabetic population (6).

PRESENCE OF INSULIN RESISTANCE BEFORE THE ONSET OF TYPE 2 DIABETES

It is interesting to note that although the incidence of people with diabetes in the UK is thought to be around 5%, the number of people with insulin resistance is nearer 25% (7). There are strong genetic determinants for the development of insulin resistance. The offspring of people with Type 2 diabetes have been shown to be more insulin resistant than those with no family history and this relationship is independent of obesity (8). Non-diabetic first-degree relatives of people with Type 2 diabetes also have similar thrombotic risk clustering to their diabetic relatives (9).

In 1990 Haffner *et al.* (10) theorised that macrovascular complications start to develop very early on, initiated by insulin resistance and/or hyperinsulinae-mia in the prediabetic state, whereas microvascular complications develop after sustained hyperglycaemia. In the Quebec heart disease study high fasting insulin concentrations were reported to be an independent predictor of ischaemic heart disease in men (11). However, a meta-analysis of a prospective population-based cohort and case-controlled studies, reported by Ruige *et al.* in 1998 (12), found a weak relationship between plasma insulin levels and CVD, suggesting that other risk factors, such as lipids, must also be involved.

NOT JUST FASTING LIPIDS BUT POSTPRANDIAL LIPID CONCENTRATIONS

Only 50% of CHD is explained by traditional risk factors such as smoking, hyperlipidaemia, hypertension and diabetes. This may be because most risk factor assessments and many public health campaigns have focused on fasting lipid levels as their main criteria rather than diets to reduce many of the postprandial metabolic disturbances attributed to insulin resistance. Much of the current work in this area is investigating the role of lipids in the postprandial state.

OBESITY AND INSULIN RESISTANCE

Obesity is the most common condition associated with insulin resistance (13). Obesity is a health problem reaching epidemic proportions in Western countries. In the UK alone some 16% of men and 18% of women are obese (14). Obesity can be defined as a body mass index (BMI) greater than $30\,kg/m^2$. Insulin resistance is frequently observed in obese subjects and constitutes an independent risk factor for the development of Type 2 diabetes and atherosclerosis. The importance of increasing visceral fat (measured by waist:hip ratio) as a risk factor for insulin resistance and cardiovascular disease has also been demonstrated (15).

Weight loss improves insulin sensitivity and any type of therapy, whether it is dietary or pharmacological, that can aid effective weight loss and/or weight maintenance will help prevent some of the deleterious metabolic changes associated with insulin resistance.

SUMMARY OF DISTURBANCES AT A CELLULAR LEVEL IN INSULIN RESISTANCE

At a molecular level cellular factors have been identified that can markedly influence insulin action either directly or indirectly. These include tumour necrosis factor (TNF)α, glucose transporters (GLUT) and peroxisome proliferator activated receptor (PPAR)γ, while increased glucose flux has been shown to induce insulin resistance in skeletal muscle. For a more detailed review see Garvey and Birnbaum (16). There is also likely to be a genetic predisposition to insulin resistance (17).

Current treatments of Type 2 diabetes have little impact on reducing insulin resistance and this may explain why treating diabetes has only marginal benefits on reducing CHD mortality. It is hoped that with the introduction of thiazolidinediones, a novel class of oral agents that reduce insulin resistance, this may change.

Environmental influences on insulin sensitivity are not yet completely understood. Exercise has a strong beneficial effect (18) and obesity a strong adverse effect. The effects of diet on insulin sensitivity are discussed later.

DYSLIPIDAEMIC LIPID PROFILE

Patients with Type 2 diabetes have an abnormal lipid profile with high levels of LDL-cholesterol and triglycerides (TG) and a low level of HDL-cholesterol. Data from the Multiple Risk Factor Intervention Trial (MRFIT) (19) suggest that although levels of total cholesterol and LDL-cholesterol do not differ significantly between patients with and without diabetes, those with diabetes have higher concentrations of atherogenic small dense LDL-cholesterol particles.

A few years ago effects on TG were seen as largely irrelevant, as it was thought that the relationship between TG levels and CHD was weak. However fasting plasma TG concentrations have recently been demonstrated to be an independent risk factor for the development of CHD (20). In a meta-analysis of 17 population-based studies, TG concentrations were particularly important in relation to CHD risk, where a 1 mmol/l increase in plasma TG increased cardiovascular risk by 32% in men and 76% in women.

DIETARY MANIPULATION

While diet is the mainstay of therapy for people with Type 2 diabetes, the ideal dietary guidelines remain unsettled. Current recommendations aim to promote good glycaemic control and maintain ideal body weight while reducing the risk of CHD through improved lipid profiles. These are very much in line with the recommendations of the Committee on Medical Aspects of Food (COMA) on diet and cardiovascular disease. In addition to this there is a move away from defined macronutrient prescription and a move towards the treatment of risk factors in the context of lifestyle, behavioural and individualised changes that the patient is willing and able to make. Cultural and ethnic background should be taken into account.

The Stanford group led by Reaven, as well as groups led by Katan, Grundy and Willet have argued for many years that guidelines for CHD and diabetes should be changed from the historic high-carbohydrate/low-fat diet philosophy. They recommend lowering the carbohydrate level and increasing energy from monounsaturated fats which do not demonstrate the postulated detrimental effects of carbohydrate on TG (21).

FAT AND INSULIN SENSITIVITY

Himsworth first made the association between increased dietary fat and insulin resistance in the 1930s and since then much has been published on these effects. In a recently published review on the subject by Storlien *et al.* (22), the premise was developed that the type of fatty acids eaten may be as important as the quantity of fat in the diet. High-fat diets, particularly high saturated fat, are associated with the development of Type 2 diabetes and glucose intolerance, while the intake of long-chain fatty acids, in particular *n*-3 fatty acids, seems protective.

In addition the San Luis Valley Diabetes Study found that high saturated fat and low starch and fibre intakes were associated with hyperinsulinaemia in a non-diabetic population (23).

It has also been demonstrated, using the euglycaemic hyperinsulinaemic clamp method, that increased monounsaturated fat improves insulin sensitivity and glycaemic control while having no adverse effects on lipids (24,25). The mechanism for this is uncertain (26).

FAT AND PLASMA LIPIDS

A high intake of saturated fatty acids has been associated with an increased incidence of CHD, presumably because a high saturated fat intake increases LDL-cholesterol and reduces HDL-cholesterol (27).

The lipid-lowering effects of monounsaturated fatty acids (MUFAs) compared to *n*-6 polyunsaturated fatty acids (PUFAs) are well studied, suggesting that PUFAs may be more potent at lowering plasma LDL-cholesterol and TG (27).

There is accumulating evidence in the literature that increasing the percentage of total energy contribution from MUFA fat has a positive effect on lipids as well as improving glycaemic control in people with Type 2 diabetes.

In a review by Garg (26) monounsaturated fat diets compared to high-carbohydrate diets reduced fasting TG and VLDL-cholesterol by 19% and 22% respectively, with a modest increase in HDL-cholesterol without adversely affecting LDL-cholesterol (25).

CARBOHYDRATE AND INSULIN SENSITIVITY

Daly *et al.* (28) have recently reviewed the evidence and clinical implications of dietary carbohydrates and insulin sensitivity. This is a controversial area. Extensive studies in animals show a detrimental effect of diets very high in fructose or sucrose, particularly in association with induction of hypertrigly-ceridaemia. The more limited results in human studies show conflicting results, partly because of heterogeneity of design. Certain groups of subjects such as the elderly, sedentary subjects, those with established coronary artery disease, males and hyperinsulinaemic subjects may be more sensitive to very high intakes of sucrose and fructose than others.

CARBOHYDRATE AND PLASMA LIPIDS

The elevation of blood lipid concentrations in response to large amounts of dietary sugars, particularly fructose and sucrose, has been recognised for many years. There are also many other variables that can influence postprandial TG concentrations, such as obesity, excessive alcohol consumption, genetic background and renal failure.

High-carbohydrate diets are reported to increase TG, mainly in short-term studies (29). However, most of these studies have been poorly controlled and have been very short term and thus the evidence is poor. Turley *et al.* (30) recently demonstrated that free-living healthy subjects randomised to a high-carbohydrate diet (59%) had no detrimental effect on fasting TG concentrations over a six-week period.

The literature contains conflicting findings, particularly in studies that contain > 20% of energy from sucrose or > 5% from fructose, where both sugars have been shown to raise TG concentrations. In studies containing amounts of sugars more typical of dietary habits in the Western world, elevated plasma TG concentrations are not usually observed (29). Interestingly, the glycaemic index of carbohydrate was significantly related to serum HDL-cholesterol in a retrospective cross-sectional study of 2200 middle-aged adults, where a low glycaemic diet was the only dietary variable related to the CHD risk factors measured (31).

OTHER NUTRITIONAL FACTORS ASSOCIATED WITH REDUCED CARDIAC RISK

FISH AND OMEGA-3 FATTY ACIDS

The cardioprotective benefits of the 'Mediterranean' diet and its reduction of mortality are strikingly evident in the results of studies such as the DART study (32) and the Lyon Diet Heart Study (33). The results of these studies are not solely due to the regular inclusion of oily fish, but this did have a key role. Oily fish such as mackerel, herring, sardines, trout and salmon are a rich source of the n-3 polyunsaturates. Eicosapentaenoic acid (EPA) and docosahexaenoic acid (DHA), the long-chain omega-3 PUFAs, are thought to be beneficial due to their anti-thrombolytic and anti-inflammatory action as well as their triglyceride-lowering effects. The UK Department of Health has recommended to the general population that they consume two portions of fish (100 g or 3–4 oz portion) a week, one of which should be oily (34). People with diabetes should be encouraged to include oily fish in the diet, ideally two to three times a week (35). Fish oils are increasingly available in capsule or liquid form. These should provide approximately 0.5–1.0 g of n-3 fatty acids per day. Vegetarians, or those allergic to fish, can optimise their n-3 intakes by using vegetable n-3 sources (rapeseed, canola, linseed and flax oils), but the conversion rate is low and other polyunsaturates can compete.

STANOLS AND STEROLS

Foods enriched with plant stanols and sterols have recently been introduced to the market. Plant sterols and stanols, which are structurally closely related to cholesterol, effectively inhibit the absorption of cholesterol. Plant sterols occur naturally in vegetable oils such as soybean and rapeseed, whereas plant stanols are found in tall oil, a side-product of paper manufacture. Manufactured products containing these products include spreads, cereal bars, cheeses, milk, ice cream and yoghurts. The optimal dose appears to be 1.6–2.0 g/day which equates to ~ 20 g spread/day. For these products to be effective the recommended intake should be consumed daily. This results in a 9–14% decrease in LDL-cholesterol (36). Moreover, these agents complement the action of the statin drugs, particularly in poor responders to drug therapy who have high rates of cholesterol absorption from the gut but low rates of cholesterol synthesis in the liver. However, concern exists regarding absorption of fat-soluble vitamins. Randomised trials have shown that plant sterols and stanols lower the blood concentration of β-carotene by about 25%, the concentration of α-carotene by about 10% and the concentration of vitamin E by about 8%. However, since these vitamins protect LDL-cholesterol from oxidation and stanols/sterols decrease the amount of LDL-cholesterol, these changes may self-adjust. Patients should be encouraged to eat foods containing stanols and/or sterols daily to reduce LDL-cholesterol.

SOYA PROTEIN, FLAVONOIDS AND PHYTO-OESTROGENS

The efficacy of soya and soya derivatives in lowering total cholesterol and LDL-cholesterol was recently supported by the US Food and Drug Administration (FDA) approving a health claim about the role of soya protein in reducing the risk of CHD. In 1999 the FDA finalised a rule that authorises the use on food labels and in food packages under FDA jurisdiction of the health claims concerning the association between soya protein and reduced risk of CHD: '*25 g of soya protein a day, as part of a diet low in saturated fat and cholesterol may reduce the risk of heart disease*' (37). Serum total cholesterol and LDL-cholesterol concentrations can be lowered by about 13%, plasma TG by 10% and HDL-cholesterol goes up by about 2% (38), and these beneficial effects are also seen in people with Type 2 diabetes (39). It is unclear if the benefits come from the main phyto-oestrogens found in soya, diadzein and genistein or from the soy protein itself. Epidemiological evidence suggests high intakes of flavonols such as onions, broccoli, apples and tea may reduce the risk of CHD or certain cancers – however, as yet, prospective data in disease prevention is lacking.

EGGS

In 2001 the American Heart Association relaxed its recommendations concerning the restriction of eggs and other high-cholesterol foods for the general healthy population, allowing people on plasma cholesterol-lowering diets five to six eggs a week. However, in a recent meta-analysis concern remains in the diabetic population where higher egg consumption was associated with an apparent increased risk of CHD (40). Further research is called for and continuing egg restriction for people with diabetes should be maintained.

GARLIC

Garlic shows some promise for improving some cardiovascular risk factors. Studies suggest small short-term benefits of garlic on some lipid and antiplatelet factors (41). However, conclusions about the true effects of garlic are limited by the marginal quality and short duration of many studies. Debate also continues regarding the quantity of garlic needed to see an effect, with some studies reporting an intake as high as three bulbs per day. The implication for clinical practice is that this may not be the most effective way to reduce lipid levels, but if the patient enjoys garlic then do not dissuade the use of it.

HOMOCYSTEINE AND FOLIC ACID

Elevated plasma homocysteine has been shown in many studies to be an independent marker for an increased risk of cardiovascular disease (42). The mean plasma homocysteine level is usually low or normal in DM patients except when nephropathy is present. Levels in that case tend to be higher than in people without diabetes. For people with diabetes an independent association with homocysteine and CVD has been shown in retrospective studies. Prospective studies showed an association between elevated homocysteine and all-cause mortality in DM patients. In general, the association between elevated levels of homocysteine and an adverse outcome was stronger for people with diabetes compared with non-diabetics.

Homocysteine is formed as a result of the breakdown of the dietary amino acid methionine. This is dependent on the presence of four B vitamins (vitamin B_{12}, vitamin B_6, folate and riboflavin). Homocysteine reference ranges still need to be clarified, as does the mechanism by which homocysteine damages the vasculature.

To try and prevent a raised homocysteine level, patients should be encouraged to have five portions of fruit and vegetables each day to ensure that adequate amounts of vitamins and minerals are consumed. The combination of vitamins that most effectively lowers homocysteine levels has yet to be discovered. If supplementation with B vitamins is going to form part of a public health strategy to prevent vascular disease, it is important, to avoid toxicity, that the lowest effective dose is found.

In the USA, grain products are fortified with folic acid at a level of 1.4 µg/g of product. Although this is primarily to prevent neural tube defects, it is also hoped that it may be beneficial for vascular disease prevention. Promotion of foods high in the appropriate B vitamins should therefore be encouraged within a healthy diet. There continues to be doubt as to whether supplementation should be encouraged until further research has been completed, and specific information on target groups such as people with diabetes is lacking.

COFFEE

The evidence remains ambiguous regarding the effect of coffee on CHD (43). The association between CHD and coffee consumption has been weakened by long-term follow-up. These findings may possibly be explained by a change in the type of coffee consumed. A lipid-rich fraction from boiled coffee seems to increase serum cholesterol concentration. When boiled coffee is filtered the lipid-rich factor is retained in the filter paper and the effect on cholesterol is reduced substantially (44).

An elevated plasma concentration of total homocysteine is considered to be a risk factor for cardiovascular disease. Heavy coffee drinking has been related to high homocysteine concentrations in epidemiologic studies and one experiment in which healthy subjects drank unfiltered boiled coffee (45).

VITAMIN E

Several observational studies have suggested that a high intake of vitamin E may slow the development and progression of atherosclerosis. Some clinical trials have also reported beneficial effects of vitamin E supplementation in the secondary prevention of cardiovascular events. However, the results of a recent large, multi-centre clinical trial reported that vitamin E supplementation was not effective in reducing the incidence of cardiovascular events in high-risk patients (46).

CHROMIUM

Within the past five years chromium has been shown to improve glucose and related variables in subjects with glucose intolerance and Type 1, Type 2, gestational and steroid-induced diabetes. Chromium is an essential nutrient involved in the metabolism of glucose, insulin and blood lipids. In some studies a suboptimal dietary intake of chromium is associated with increased risk factors associated with diabetes and cardiovascular diseases (47). Minerals such as magnesium, calcium, potassium, zinc and vanadium also appear to have associations with insulin resistance or its management. It is interesting to note that high fibre and wholegrain intakes are also associated with increased intakes of these nutrients in the diet, and this may go some way to explaining the improvements in glycaemic control seen on this type of diet.

Additional studies are urgently needed to elucidate the mechanism of action of these trace elements and their role in the prevention and control of diabetes. However, until this time the benefit from chromium supplementation in diabetic individuals has not been conclusively demonstrated.

SUMMARY

The balance of evidence suggests that dietary fats, particularly saturated fat, are likely to reduce insulin sensitivity but the effects of dietary carbohydrates on insulin sensitivity are more controversial.

The lipid-lowering effects of MUFAs compared to n-6 PUFAs are well studied, suggesting that MUFAs may be more potent at lowering plasma LDL-cholesterol and TG, whereas saturated fat increases LDL-cholesterol. There is concern that an intake above 55% from carbohydrate exaggerates the postprandial TG response.

REFERENCES

1. The Kings Fund Policy Institute. Counting the cost: the real impact of non insulin dependent diabetes. A Kings Fund Report commissioned by The British Diabetes Association, 1996.
2. Haffner SM. Coronary heart disease in patients with diabetes. *N Engl J Med* 2000; 342: 1040–1042.
3. Reaven GM. Banting lecture 1988. Role of insulin resistance in human disease. *Diabetes* 1988; 37: 1595–1607.
4. Reaven GM. The fourth musketeer – from Alexandre Dumas to Claude Bernard. *Diabetologia* 1995; 38: 3–13.
5. Tunstall PH, Kuulasmaa K, Mahonen M, Tolonen H, Ruokokoski E, Amouyel P. Contribution of trends in survival and coronary-event rates to changes in coronary heart disease mortality: 10-year results from 37 WHO MONICA Project populations. *Lancet* 1999; 353: 1547–1557.
6. Gu K, Cowie CC, Harris MI. Diabetes and decline in heart disease mortality in US adults. *J Am Med Assoc* 1999; 281: 1291–1297.
7. Hansen BC. *Insulin Resistance and Disease*. London: Baillière's Clinic in Endocrinology and Metabolism, 1994.
8. Laws A, Reaven G. Insulin resistance and risk factors for coronary heart disease. In: *Clinical Endocrinology and Metabolism – Insulin Resistance and Disease*, ed. E Ferrannini. London: Baillière's Clinic in Endocrinology and Metabolism, 1994: 1063–1077.
9. Mansfield MW, Heywood DM, Grant PJ. Circulating levels of Factor VII, fibrinogen and von Willebrand factor and features of insulin resistance in first-degree relatives of patients with NIDDM. *Circulation* 1996; 94: 2171–2176.
10. Haffner SM, Stern MP, Hazuda HP. Cardiovascular risk factors in confirmed prediabetic individuals. Does the clock for coronary heart disease start ticking before the onset of clinical diabetes? *J Am Med Assoc* 1990; 263: 2893–2898.
11. Despres JP, Lamarche B, Mauriege P, Cantin B, Dagenais GR, Moorjani S, Lupien PJ. Hyperinsulinemia as an independent risk factor for ischemic heart disease. *N Engl J Med* 1996; 334: 952–957.
12. Ruige JB, Assendelft WJJ, Dekker JM, Kostense PJ, Heine RJ, Bouter LM. Insulin and risk of cardiovascular disease: a meta-analysis. *Circulation* 1998; 97: 996–1001.
13. Groop LC, Bonadonna RC, Simonson DC, Petrides AS, Shank M, DeFronzo RA. Effect of insulin on oxidative and non-oxidative pathways of free fatty acid metabolism in human obesity. *Am J Physiol* 1992; 263: E79–E84.
14. HMSO. Health Survey for England, 1996.
15. McKeigue PM, Shah B, Marmot MG. Relation of central obesity and insulin resistance with high diabetes prevalence and cardiovascular risk in South Asians [see comments]. *Lancet* 1991; 337: 382–386.
16. Garvey WT, Birnbaum MJ. Cellular insulin action and insulin resistance. In: *Clinical Endocrinology and Metabolism – Insulin Resistance and Disease*, ed. E Ferrannini. London: Baillière's Clinic in Endocrinology and Metabolism, 1993: 785–875.

17. Pedersen O. Genetics of insulin resistance. *Exp Clin Endocrinol Diabetes* 1999; 107: 113–118.
18. Richter E, Mikines K, Galbo H, Kiens B. Effect of exercise on insulin action in skeletal muscle. *J Appl Physiol* 1989; 66: 876–885.
19. Multiple Risk Factor Intervention Trial. Risk factor changes and mortality results. Multiple Risk Factor Intervention Trial Research Group 1982. *J Am Med Assoc* 1997; 277: 582–594.
20. Hokanson JE, Austin MA. Plasma triglyceride level is a risk factor for cardiovascular disease independent of high-density lipoprotein cholesterol level: a meta-analysis of population based prospective studies. *J Cardiovasc Risk* 1996; 3: 213–219.
21. Katan MB, Grundy SM, Willett WC. Should a low-fat, high-carbohydrate diet be recommended for everyone? Beyond low fat diets. *N Engl J Med* 1997; 337: 563–567.
22. Storlien LH, Baur LA, Kriketos AD, Pan DA, Cooney GJ, Jenkins AB, Calvert GD, Campbell LV. Dietary fats and insulin action. *Diabetologia* 1996; 39: 621–631.
23. Marshall JA, Hamman RF, Baxter J. High-fat, low-carbohydrate diet and the etiology of non-insulin-dependent diabetes mellitus: the San Luis Valley Diabetes Study. *Am J Epidemiol* 1991; 134: 590–603.
24. Garg A, Grundy SM, Unger RH. Comparison of effects of high and low carbohydrate diets on plasma lipoproteins and insulin sensitivity in patients with mild NIDDM. *Diabetes* 1992; 41: 1278–1285.
25. Parillo M, Rivellese AA, Ciardullo AV, Capaldo B, Giacco A, Genovese S, Riccardi G. A high-monounsaturated-fat/low-carbohydrate diet improves peripheral insulin sensitivity in non-insulin-dependent diabetic patients. *Metabolism* 1992; 41: 1373–1378.
26. Garg A. High-monounsaturated-fat diets for patients with diabetes mellitus: a meta-analysis. *Am J Clin Nutr* 1998; 67 (Suppl 3): S577–S582.
27. Mensink RP, Katan MB. Effect of dietary fatty acids on serum lipids and lipoproteins. A meta-analysis of 27 trials. *Arterioscler Thromb* 1992; 12: 911–919.
28. Daly ME, Vale C, Walker M, Alberti KG, Mathers JC. Dietary carbohydrates and insulin sensitivity: a review of the evidence and clinical implications. *Am J Clin Nutr* 1997; 66: 1072–1085.
29. Frayn FN, Kingman SN. Dietary sugar and lipid metabolism in humans. *Am J Clin Nutr* 1995; 62: 250S–263S.
30. Turley ML, Skeaff CM, Mann JI, Cox B. The effect of a low-fat, high-carbohydrate diet on serum high density lipoprotein cholesterol and triglyceride. *Eur J Clin Nutr* 1998; 52: 728–732.
31. Frost G, Leeds AA, Dore CJ, Madeiros S, Brading S, Dornhorst A. Glycemic index as a determinant of serum HDL-cholesterol concentration. *Lancet* 1999; 353: 1045–1048.
32. Burr ML, Fehily AM, Gilbert JF, Rogers S, Holliday RM, Sweetnam PM, Elwood PC, Deadman NM. Effects of changes in fat, fish, and fibre intakes on death and myocardial reinfarction: diet and reinfarction trial (DART). *Lancet* 1989; 2: 757–761.
33. De Loregil M, Salen P, Martin JL, Monjaud I, Delaye J, Mamelle N. Mediterranean diet, traditional risk factors and the rate of cardiovascular complications after myocardial infarction; final report of the Lyon Diet Heart Study. *Circulation* 1999: 779–785.
34. Nutritional Aspects of Cardiovascular Disease. Department of Health RHSS 46. London: HMSO, 1994.

35. The Diabetes and Nutrition Study Group of the European Association for the Study of Diabetes. Recommendations for the nutritional management of patients with diabetes mellitus. *Eur J Clin Nutr* 2000; 54: 353–355.
36. Law M. Plant sterol and stanol margarines and health. *Br Med J* 2002; 320: 861–864.
37. Department of Health and Human Services, Food and Drug Administration. 21 CFR Part 101: Food labelling: Health claims: Soy protein and coronary heart disease: Final rule, October 26, 1999. Federal Register Part II.
38. Vitolins MZ, Anthony M, Burke GL. Soy protein isoflavones, lipids and arterial disease. *Curr Opin Lipidol* 2001; 12: 433–437.
39. Hermansen K, Sondergaard MD, Hoie L, Carstensen M, Brock B. Beneficial effects of a soy-based dietary supplement on lipid levels and cardiovascular risk markers in type 2 diabetic subjects. *Diabetes Care* 2001; 24: 228–233.
40. Hu FB, Stampfer MJ, Rimm EB, Manson JE, Ascherio A, Colditz GA, Rosner BA, Spiegelman D, Speizer FE, Sacks FM, Hennekens CH, Willett WC. A prospective study of egg consumption and risk of cardiovascular disease in men and women. *J Am Med Assoc* 1999; 281: 1387–1394.
41. Ackermann RT, Mulrow CD, Ramirez G, Gardner CD, Morbidoni L, Lawrence VA. Garlic shows promise for improving some cardiovascular risk factors. *Arch Intern Med* 2001; 161: 813–824.
42. Audelin MC, Genest J Jr. Homocysteine and cardiovascular disease in diabetes mellitus. *Atherosclerosis* 2001; 159: 497–511.
43. Greenland S. A meta-analysis of coffee, myocardial infarction and coronary death. *Epidemiology* 1993; 4: 366–374.
44. Stensvold I, Tverdal A, Jacobsen BK. Cohort study of coffee intake and death from coronary heart disease over 12 years. *Br Med J* 1996; 312: 544–555.
45. Urgert R, van Vliet T, Zock PL, Katan MB. Heavy coffee consumption and plasma homocysteine: a randomized controlled trial in healthy volunteers. *Am J Clin Nutr* 2000; 72: 1107–1110.
46. de Gaetano G. Low-dose aspirin and vitamin E in people at cardiovascular risk: a randomised trial in general practice. Collaborative Group of the Primary Prevention Project. *Lancet* 2001; 357: 1134.
47. Andersen RA. Chromium in the prevention and control of diabetes. *Diabetes Metab* 2000; 26: 22–27.

10

Nutritional Management of the Elderly Person with Diabetes

MARY HICKSON AND LUCY WRIGHT

Charing Cross Hospital, London, UK

INTRODUCTION

Diabetes is a common chronic disease of older people and is found with increasing frequency with advancing years (1). The true prevalence can only be estimated as probably half of all cases are undiagnosed (2). When the diagnosis is made it is often at a time of an intercurrent illness or a stressful life event. Today the majority of people with Type 2 diabetes could be considered elderly with most being over 60 years of age (3,4). In Western societies, where the population is increasingly aged, the prevalence of diabetes is set to rise further. Population changes in the level of background obesity and increased assimilation of people from ethnic groups with a higher rate of diabetes (3) will also contribute to this rise. Nevertheless diabetes in the older age group is still heterogeneous, consisting of:

- A small but increasing population of elderly patients with Type 1 diabetes;
- Elderly patients with established Type 2 diabetes;
- Elderly patients with newly diagnosed Type 2 diabetes;
- Transient forms of diabetes secondary to an intercurrent or underlying disease or treatment.

The dietary and medical management of elderly individuals with diabetes will depend on the aetiology of their glucose intolerance as well as their other medical and physical co-morbidities.

Nutritional Management of Diabetes Mellitus. Edited by G. Frost, A. Dornhorst and R. Moses
© 2003 John Wiley & Sons, Ltd. ISBN 0 471 49751 7

The clinical presentation of Type 2 diabetes in older age is often insidious and unlike the acute symptoms frequently seen in younger individuals. A gradual and unrecognised rise in blood glucose can occur over many years and be accentuated by some of the physiological changes associated with ageing:

- Increased fasting hepatic glucose production,
- Decrease in beta cell mass,
- Changes in beta cell secretory function,
- Change in body composition,
- Increase in insulin resistance.

While all these physiological changes occur with advancing age, the contribution that each can make to the development of overt diabetes will vary between subjects. Unlike other age groups, Type 2 diabetes is not uncommon among lean elderly individuals who are often characterised by a marked reduction in insulin secretory function. By contrast, obese elderly Type 2 patients are more typically insulin-resistant (5,6).

Most diabetes associated complications are dependent on a product of the duration of diabetes and the glycaemic control. Concerns about the development of microvascular complications need to be balanced against the likely life expectancy of an elderly individual who develops Type 2 diabetes in later life. In some cases it may be more appropriate to focus on ameliorating glycaemic symptoms, if any, and promoting general well-being rather than striving for euglycaemia. The older people who develop diabetes in their later years have different clinical needs than a similar aged person with diabetes of many years' duration. Elderly patients with Type 2 diabetes of longer duration are more likely to have diabetic micro- and macrovascular complications and a more aggressive approach to their glycaemic control may be warranted (7,8,9). As improving glycaemic control has been shown to improve cognition, one should continue to strive for acceptable glycaemic control whenever possible and appropriate (10).

Type 2 diabetes is associated with significant co-morbidities (11,12), many of which lead to physical and mental disability (13,14). All management plans have to take an holistic approach, as any one of the co-morbidities may take precedence over the actual management of the diabetes.

With no specific dietary diabetic guidelines for the older age group, advice has usually been based around the same recommendations as for all adults with diabetes. Clearly these need to be individually modified and at times liberally interpreted. Important factors to consider when giving dietary advice to this age group are:

- Functional and mental ability,
- Polypharmacy,

- Co-morbidities,
- Dependency on others.

CURRENT DIETARY RECOMMENDATIONS AS APPLICABLE TO THE OLDER PERSON WITH DIABETES

Current European recommendations are based on studies in younger age groups, which have then been extrapolated to the elderly. The quality of evidence for the specific effects of dietary intervention in older age groups is poor.

The most recent European recommendations for adults with diabetes are shown in Table 10.1 (15). They emphasise energy balance and weight control, and recognise a wide variation in carbohydrate intake as being compatible with good diabetic control. The target of nutritional management is to help optimise glycaemic control and reduce the risk of cardiovascular disease and nephropathy. However, the quality of life of the individual person must be considered when defining nutritional objectives and health care providers must achieve a balance between the demands of metabolic control, risk factor management, patient well-being and safety. Compliance with all treatment modalities is likely to be compromised by increasing physical and mental disabilities, which occur more frequently in the ageing population.

If beneficial changes to the diet of an elderly person with diabetes are to be achieved, access to dietetic services is needed. The following topics should be considered: body weight, physical activity and the specific micronutrient composition of the diet including carbohydrates, protein, alcohol, sodium, vitamins and minerals.

BODY WEIGHT

The National Diet and Nutrition Survey of people aged 65 years and over (16) showed that two-thirds of free-living elderly were overweight or obese. While only 3% of men and 6% of women in the community were underweight, this figure rose to 17% for the elderly in institutions. Undernutrition in acutely ill hospitalised elderly patients has been estimated at 26% (17).

A BMI range of $24-29 \, \text{kg/m}^2$ has been suggested as appropriate for the elderly population (18), especially for individuals above 70 years of age, as this higher than conventional BMI range has been associated with lower mortality rates. Morley suggested weight reduction only be considered in patients 20% above their desirable body weight (19) and then a BMI of 29 may be a safer and more realistic target for older people to achieve.

Weight loss of between 5-10% from initial body weight is known to benefit blood pressure, glycaemic control and lipid profiles, with a 10% weight loss

Table 10.1 Summary of the European recommendations, 1999

	Recommendation
Total dietary energy	No specific recommendation unless the person is overweight or gaining weight, when a reduction in total energy intake is advised
Body weight	Ideally BMI 19–25. Those overweight should be encouraged to lose weight. Weight gain should be avoided
Activity	All should be encouraged to engage in moderate activity for 20–30 min most days
Carbohydrate	Acceptable range 45–60% of total energy
	A combined intake of 60–70% of total energy is recommended for carbohydrate and monounsaturated with *cis* configuration fatty acids. The proportions will vary according to the individual's clinical state and preferences
	Carbohydrates rich in fibre or having a low glycaemic index are particularly recommended
	Sucrose intake should not exceed 10% of total energy
Fat	Acceptable range 25–35% of total energy
	Saturated and *trans*-unsaturated fatty acids to provide less than 10% of total energy
	Polyunsaturated fatty acids not to exceed 10% of total energy
	Monounsaturated fatty acids with *cis* configuration in combination with carbohydrate should provide 60–70% total energy
	One portion of oily fish/week plus other plant sources are recommended for *n*-3 fatty acids
Protein	Intake should be between 10–20% of total energy
Cholesterol	Should not exceed 300 mg/day
Dietary supplements	Fish oils or their derived preparations and pharmacological doses of vitamins are not recommended
Vitamins and antioxidant nutrients	Foods naturally rich in dietary antioxidants and other vitamins should be encouraged
Fruit and vegetables	Five portions a day
Folate	Regular consumption of foods with readily bioavailable folate (citrus fruits and legumes)
Sodium	Restrict salt intake to less than 6 g/day
Alcohol	Recommendations for the general public apply. Recommends 15 g for women and 30 g for men per day as acceptable for most
	When using insulin or sulphonylureas it is advised to consume alcohol with carbohydrate-containing foods
'Diabetic' foods	These are not recommended
	Non-nutritive sweeteners can be useful in drinks

required to provide long-term improvements in patients with Type 2 diabetes (20). Even though weight loss will improve glycaemic control and symptoms (20), weight loss in this group can be hard to achieve due to decreased activity levels.

Over the age of 65 years there is an age-related loss in body fat and lean body mass, reversing the tendency to increased fat deposition in middle age. During these years the number of underweight individuals increases, particularly in institutions and in the presence of acute illness. It is extremely important to identify these underweight and malnourished individuals when providing dietary advice. Factors influencing undernutrition are discussed later in this chapter.

ACTIVITY

As people get older activity levels generally fall. The presence of co-morbidities such as arthritis can significantly affect functional ability, which in turn further limits physical activity. This fall in activity contributes to being overweight and makes losing weight harder. The benefits of exercise for all people with diabetes are well documented and are irrespective of body weight or age. Exercise will lead to an improvement in metabolic and cardiovascular risk factors as well as improving strength, flexibility, balance and function (21).

The recommendation of 30 min moderate activity on most days is achievable for many older people – it does not have to be 30 continuous minutes and can consist of any light activity, e.g. walking (22). Moderate intensity has a very different meaning at the age of 70 years compared to the age of 30 years, and in general individuals should be encouraged to do what they can achieve, do it regularly and gradually build up in intensity and frequency. Even very frail older people can manage certain activities and over time should be able to gradually improve their strength. For some older adults whose mobility is severely restricted, activities may need to be adapted to the individual's abilities, e.g. chair, arm and non-weight-bearing exercises. Some types of very strenuous activity are contraindicated, for example in patients with known ischaemic heart disease or severe retinopathy (23).

CARBOHYDRATES

Fibre is a particularly important component to encourage in an older person's diet. Constipation is common and increasing fibre intake can reduce laxative use and improve bowel function. However, fibrous foods tend to have a greater satiating effect and should be advised with caution for those with depressed appetites.

Foods with a low glycaemic index (GI) should also be encouraged to improve glycaemic control in patients with diabetes. However, the compliance to dietary advice in general is often poor and providing more complex advice around GI foods may not necessarily achieve the level of compliance required to be beneficial.

PROTEIN

The European Association for the Study of Diabetes recognised that the recommendations for the protein content of the diet are based on incomplete evidence. Concerns exist about the development of nephropathy with a high protein intake (24,25). Overall the incidence of nephropathy in the elderly population has increased over the last 20 years. One possible explanation is that the improved treatment of coronary heart disease and hypertension has resulted in more patients with Type 2 diabetes living long enough to develop nephropathy and end-stage renal failure (ESRF).

In a recent review of the literature that looked at protein ranges between 0.3–0.8 g/kg bw/day, high protein intakes contributed to the development of nephropathy (24–26). Reducing protein intake appears to slow the progression to renal failure, however the level of restriction that is both effective and acceptable to patients is unknown. The current literature is based mainly on individuals with Type 1 diabetes and often uses proxy indicators such as creatinine clearance rather than hard clinical end-points such as time to dialysis or death from ESRF. In another meta-analysis of the literature dietary protein restriction was shown to have only a relatively weak effect on slowing the rate of decline in renal function (27).

Current European recommendations suggest that patients with diabetes, who exhibit evidence of microalbuminuria or established nephropathy should have a protein intake at the lower end of the normal range (0.7–0.9 g/kg bw/day). This level is compatible with the current medical literature and the 1985 WHO guidelines (28,29). Protein intakes below this increase the risk of malnutrition during chronic illness or catabolic states. While not commonly a problem, in some elderly patients with diabetes the balance between the risk of malnutrition and the possible benefits of a reduced protein intake to delay nephropathy need to be carefully assessed.

ALCOHOL

Older people are more susceptible to the effects of alcohol and are likely to develop problems at relatively lower levels of consumption. The reduction in body water content and lean body mass with advancing age results in a smaller volume of distribution for the alcohol (30). Higher peak blood alcohol concentrations occur in older than younger subjects matched for body size and sex, yet ethanol clearance does not appear to be altered by age (31).

Moderate intakes of alcohol appear to benefit blood pressure, glycaemic control and reduce the risk of thrombosis (32). Alcohol can also act as an appetite stimulant and this can be beneficial. Large intakes however have been shown to increase the risk of stroke, hypertension, hypoglycaemia and both lactic and ketoacidosis (33). Patients should be encouraged to limit their intake to 1–2 units per day for women, or 2–3 units per day for men. Due to the age-related body composition changes, the lower end of these ranges is probably preferable.

SODIUM

Taste and smell declines with age, beginning around 60 years but becoming more marked above 70 years (34). Salt and monosodium glutamate are commonly used as taste enhancers and can improve dietary intake in elderly people (35). However, sodium intake is linked with the development or exacerbation of hypertension (36), and when salt intake is reduced blood pressure can fall (37). A balance between using flavour enhancers to encourage dietary intake for underweight people, while not exacerbating hypertension, needs to be made.

VITAMIN AND MINERALS

The National Diet and Nutrition Survey of people aged 65 years and over provides valuable data on the current eating practices and nutritional status of elderly people in the UK (16). Areas of concern highlighted in this report were the inadequate intakes of folate, vitamin D, vitamin C, vitamin K, iron and magnesium. Of the survey population 10–40% were shown to have multiple vitamin deficiencies and 10% were anaemic. Levels of deficiencies were higher when an individual was receiving institutionalised care.

The micronutrient status of elderly individuals with diabetes is controversial. The literature is limited and recommending any intervention should be done with caution until further research is undertaken. The literature on selected vitamins and minerals such as chromium, B vitamins and selenium in diabetes has been reviewed (38). The authors conclude that micronutrient supplementation for people with diabetes should be individualised and based on clinical findings, dietary history and laboratory results.

Some of the questions surrounding certain nutrient supplementation are particularly relevant to the management of the older patient with diabetes. These include vitamins for wound healing and bone health. Pressure sores develop in 4–10% of newly hospitalised patients, increasing to 14% in long-term elderly care (39). Patients with diabetes are a vulnerable group with poor wound healing. To date there is insufficient evidence to support the routine supplementation of micronutrients for wound or leg ulcer healing using either multivitamins or vitamin C with or without zinc. Improved healing of leg ulcers and wounds has been reported following three months' zinc supplementation given as 70 mg of zinc three times a day (38). However a review on nutrition and wound healing by Albina concluded that while supplementation of hospitalised patients with zinc and vitamin C may be reasonable (40), routine use of vitamin C supplementation alone is unlikely to be beneficial (41). The UK Department of Health currently recommends a reference nutrient intake of 40 mg of vitamin C daily (42), but not routine supplementation. These vitamin C requirements are based on the prevention of scurvy, and further research on the benefits of higher intakes is still required.

All elderly people are at risk of fractures due to falls and osteoporosis, but when diabetes is present this risk may be further increased by peripheral neuropathy, autonomic neuropathy, hypoglycaemic episodes and poor eyesight.

In 1998 the Department of Health recommended the reference nutrient intake for calcium for people over 50 years of age to be 700 mg daily (43), with this being obtained from milk and milk-based foods. The National Osteoporosis Society (NOS) has set its recommended daily calcium intake higher in order to meet individual rather than population needs. The NOS recommend a level of 1500 mg for people over 60 years of age.

Older people are vulnerable to vitamin D deficiency due to an age-related decline in vitamin D synthesis and less sunlight exposure. Sunlight on the skin in the UK from May to September should be sufficient for vitamin D synthesis for most adults. The Department of Health suggests that the face and arms be exposed for 30 min per day (43). Vitamin D supplementation should be considered for all elderly housebound individuals and other groups unable to achieve this exposure. A daily vitamin D intake of 10 µg is recommended and if dietary intake is less, vitamin D by tablet or as a six-monthly injection is required.

Further research is needed to clarify the assessment of vitamin and mineral status in elderly patients with diabetes and to develop appropriate guidelines on the need for supplementation.

OTHER CONTRIBUTING FACTORS TO NUTRITIONAL HEALTH IN THE ELDERLY PATIENT WITH DIABETES

Undernutrition is as much a concern in older patients with diabetes as obesity (44). There are lifestyle changes and functional and cognitive problems that can cause inadequate dietary intake in these patients, as addressed below.

ORAL HEALTH

Diabetes adversely affects oral health, increasing the risk of gingivitis and other oral infections. Gingivitis is a major cause of tooth loss and pain that can affect oral intake. Saliva flow protects against dental caries but age, drugs and diseases can reduce this. Poor oral and dental health is linked with chewing difficulties that can cause malnutrition, poor general health and reduced quality of life (45,46).

Population changes in oral health and dentition over the last 30 years have resulted in fewer older people with no natural teeth – declining from 37% in 1968 to 12% in 1998 and predicted to fall to around 2% by 2018 (47). There are dietary implications for those with no teeth or partial dentures, as difficulties in eating can lead to a reduction in the variety of food choices and an overall reduction in nutrient intake. A 15% drop in energy intake has been reported in free-living elderly people without any natural teeth. Full dentures, in particular, can lead to a reduction in food consumption due to the mouth feeling full, a greater time needed to eat causing embarrassment and changes in food flavours (48).

All patients need to be encouraged to maintain good oral hygiene, with special attention given to those with dry mouths or who eat more frequently due to a small appetite or, in the case of a person with Type 1 diabetes, due to the need for frequent snacks. Dental advice is required for patients with chewing difficulties, pain and other oral health problems. However, it should be recognised that elderly patients may have mobility problems getting to a dentist. In addition, many elderly patients have perceived barriers to dental care, the major ones being fear and costs (47).

SENSORY LOSSES

Loss of taste and smell can influence the enjoyment of food and decrease motivation to eat and drink. Such sensory losses occur naturally as a function of age (49) as well as with certain diseases, such as cancer. Adding ready-to-use flavour enhancers containing monosodium glutamate (MSG) may improve dietary intake and thus reverse weight loss, improve immunity, functional status and quality of life (34,50,51).

When the thirst sensation is decreased, dehydration can occur. Many elderly patients deliberately reduce their fluid intake to reduce their urine frequency, which may be increased due to glycosuria and prescribed diuretics. The recommended minimum daily fluid intake is 1500 ml (approximately 7–8 cups/ glasses), but this will be higher for patients with poorly controlled diabetes since urinary output is increased (52).

SOCIAL FACTORS

Eating is not just a feeding process, but an important social event. Food choices and access to food can be affected by numerous factors including bereavement, immobility and isolation. All can affect the motivation to eat and enjoy food. The ability to shop and prepare meals decreases with age (16), with 30% of men and 50% of women reported as housebound or requiring assistance to shop when over 85 years of age (53). The available and discretionary income may also fall with age. It is therefore difficult for many elderly patients to follow a prescribed diabetic diet especially as many luncheon clubs, community meals, day centres and ready meals do not cater specifically for people with diabetes.

PHYSICAL FACTORS

Functional limitations such as mobility and illness affect nutritional status. Elderly people with diabetes have increased levels of disability and immobility that affect all aspects of daily living, including shopping, meal preparation and leisure activities (54).

Patients with diabetes are at an increased risk of a stroke and any resultant neurological deficit can lead to eating problems and malnutrition (55,56). The most frequently encountered eating problems are hoarding food in the mouth, poor lip seal leading to leakage of food, dysphagia and chewing problems. Careful observation at mealtimes, and assessment by a speech therapist if necessary, will enable identification of specific eating problems. For some patients, eating in front of people can be a traumatic and embarrassing event, further reducing food intake.

PSYCHOLOGICAL AND COGNITIVE FUNCTION

Any level of psychological or cognitive deficit may lead to a poor or erratic diet affecting both nutritional state and glycaemic control. Memory lapses can result in missed meals and medication or an inadvertent repeated dose of some medications leading to, amongst other things, hypoglycaemia. Cognitive function is also impaired in people with diabetes due to increased incidence of cerebrovascular disease and depression (57,58). Psychological problems are both a predictor of mortality and of hospital admissions (59). Food intake can be markedly reduced in the presence of dementia. VOICES (Voluntary Organisations Involved in Caring in the Elderly Sector) produced a report in 1998 regarding the specific nutritional needs of elderly people with dementia (60).

Cognitive deterioration in patients with diabetes may be made worse by nutritional deficiencies (61) and poor glycaemic control. Cognitive function with documented improvements in problem solving, attention, concentration, memory and learning ability have been reported with better glycaemic control (10).

Figure 10.1 summarises many of these factors and offers strategies for their treatment.

OTHER CONSIDERATIONS WHEN ADVISING OLDER PEOPLE WITH DIABETES

DELAYED GASTRIC EMPTYING

Hyperglycaemia delays gastric emptying (62) as do multiple other factors, many of which remain poorly understood. Physiological inhibitory pathways exist that control gastric emptying and involve small intestinal receptors that are stimulated by nutrients in the lumen of the gut. Posture, meal size and meal composition all influence gastric emptying through activating these receptors. Dietary fat empties at a slower rate than protein or carbohydrate and liquids empty faster than solids.

A modest degree of gastroparesis occurs with ageing. However, this is much commoner in people with diabetes; upto half of all patients with long-standing diabetes (both Type 1 and 2) have some evidence of delayed gastric emptying (62). Gastroparesis affects both glycaemic control as well as oral hypo-glycaemic drug absorption, and in elderly people may precipitate post-prandial events, which may lead to loss of consciousness and falls.

Delayed gastric emptying can be asymptomatic, making the diagnosis difficult. Symptoms, if present, include nausea, vomiting and abdominal fullness. However, none of these symptoms correlate well with gastric emptying. Patients presenting with gastrointestinal symptoms, who already have diabetic complications, in particular autonomic neuropathy, are major candidates for this condition or other disorders of gut motility. Hyper-glycaemia may contribute to these symptoms as it has been reported to increase the perception of sensations arising from the gut (63).

Delays in gastric emptying can reduce the rate of drug transit and slow the rate of absorption. A few studies have been conducted in patients with diabetes that demonstrate a correlation between the absorption of glibenclamide and glipizide and gastric emptying time (62). With drugs that have a long half-life and are given long-term, this effect would not be expected to lead to significant alterations in blood concentrations of the drug.

Gastric emptying can affect glycaemic profiles. Rapid gastric emptying can cause glycaemic spikes and a worsening of control. On the other hand, when gastric emptying is delayed a mismatch with the onset of hypoglycaemic drug action and glucose absorption can occur, leading to hypoglycaemia.

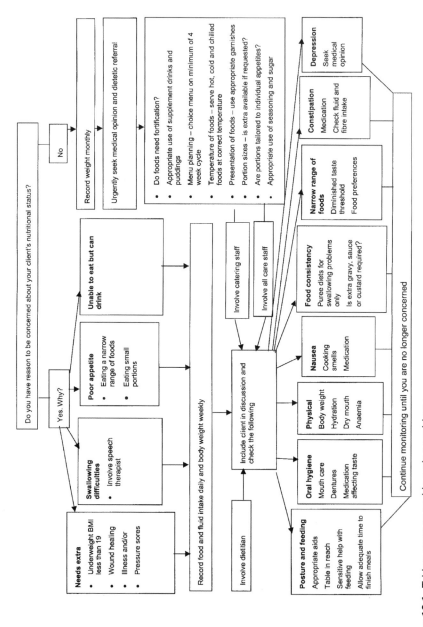

Figure 10.1. Taking steps to tackle eating problems
Source: Reproduced from the British Dietetic Association's Nutrition Advisory Group for Elderly People (64).

The most successful treatment for gastroparesis remains pharmacological. Dietary advice should focus on preventing weight loss and malnutrition. Eating and drinking separately and advice encouraging small frequent meals and snacks can improve symptoms. Supplements may be needed if specific nutrients are deficient or malabsorption is present.

RISK OF HYPOGLYCAEMIA

The risk of, and fear of, hypoglycaemia is a major reason why diabetes is undertreated in older people. The Diabetes Control and Complications Trial in Type 1 diabetes and the UKPDS trial in Type 2 diabetes clearly demonstrated that secondary complications could be decreased by tight glycaemic control, but this increased the risk of hypoglycaemia (65,66). Hypoglycaemia is a particular problem in older patients with Type 1 diabetes as hypoglycaemic awareness decreases with duration of diabetes and advancing age. In addition, older patients with Type 2 diabetes treated with hypoglycaemic drugs are particularly prone to hypoglycaemia if dietary intake is variable. General frailty, polypharmacy, renal impairment and frequent hospitalisations are all risk factors for hypoglycaemia (67). Hypoglycaemic symptoms are frequently unrecognised and, when they are recognised, may not be treated appropriately.

There are no established glycaemic goals for the older patient. Sinclair has recommended pre-meal targets of 6–8 mmol/l and 7–9 mmol/l at bedtime, with less stringent levels for individuals with recurrent hypoglycaemia (68). The St Vincent Joint Task Force for Diabetes final report emphasises selecting glycaemic targets on an individual basis and focusing management goals on elevated lipids and blood pressure (69).

Dietary management on how to avoid hypoglycaemia is discussed in detail elsewhere in this book. As for any hypoglycaemic episode, rapidly absorbed carbohydrate should be consumed, followed by longer lasting carbohydrate. Education of elderly patients and their carers on how to avoid hypoglycaemia is important, and emphasis should be placed on regular meals and ensuring adequate carbohydrate with each meal.

MEDICATION

The choice of a single oral agent for the elderly individual with Type 2 diabetes is made predominately on the basis of weight, clinical assessment of insulin resistance and renal function. Lean patients with Type 2 diabetes are more likely to need an agent to increase their circulating insulin levels (e.g. sulphonylureas or insulin) while obese patients may require an agent to reduce insulin resistance (e.g. metformin or a glitazone).

Sulphonylureas with a long biological action, such as glibenclamide, increase the risk of hypoglycaemia in elderly people (70). Reduced renal function delays the excretion of some active drug metabolites and increases the risk of hypoglycaemia. Sulphonylureas with shorter biological actions, such as glicazide or the older tolbutamide (metabolised by the liver) are associated with less hypoglycaemia. Metformin is effective in obese older patients as it indirectly increases insulin sensitivity, promotes weight loss and is not associated with hypoglycaemia when given as monotherapy. Renal function should be monitored in patients taking metformin (71) and not used when renal impairment is present or if there is severe anorexia. Age should not be a barrier to starting insulin and is often required for elderly patients with Type 2 diabetes, who can usually cope well with the new insulin pen devices (68).

Elderly people are at risk for drug–nutrient interaction, a problem which has been reviewed by Lewis et al. (72) and Roe (73). Drugs can interfere with nutrient intake, absorption, metabolism and excretion. Foods can interact with drugs, altering their absorption and action. For example, bulking agents, such as methylcellulose, can decrease appetite by creating a feeling of fullness. Metformin reduces vitamin B_{12} absorption, diuretics increase urinary loss of potassium and magnesium and warfarin can affect vitamin K metabolism. Food in general may decrease the absorption and absorptive rate of aspirin, while fibre can specifically reduce the absorption of digoxin. It is important to be aware of these interactions and to ensure sufficient intake of nutrients to prevent any potential nutritional deficiencies.

ACUTE INTERCURRENT ILLNESS

As with any adult with diabetes who becomes ill, older people should be encouraged to take regular carbohydrate and sufficient drinks while continuing their medication. As their appetite may be reduced, small frequent drinks may be more tolerable and acceptable. Older people should be advised to prepare for illness by keeping suitable foods stored for such an eventuality, e.g. long-life or dried milk, tinned milk puddings, fortified drinks, tinned and dried foods, UHT fruit juice, porridge oats or other cereals, etc.

GUIDELINES FOR PRACTICE IN NURSING AND RESIDENTIAL HOMES

Results from studies of the prevalence of diabetes in nursing and residential homes range from 7.2–17.5%, see Table 10.2.

When self-reporting questionnaires are used to obtain prevalence figures in residential care an underestimate of the true prevalence occurs, as diabetes is often undiagnosed. Available prevalence studies show that diabetes is more common among the ageing population in care than in the community.

The three UK studies indicate that the majority of patients are treated using diet and tablets, followed by diet alone and finally diet and insulin. The most recent study carried out in Sheffield also investigates the patterns of diabetes

Table 10.2 Studies examining the prevalence of diabetes in care homes

Study	Year	Method	Rate (%)
South Glamorgan (74)	1997	Questionnaire	7.2
Liverpool (75)	1998	Questionnaire	9.9
Canada (76)	1998	Questionnaire and random venous glucose sampling	17.5
Sheffield (77)	2000	Questionnaire	8.8

care and the level of training received by the staff in these institutions. Their results show that very few homes in the area employ staff with specialised training in diabetes care and that diabetes management is poorly structured. They also show that the majority of homes do not give patients the choice to manage their own treatment, being instead encouraged to follow the routine within the establishment. Similar results were found by Tong *et al.* (78) in 1994, where those in care homes received fewer services than those in their own homes in terms of annual review and access to therapists (chiropodist, dietitian and optician).

Looking more specifically at dietary care there are two interesting American studies. One investigated the benefits of a 'diabetic' diet for nursing home residents and found only insignificant differences in glucose control (fasting glucose increased on average only 0.6 mmol/l) when patients followed the normal diet instead of the 'diabetic' diet (79). Both diets met the recommended dietary allowances for the age group and body weight did not change significantly despite a slightly increased calorie intake on the normal diet. This raised the question as to whether care homes need to routinely provide special 'diabetic' diets. However this study was only short in duration (16 weeks, eight weeks on either diet), and the participants were all in good health, maintained good glycaemic control before entry to the study and were not obese. The second study by Funnell and Herman investigated local standards of care for nursing home patients with diabetes (80). This was conducted using a questionnaire and chart review of a sample of the patients with diabetes. The results showed that although most homes had some diabetes care orders and protocols, in general the care did not meet local or national standards. Care practices were closer to national standards if dietitians participated in meal planning and written institutional policies existed. These results highlight the need for dietetic input into residential and nursing homes to provide education as well as assessing and monitoring patients.

In 1999 the British Diabetic Association (now Diabetes UK) produced guidelines of practice for residents with diabetes in care homes (81). This comprehensive report is the only document currently available providing a framework for standards of diabetes care within care homes. It aims to identify major issues relating to the nature and delivery of diabetes care within care homes and to determine the current evidence base in the published literature. The report emphasised the need to monitor weight, provide each patient with an individualised diet and nutritional plan for their care, and obtain the input of a state registered dietitian.

The report's recommendations concerning diet and nutritional care included the following.

1. Each resident should expect to have:
   - The opportunity to play an active role in self-diabetes care according to their abilities.
   - An individualised dietary and nutritional plan as part of the overall care plan.
   - Access to community health professionals including a community dietitian.
2. Each care home should expect:
   - Training for staff and catering staff on diet and diabetes, which is jointly funded through the health and social care budget at a district, regional and national level.
3. Each district should have at least one community dietitian whose primary responsibility is the provision of dietary and nutritional support for residents within care homes.

Individualised care and choice about treatment are also reflected in the National Service Framework for Older People for England, although no specific recommendations are given regarding diabetes. The Caroline Walker Trust and VOICES have both produced reports providing detailed guidelines for the nutrient provision in care homes. One report covers the general care home population and the other is specifically for residents who have dementia (see 'Useful resources' section for details).

The need for skilled individualised nutritional care is highlighted by the number of factors that can contribute to nutritional problems, as listed in Table 10.3.

GUIDELINES FOR PRACTICE IN HOSPITAL

Two-thirds of hospitalised patients with diabetes are aged 65 years or older (82) and these patients have more hospital admissions and stay longer than non-diabetic patients (83). There is evidence that undernutrition is prevalent on admission in this patient group and that this can worsen during the hospital stay (84). Contributing factors are listed in Table 10.3.

Two reports entitled 'Hungry in Hospital' (85) and 'Not because they are old' (86) document the inadequacy of the meal service to elderly patients in

Table 10.3 Factors contributing to management difficulties in care home residents with diabetes

- Loss of appetite.
- Poor food intake, exacerbated by reduced food choice or unnecessary food restrictions, inflexibility of meal times, reduced food availability, poor knowledge of care home staff.
- Weight loss, which may be unidentified due to lack of routine weighing.
- Difficulties feeding self or unable to feed self.
- Poor glycaemic control related to poor intake.
- Physical impairments, such as reduced dexterity, poor mobility, etc.
- Cognitive impairments, e.g. acute confusion, depression, dementia.
- Communication difficulties, e.g. dysphasia and dysarthria, confusion, deafness.
- Multiple co-morbidities.
- Polypharmacy.
- Dysphagia, which may lead to need for modified texture diet further restricting food choice and palatability.
- Increased incidence of infections, leg ulceration and pressure sores with corresponding increases in nutritional requirements.
- Sensory impairments such as vision, taste, smell and hearing.

hospital. Improving hospital food in the UK was the objective of the 'Better Hospital Food' campaign, launched in 2001 and aimed at creating new NHS hospital menus to encourage patients to eat more. It is hoped that the quality and style of hospital food can be improved using standardised recipes and ward housekeepers. The British Association for Enteral and Parenteral Nutrition has produced a report putting forward food as treatment, summarised in Table 10.4.

If dietary measures are not enough, prescribed nutritional supplements may be used. The use of oral supplements and sip feeds has recently been reviewed (88). Nutritional supplement preparations are suitable for patients with diabetes under medical supervision, the principal aim being to ensure an adequate energy intake. Once the person has recovered their appetite, long-term

Table 10.4 Key areas for improvements to the hospital meal service (87)

- Staff training on the importance of nutrition in hospital.
- Staffing on wards, e.g. clear definitions of roles and responsibilities of staff at mealtimes, additional staff at mealtimes.
- Nutrient content of meals, e.g. energy-dense meals for the acutely ill or undernourished.
- Individual nutrition screening of all patients to provide baseline information such as physical problems, weight changes, food and fluid intake.
- Improved distribution and service such as timing of meals.
- Increasing the budget for hospital food.
- Regular auditing of nutrition screening and assessment of nutritional care.

plans to maintain adequate food intake may need to be devised. Enteral feeding has been used successfully in the management of dysphagia following stroke and in supplementing oral feeding in undernourished old people (89).

AREAS FOR FUTURE RESEARCH

The benefits of striving for optimal glycaemic control in older people to prevent long-term complications needs to be balanced against the short-term risks and consequences of hypoglycaemia (7). Further research is needed to establish under what circumstances intensive treatment to achieve good glycaemic control is justified, and whether optimising blood pressure and lipid profiles has a greater influence on morbidity and mortality.

SUMMARY

It is important that dietetic advice to elderly patients with diabetes is tailored to the individual and their specific nutritional needs. As chronological age is often a poor indicator of the ageing process, an individual's physical and mental profile needs to be assessed and addressed. Advising older patients requires balancing health needs with quality of life issues.

USEFUL RESOURCES

The British Dietetic Association's Nutritional Advisory Group for Elderly People (NAGE) publishes a range of resources to assist in the dietary management of older people. Further information can be obtained from the British Dietetic Association, 5th Floor, Charles House, 148/9 Great Charles Street, Birmingham B3 3HT or on the web site at www.bda.uk.com.

Diabetes UK provides a range of resources for patients and health care professionals and can be contacted at 10 Queen Anne Street, London W1G 9HL or www.diabetes.org.uk.

The Caroline Walker Trust distributes two guidelines relating to care of older people: Eating Well for Older People and Eating Well for Older People with Dementia. Further information can be obtained from 22 Kindersley Way, Abbots Langley, Hertfordshire WD5 0DQ or www.cwt.org.uk.

REFERENCES

1. Sinclair AJ. Diabetes in the elderly: a perspective from the United Kingdom. *Clin Geriatr Med* 1999; 15: 225–237.

2. Harris MI, Flegal KM, Cowie CC, Eberhardt MS, Goldstein DE, Little RR, Wiedmeyer HM, Byrd-Holt DD. Prevalence of diabetes, impaired fasting glucose, and impaired glucose tolerance in U.S. adults. The Third National Health and Nutrition Examination Survey, 1988–1994. *Diabetes Care* 1998; 21: 518–524.
3. Cohen DL, Neil HA, Thorogood M, Mann JI. A population-based study of the incidence of complications associated with type 2 diabetes in the elderly. *Diabet Med* 1991; 8: 928–933.
4. Walters DP, Gatling W, Mullee MA, Hill RD. The prevalence of diabetic distal sensory neuropathy in an English community. *Diabet Med* 1992; 9: 349–353.
5. Meneilly GS, Tessier D. Diabetes in elderly adults. *J Gerontol A: Biol Sci Med Sci* 2001; 56: M5–M13.
6. Arner P, Pollare T, Lithell H. Different aetiologies of type 2 (non-insulin-dependent) diabetes mellitus in obese and non-obese subjects. *Diabetologia* 1991; 34: 483–487.
7. Sinclair AJ, Meneilly GS. Re-thinking metabolic strategies for older people with type 2 diabetes mellitus: implications of the UK Prospective Diabetes Study and other recent studies. *Age Ageing* 2000; 29: 393–397.
8. Groeneveld Y, Petri H, Hermans J, Springer MP. Relationship between blood glucose level and mortality in type 2 diabetes mellitus: a systematic review. *Diabet Med* 1999; 16: 2–13.
9. Muggeo M, Zoppini G, Bonora E, Brun E, Bonadonna RC, Moghetti P, Verlato G. Fasting plasma glucose variability predicts 10-year survival of type 2 diabetic patients: the Verona Diabetes Study. *Diabetes Care* 2000; 23: 45–50.
10. Meneilly GS, Cheung E, Tessier D, Yakura C, Tuokko H. The effect of improved glycemic control on cognitive functions in the elderly patient with diabetes. *J Gerontol* 1993; 48: M117–M121.
11. Gu K, Cowie CC, Harris MI. Mortality in adults with and without diabetes in a national cohort of the U.S. population, 1971–1993. *Diabetes Care* 1998; 21: 1138–1145.
12. Sinclair AJ, Robert IE, Croxson SC. Mortality in older people with diabetes mellitus. *Diabet Med* 1997; 14: 639–647.
13. Volpato S, Blaum C, Resnick H, Ferrucci L, Fried LP, Guralnik JM. Comorbidities and impairments explaining the association between diabetes and lower extremity disability: The Women's Health and Aging Study. *Diabetes Care* 2002; 25: 678–683.
14. Strachan MW, Deary IJ, Ewing FM, Frier BM. Is type II diabetes associated with an increased risk of cognitive dysfunction? A critical review of published studies. *Diabetes Care* 1997; 20: 438–445.
15. The Diabetes and Nutrition Study Group of the European Association for the Study of Diabetes. Recommendations for the nutritional management of patients with diabetes mellitus. *Eur J Clin Nutr* 2000; 54: 353–355.
16. Finch S, Doyle W, Lowe C, Bates CJ, Prentice A, Smithers G, Clarke P. National Diet and Nutrition Survey: people aged 65 years and over. Vol. 1. Report of the diet and nutrition survey. London: The Stationary Office, 1998.
17. Potter J, Klipstein K, Reilly JJ, Roberts M. The nutritional status and clinical course of acute admissions to a geriatric unit. *Age Ageing* 1995; 24: 131–136.
18. Flodin L, Svensson S, Cederholm T. Body mass index as a predictor of 1 year mortality in geriatric patients. *Clin Nutr* 2000; 19: 121–125.
19. Morley JE, Perry HM 3rd. The management of diabetes mellitus in older individuals. *Drugs* 1991; 41: 548–565.
20. Lee A, Dundoo G. Obesity in the elderly. In: *Endocrinology of Aging*, eds JE Morley and L van den Berg. Totowa: Humana Press, 2000: 205–220.
21. American College of Sports Medicine Position Stand. Exercise and physical activity for older adults. *Med Sci Sports Ex* 1998; 30: 992–1008.

22. Christmas C, Andersen RA. Exercise and older patients: guidelines for the clinician. *J Am Geriatr Soc* 2000; 48: 318–324.

23. American Diabetes Association. Diabetes mellitus and exercise. *Diabetes Care* 1997; 20: 1908–1912.

24. Kupin WL, Cortes P, Dumler F, Feldkamp CS, Kilates MC, Levin NW. Effect on renal function of change from high to moderate protein intake in type I diabetic patients. *Diabetes* 1987; 36: 73–79.

25. Toeller M, Buyken A, Heitkamp G, Bramswig S, Mann J, Milne R, Gries FA, Keen H. Protein intake and urinary albumin excretion rates in the EURODIAB IDDM Complications Study. *Diabetologia* 1997; 40: 1219–1226.

26. Waugh NR, Robertson AM. Protein restriction for diabetic renal disease. *Cochrane Database Syst Rev* 2000; 2: CD002181.

27. Kasiske BL, Lakatua JD, Ma JZ, Louis TA. A meta-analysis of the effects of dietary protein restriction on the rate of decline in renal function. *Am J Kidney Dis* 1998; 31: 954–961.

28. Food and Agriculture Organisation, World Health Organization, and United Nations University. Energy and Protein Requirements. Report of a Joint Expert Consultation, 724. WHO Technical Report Series. Geneva: WHO, 1985.

29. Millward DJ. Optimal intakes of protein in the human diet. *Proc Nutr Soc* 1999; 58: 403–413.

30. Dufour M, Fuller RK. Alcohol in the elderly. *Ann Rev Med* 1995; 46: 123–132.

31. Vestal RE, McGuire EA, Tobin JD, Andres R, Norris AH, Mezey E. Aging and ethanol metabolism. *Clin Pharmacol Ther* 1977; 21: 343–354.

32. Bell DS. Alcohol and the NIDDM patient. *Diabetes Care* 1996; 19: 509–513.

33. Swade TF, Emanuele NV. Alcohol and diabetes. *Compr Ther* 1997; 23: 135–140.

34. Schiffman SS. Taste and smell losses in normal aging and disease. *J Am Med Assoc* 1997; 278: 1357–1362.

35. Schiffman SS. Intensification of sensory properties of foods for the elderly. *J Nutr* 2000; 130 (Suppl 4S): S927–S930.

36. Elliott P, Stamler J, Nichols R, Dyer AR, Stamler R, Kesteloot H, Marmot M. Intersalt revisited: further analyses of 24 hour sodium excretion and blood pressure within and across populations. Intersalt Cooperative Research Group. *Br Med J* 1996; 312: 1249–1253.

37. Cappuccio FP, Markandu ND, Carney C, Sagnella GA, MacGregor GA. Double-blind randomised trial of modest salt restriction in older people. *Lancet* 1997; 350: 850–854.

38. Mooradian A, Failla M, Hoogwerf BJ, Maryniuk M, Wylie-Rosett J. Selected vitamins and minerals in diabetes. *Diabetes Care* 1994; 17: 464–479.

39. Collins C. A practical guide to nutrition and pressure sores. *Compl Nutr* 2001; 1: 25–27.

40. Albina JE. Nutrition and wound healing. *J Parent Ent Nutr* 1994; 18: 367–376.

41. North G, Booth A. Why appraise the evidence? A case study of vitamin C and the healing of pressure sores. *J Human Nutr Diet* 1999; 12: 237–244.

42. Department of Health. Dietary Reference Values for Food, Energy and Nutrients for the United Kingdom. Report on Health and Social Subjects No. 41. Report of the Panel on Dietary Reference Values of the Committee on Medical Aspects of Food Policy. London: HMSO, 1991.

43. Department of Health. Nutrition and Bone Health. Report of the Working Group of the Committee on Medical Aspects of Food Policy. Report on Health and Social Subjects. London: The Stationery Office, 49, 1998.

44. Gilden JL. Nutrition and the older diabetic. *Clin Geriatr Med* 1999; 15: 371–390.

45. Mojon P, Budtz-Jorgensen E, Rapin CH. Relationship between oral health and nutrition in very old people. *Age Ageing* 1999; 28: 463–468.
46. Nakanishi N, Hino Y, Ida O, Fukuda H, Shinsho F, Tatara K. Associations between self-assessed masticatory disability and health of community-residing elderly people. *Commun Dent Oral Epidemiol* 1999; 27: 366–371.
47. Office for National Statistics. Adult Dental Health Survey: oral health in the United Kingdom 1998. London, 1999.
48. Steele JG. National Diet and Nutrition Survey: people aged 65 years and over. Vol. 2. Report of the Oral Health Survey. London: The Stationery Office, 1998.
49. Kaneda H, Maeshima K, Goto N, Kobayakawa T, Ayabe-Kanamura S, Saito S. Decline in taste and odor discrimination abilities with age, and relationship between gustation and olfaction. *Chem Senses* 2000; 25: 331–337.
50. Schiffman SS. The use and utility of glutamates as flavoring agents in foods. *Am Soc Nutr Sci* 2000: S927–S930.
51. Mathey MF, Siebelink E, de Graaf C, van Staveren WA. Flavor enhancement of food improves dietary intake and nutritional status of elderly nursing home residents. *J Gerontol A: Biol Sci Med Sci* 2001; 56: M200–M205.
52. Euronut/SENECA. Nutrition and the elderly in Europe. First European Congress on Nutrition and Health in the Elderly, The Netherlands, December 1991. *Eur J Clin Nutr* 1991; 45 (Suppl 3): 1–196.
53. Department of Health. The Health of Elderly People: an epidemiological overview. Central Health Monitoring Unit Epidemiological Overview Series, 1. London: HMSO, 1992.
54. Sinclair AJ, Bayer AJ. All Wales Research in Elderly (AWARE) Diabetes Study. Department of Health Report. 121/3040. London: UK Government, 1998.
55. Gariballa SE, Parker SG, Taub N, Castleden CM. Influence of nutritional status on clinical outcome after acute stroke. *Am J Clin Nutr* 1998; 68: 275–281.
56. Axelsson K, Norberg A, Asplund K. Eating after a stroke – towards an integrated view. *Int J Nurs Stud* 1984; 21: 93–99.
57. Peyrot M, Rubin RR. Levels and risks of depression and anxiety symptomatology among diabetic adults. *Diabetes Care* 1997; 20: 585–590.
58. Boston PF, Dennis MS, Jagger C. Factors associated with vascular dementia in an elderly community population. *Int J Geriatr Psychiatry* 1999; 14: 761–766.
59. Rosenthal AJ, Fajardo M, Gilmore S. Hospitalisation and mortality of diabetes on older adults: a three year prospective study. *Diabetes Care* 1998; 21: 231–235.
60. VOICES. Eating Well for Older People with Dementia. London: Voluntary Organisations Involved in Caring in the Elderly Sector, 1998.
61. Ortega RM, Requejo AM, Andres P, Lopez-Sobaler AM, Quintas ME, Redondo MR, Navia B, Rivas T. Dietary intake and cognitive function in a group of elderly people. *Am J Clin Nutr* 1997; 66: 803–809.
62. Kong MF, Horowitz M. Gastric emptying in diabetes mellitus: relationship to blood-glucose control. *Clin Geriatr Med* 1999; 15: 321–338.
63. Rayner CK, Samsom M, Jones KL, Horowitz M. Relationships of upper gastrointestinal motor and sensory function with glycemic control. *Diabetes Care* 2001; 24: 371–381.
64. NAGE. Taking steps to tackle eating problems, Birmingham, 1994.
65. UK Prospective Diabetes Study (UKPDS) Group. Intensive blood-glucose control with sulphonylureas or insulin compared with conventional treatment and risk of complications in patients with type 2 diabetes (UKPDS 33). *Lancet* 1998; 352: 837–853.

66. The Diabetes Control and Complications Trial Research Group. The effect of intensive treatment of diabetes on the development and progression of long term complications in insulin-dependent diabetes mellitus. *N Engl J Med* 1993; 329: 977–986.
67. Shorr RI, Wayne A, Daugherty JR, Griffin MR. Incidence and risk factors for serious hypoglycaemia in older persons using insulin or sulfonylureas. *Arch Intern Med* 1997; 157: 1681–1686.
68. Sinclair AJ. Insulin regimens for older people with type 2 diabetes. *Mod Diabetes Manag* 2000; 1: 14–16.
69. Hendra TJ, Sinclair AJ. Improving the care of elderly diabetic patients: the final report of the St Vincent Joint Task Force for Diabetes. *Age Ageing* 1997; 26: 3–6.
70. Asplund K, Wiholm BE, Lithner F. Glibenclamide associated hypoglycaemia: a report on 57 cases. *Diabetologia* 1983; 24: 412–417.
71. Lee A, Morley JE. Metformin, anorexia and weight loss. *Obes Res* 1998; 6: 47–53.
72. Lewis CW, Frongillo EA, Roe DA. Drug–nutrient interactions in three long-term care facilities. *J Am Diet Assoc* 1995; 95: 315.
73. Roe DA. Medications and nutrition in the elderly. *Prim Care* 1994; 21: 135–147.
74. Sinclair AJ, Allard I, Bayer A. Observations of diabetes care in long-term institutional settings with measures of cognitive function and dependency. *Diabetes Care* 1997; 20: 778–784.
75. Benbow SJ, Walsh N, Gill GV. Diabetes in institutionalised people: a forgotten population? *Br Med J* 1998; 314: 1868–1869.
76. Rockwood K, Tan M-H, Phillips S. Prevalence of diabetes mellitus in elderly people in Canada: report from the Canadian Study of Health and Aging. *Age Ageing* 1998; 27: 573–577.
77. Taylor CD, Hendra TJ. The prevalence of diabetes mellitus and quality of diabetic care in residential and nursing homes. A postal survey. *Age Ageing* 2000; 29: 447–450.
78. Tong P, Baillie SP, Roberts SH. Diabetes care in the frail elderly. *Pract Diabetes* 1994; 11: 163–164.
79. Coulston AM, Mandelbaum D, Reaven GM. Dietary management of nursing home residents with non-insulin-dependent diabetes mellitus. *Am J Clin Nutr* 1990; 51: 67–71.
80. Funnell MM, Herman WH. Diabetes care policies and practices in Michigan nursing homes, 1991. *Diabetes Care* 1995; 18: 862–866.
81. British Diabetic Association. Guidelines of Practice for Residents with Diabetes in Care Homes. London: British Diabetic Association, 1999.
82. Harrower AD. Prevalence of elderly patients in a hospital diabetic population. *Br J Clin Pract* 1980; 34: 131–133.
83. Currie CJ, Willimas DRR, Peters JR. Patterns of in- and out-patient activity for diabetes: a district survey. *Diabet Med* 1996; 13: 273–280.
84. Corish CA, Kennedy NP. Protein–energy undernutrition in hospital in-patients. *Br J Nutr* 2000; 83: 575–591.
85. Association of Community Health Councils for England and Wales. Health News Briefing – Hungry in Hospital? Association of Community Health Councils for England and Wales, 1997.
86. Health Advisory Service. Not Because They are Old. London, 1998.
87. Allison SP. Hospital Food as a Treatment. Maidenhead, BAPEN, 1999.
88. Green CJ. Existence, causes and consequences of disease-related malnutrition in the hospital and the community, and clinical and financial benefits of nutritional intervention. *Clin Nutr* 1999; 18: 3–28.
89. Bastow MD, Rawlings J, Allison SP. Benefits of supplementary tube feeding after fractured neck of femur: a randomised controlled trial. *Br Med J Clin Res Ed* 1983; 287: 1589–1592.

11

The Role of Carbohydrate in the Management of Diabetes

JANETTE C. BRAND-MILLER AND SUSANNA H. A. HOLT

University of Sydney, Sydney, Australia

INTRODUCTION

Diet is said to be the 'cornerstone' of management of diabetes, yet the recommended dietary guidelines remain controversial and relatively few patients succeed in being well controlled on diet alone (1). This may imply that dietary treatment is not sufficient in itself or the dietary changes are too difficult to comply with or even that the wrong type of diet is being recommended. Many experts argue against the current dietary recommendations for diabetes, with both the quantity and quality of carbohydrate being at the centre of the controversy. This chapter is designed to critically address the issues of how much and what type of carbohydrate should be recommended for people with diabetes. It takes an evidence-based approach, giving greater weight to the results obtained from randomised controlled intervention studies.

Important questions addressed in this chapter include:

- What is the scientific basis for recommending high-carbohydrate diets?
- What are the potential adverse effects of high-carbohydrate diets?
- What is the scientific basis for recommending diets high in monounsaturated fat (MUFA)?
- What is the scientific basis for recommending low glycaemic index diets?
- What is the optimal diet for improving insulin sensitivity?
- What is the optimal diet for weight loss?
- What is the evidence for a restricted versus liberal intake of sucrose?

Nutritional Management of Diabetes Mellitus. Edited by G. Frost, A. Dornhorst and R. Moses
© 2003 John Wiley & Sons, Ltd. ISBN 0 471 49751 7

THE OBJECTIVES OF THE DIETARY MANAGEMENT OF DIABETES

The goals of dietary management are clear (beyond dispute) and they apply equally to both Type 1 and Type 2 diabetes. They should achieve:

- Near normal blood glucose with minimal risk of hypoglycaemia;
- Reduced risk of microvascular and macrovascular complications (as assessed by a variety of direct and surrogate measures, including blood lipids, clotting factors, blood pressure);
- Weight loss in overweight patients;
- Normal growth and development in children;
- Healthy outcomes for mother and child in diabetic pregnancy.

Dietitians have the enormous challenge of not only achieving all of the above, but tailoring each person's diet to suit their individual taste preferences and lifestyle.

GOOD GLYCAEMIC CONTROL IMPROVES PROGNOSIS

Good glycaemic control as indicated by near-normal HbA_{1c} levels has been shown to reduce the risk of developing microvascular complications in both Type 1 and Type 2 diabetes (2,3). In addition, there is increasing evidence that it also reduces the development and progression of macrovascular disease (1,4,5). People with diabetes are two to four times more likely to die of coronary heart disease than people without diabetes, even when total cholesterol level and blood pressure are the same. Thus, preventing the excess cardiovascular morbidity and mortality associated with diabetes is arguably the most pressing treatment goal. However, this does not mean that normalising blood lipid or clotting factors is more important than normalising blood glucose. Indeed, high blood glucose levels are now recognised to contribute directly to the pathogenesis of macrovascular disease in both diabetic and non-diabetic subjects (6,7).

Until recently, HbA_{1c} levels were thought to be mainly influenced by fasting and pre-prandial blood glucose levels. However, human beings spend much of their time in the post-prandial state and therapies which specifically reduce post-prandial glycaemia may be superior for improving overall glycaemic control and reducing the risk of complications (8,9). The degree of post-prandial glycaemia appears to adversely alter vascular function and directly contribute to thickening of the intima wall (10). For this reason, both the amount and type of carbohydrate are probably more important than presently recognised.

HISTORICAL PERSPECTIVES ON CARBOHYDRATE

Before the discovery of insulin in 1922, diets prescribed for diabetes were very low in carbohydrate, around 5% of energy, and very high in fat, around 75% [reviewed by Truswell (11)]. Even after the advent of insulin, doctors were cautious and very low carbohydrate diets continued. By 1930, diet prescriptions of carbohydrate had risen to 15% of energy. In the 1940s and 1950s, carbohydrate allowances had come up to 25–30% of energy and carbohydrate exchange lists came into use. There was little questioning of the principle that carbohydrates were bad for people with diabetes and focus was on the insulin treatment.

By the 1970s pharmaceutical treatments had expanded with the introduction of oral hypoglycaemic drugs and the average carbohydrate intake rose to about 40% energy. Prohibition of sucrose was now the main message. With extreme caution, several experimental studies compared higher carbohydrate diets (>50% energy) with the traditional diabetes diet and found improved glucose tolerance or insulin sensitivity (12–14). In the late 1970s, there was a revolution in thinking about diabetic diets and a spurt of experimental studies indicated that high-carbohydrate diets were no worse, if not better, for people with diabetes because they lowered blood cholesterol levels (see below). By then, low-fat, high-carbohydrate diets were being recommended for the prevention and treatment of cardiovascular disease in the general population.

Since 1980, dietary recommendations for people with diabetes have unanimously emphasised reducing saturated fat intake. However, if saturated fat intake is reduced, the energy has to be replaced by some other nutrient. Because there are concerns about potential adverse effects of high-protein diets on renal and bone health, the choice is either more carbohydrate or more unsaturated fat. And here lies the controversy. Since carbohydrate is the main glycaemic element in the diet (being the main precursor of blood glucose), an increase in dietary carbohydrate might be expected to result in greater post-prandial glycaemia and compromise diabetes control. An increase in fat, on the other hand, might promote weight gain and decrease insulin sensitivity.

CURRENT RECOMMENDATIONS FOR CARBOHYDRATE INTAKE

For the past 20 years, most diabetes associations around the world have recommended high-carbohydrate diets that are low in fat and high in fibre for people with diabetes (15,16). The British Diabetic Association's recommendations state that carbohydrate should provide 50–55% of the total energy content of the diet while fat should contribute 30–35% of energy intake, of which <10% should be saturated fat, <10% polyunsaturated fat (PUFA) and

10–15% monounsaturated fat (MUFA) (17). However, there is concern in some quarters that 50–55% of the total energy intake as carbohydrate may have adverse effects on blood triglyceride (TG), HDL-cholesterol and glucose levels compared with high-fat diets (>35% total energy) enriched with MUFA (18,19). During the 1990s, this issue has been the focus of much research. On the basis of the resulting evidence, the American Diabetes Association's guidelines now recommend that 60–70% of energy be divided between carbohydrate and monounsaturated fat, depending on patient preference and the appropriate nutritional goals for their medical status (20).

WHAT IS THE SCIENTIFIC BASIS FOR RECOMMENDING HIGH CARBOHYDRATE INTAKE?

There is no doubt that the goal of increasing carbohydrate intake was actually to reduce fat consumption, especially saturated fat. People with diabetes were no longer dying of diabetic ketoacidosis but coronary heart disease. In fact, some experts suspected that the prescribed high-fat (and high saturated fat) diabetic diets might actually be partly responsible for the heightened risk of cardiovascular disease among people with diabetes. Several well-designed intervention studies in diabetic subjects were undertaken and showed that high-carbohydrate diets (55–70% energy) could result in lower blood cholesterol and TG levels with no deterioration in glycaemic control compared to traditional 'diabetic' diets containing less carbohydrate and more saturated fat (12–14, 21–25). Indeed, much to their surprise, HbA_{1c}, glucose tolerance and fasting glucose were often improved following treatment with a high-carbohydrate diet. This implied that insulin sensitivity was improved on a higher carbohydrate intake as had been earlier demonstrated in non-diabetic subjects (26). Thus, in the 1980s, diabetes associations in the United States, Canada, Australia and Britain independently agreed that there was sufficient evidence to advocate an increase in the carbohydrate content of the diabetic diet.

It is important to note that these early studies used high-carbohydrate diets that were heavily based on wholegrain cereals, vegetables and legumes that concomitantly contained very large amounts of fibre (upwards of 75 g per day). This is more than three times that normally consumed and presented a very real challenge for the average person with diabetes. In addition, unless the fibre was of the soluble, viscous or leguminous type, then post-prandial blood glucose peaked at higher levels on the high-carbohydrate diet (27). Not surprisingly, some degree of weight loss was seen after subjects completed the high-fibre, high-carbohydrate dietary treatments, but not after the low-carbohydrate, high-fat diets. We now know that energy restriction *per se*, even before significant weight loss is evident, improves all aspects of diabetes control (28). A deficit of calories, rather than a high-carbohydrate intake, may well have explained much of the improved profile. Even without weight loss, consistent benefits of high-carbohydrate diets have been reported only when the diets incorporate relatively unrefined, high-fibre foods (legumes, wholegrains, cruciferous vegetables, fruit) – resulting in meals that are somewhat different from those eaten by the general population.

Because very high fibre intakes are perceived as being unpalatable and hard to achieve, many health professionals took the view that simply increasing total carbohydrate intake was the main priority because this achieved the objective of lowering saturated fat. The American Diabetes Association, for example, presently recommends a moderate intake of dietary fibre of 20–35 g per day to help lower LDL-cholesterol and does not consider that dietary fibre offers significant benefits for glycaemic control (20).

WHAT ARE THE POTENTIAL ADVERSE EFFECTS OF HIGH-CARBOHYDRATE DIETS?

During the 1980s and 1990s, a number of controlled intervention studies in healthy individuals who maintained their body weight showed that high-carbohydrate diets often resulted in higher blood TG levels and lower HDL-cholesterol levels – changes that are atherogenic and increase the risk of coronary heart disease – despite improved total and LDL-cholesterol levels (29). These findings sparked particular concern for people with diabetes because their lipid abnormalities tended to be higher TG and lower HDL-cholesterol level rather than the high total and LDL-cholesterol typically observed in non-diabetic individuals (18). Hence the magnified risk of atherosclerosis in people with diabetes might be related to blood lipid risk factors that are specifically worsened by high-carbohydrate diets.

The biochemical mechanisms responsible for increased plasma TG levels following low-fat, high-carbohydrate diets remain uncertain but are clearly different to those responsible for elevated TG levels following increased fat intakes. Parks *et al.* (30) demonstrated that high-carbohydrate diets reduce the clearance of VLDL-TG from the plasma, but do not increase VLDL-TG secretion or *de novo* lipogenesis in the liver as had been postulated.

The mechanisms by which high-carbohydrate diets decrease HDL-cholesterol are also unknown and should be a priority in future research. In two recent cross-sectional studies of healthy adults, a significant inverse association was found between serum HDL-cholesterol concentration and dietary GI for both men and women (the higher the GI rating of the diet, the lower the HDL concentration) (31,32). In fact, the glycaemic index of the diet was the only dietary variable significantly related to serum HDL-cholesterol. These findings suggest that post-prandial glucose and insulin responses may directly influence HDL levels.

THE SCIENTIFIC BASIS FOR RECOMMENDING HIGH-MUFA DIETS FOR DIABETES

Many diabetes experts argue in favour of allowing a higher MUFA intake for people with diabetes, on the grounds that high-carbohydrate diets can increase blood glucose, insulin and TG levels and reduce HDL-cholesterol levels. A meta-analysis of nine studies with a total of 133 subjects comparing these two approaches to diet therapy in patients with diabetes revealed that high-MUFA diets (22–33% of energy intake; total fat = 37–50% energy) improved lipoprotein profiles as well as glycaemic control (19). Compared to high-carbohydrate diets (50–60% energy intake), high-MUFA diets reduced fasting TG and VLDL-cholesterol levels by about 20% and caused a modest increase in HDL-cholesterol (4%) but had no effect on LDL-cholesterol. There was no evidence that high-MUFA diets induced weight gain in these tightly controlled studies. However, there are several limitations that need to be raised before deciding whether they provide sufficient evidence to formulate recommendations for therapeutic diets:

- None of the studies controlled for/considered the confounding effects of the glycaemic index of the high-carbohydrate diets.
- The diets contained relatively small amounts of fibre (< 30 g/day, mostly in processed form).
- The studies were conducted under tightly controlled conditions, not allowing spontaneous weight loss/weight gain to occur.
- Most of the studies were of very short duration (two to four weeks), the longest being six weeks.
- A third of the studies were conducted by the same research group.
- Improvement in glycaemic control was assessed on the basis of urinary glucose and fasting, pre-prandial, post-prandial or 24-h blood glucose and insulin profiles.
- Notably, in the six studies that assessed HbA_{1c} or fructosamine (the best markers of long-term glycaemic control), none of the changes were significant.

Thus we lack the evidence that high-MUFA diets improve overall diabetes control by the most valid measure of disease risk (i.e. HbA_{1c}). This contrasts with the consistent effect of low-GI, high-fibre, carbohydrate-rich diets in lowering HbA_{1c} (see below). Furthermore, the positive effects of high-MUFA diets on blood lipids are often seen only when the high-MUFA diet is extremely high in fat (as much as 45–50% of energy) and very low in carbohydrate (about 35% of energy) (33). In studies with smaller and more realistic dietary changes, the effects of MUFA on blood lipids are more modest. One can question the effect of such a very high-fat diet on insulin sensitivity, weight control and ability of patients to comply. In fact, the largest study of this kind suggests that the beneficial effects of MUFA on insulin sensitivity disappear when fat intake exceeds 38% total energy (33).

These studies confirm that there are definitive adverse risks associated with *low-fibre*, high-carbohydrate diets. However, they do not prove that the original recommendation to increase both carbohydrate and fibre was wrong, nor do they allow us to say whether a diet rich in monounsaturated fat is better than a high-fibre, high-carbohydrate diet.

THE EVIDENCE THAT LOW GLYCAEMIC INDEX, HIGH-CARBOHYDRATE DIETS ARE SUPERIOR

It is now well established that both the type and amount of carbohydrate influences the degree of post-prandial glycaemia (34). The type of carbohydrate is best described by its glycaemic index, a ranking of foods according to their immediate effect on blood glucose levels (Figure 11.1). Per gram of carbohydrate a food with a GI of 80 (e.g. potato) has twice the glycaemic impact of a food with a GI of 40 (e.g. pasta) and this applies even in mixed meals (35,36) (Figure 11.2). The proportions of starch, sugar, fat or fibre in foods are not a good guide to GI. Many common starchy foods (even wholemeal versions) such as bread, rice and breakfast cereals have surprisingly high GI values, while foods containing sugars often have a relatively low GI (37). Reducing the overall GI of the diet involves substitutions within those food groups that contribute most of the dietary carbohydrate (Table 11.1).

The GI of foods is highly relevant to the management of Type 1 and Type 2 diabetes. In nine well-designed long-term studies in diabetic subjects, low-GI diets (GI values $<55\%$) were shown to reduce glycosylated proteins (HbA$_{1c}$ and/or fructosamine) by an average of almost 11% over periods ranging from two to 12 weeks (38). At the end of the low-GI, high-carbohydrate diet, urinary C-peptide levels (a measure of endogenous insulin demand) fell by an average of 20%, daytime blood glucose levels decreased by 16%, and total cholesterol and TG were reduced by 6% and 9%, respectively (39). Triglyceride levels fell to a much larger extent (by up to 20%) in patients with overt hypertriglyceridemia. In a recent, randomised, cross-over study, clotting factors were normalised in patients with Type 2 diabetes by a low-GI, high-carbohydrate diet, but unchanged by a high-GI diet containing similar amounts of energy, protein, fat, carbohydrate, starch and fibre (40).

Studies comparing the effects of high-GI versus low-GI carbohydrate-rich diets have been longer (four to 12 weeks) than the high-MUFA studies, and unlike the latter, have been able to document beneficial changes in HbA$_{1c}$ and/or fructosamine levels. In the few studies that have directly compared high-carbohydrate, low-GI diets with high-MUFA diets, HDL levels were increased on both (compared to the

- A physiological classification of food carbohydrates
  - Based on the incremental area under the blood glucose curve
  - Comparing equal amounts of carbohydrate
  - Reference food: glucose or white bread, GI = 100

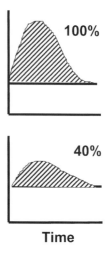

Figure 11.1 The derivation of the glycaemic index

high-carbohydrate, high-GI diet) but insulin secretory function and sensitivity appeared to be better only on the low-GI diet (41,42). Reductions in HbA_{1c} or fructosamine levels of 10% on the low-GI diets have been criticised as being 'modest', yet changes of this magnitude are commonly seen with oral hypoglycaemic drugs. Furthermore, these 'modest' changes were achieved in patients in free-living conditions, not in a controlled metabolic ward situation. Although the high- and

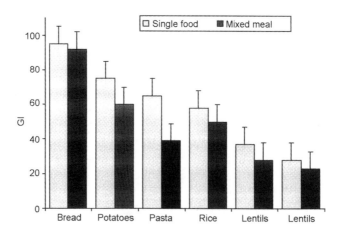

Figure 11.2 The GI of single foods predicts the GI of mixed meals in subjects with Type 2 diabetes
Source: Redrawn from Bornet *et al.* (35).

Table 11.1 A low-GI diet is achieved by substituting high-GI foods with GI alternatives. Breads, breakfast cereals and potatoes contribute the majority of carbohydrate in Western diets. Changes within these food groups have the biggest impact on the diet's overall GI

High-GI food	Low-GI alternative
Bread, ordinary wholemeal or white	Bread containing a high proportion of wholegrains ('granary' breads), sour dough breads, stone ground breads
Most breakfast cereals	Unrefined cereal such as oats (muesli or porridge). Some processed cereals (e.g. All-Bran)
Potato (all varieties)	Sweet potatoes, pasta, noodles, legumes
Most varieties of rice	Basmati or other high amylose rices
Cakes, biscuits and muffins	Versions made with fruit, oats, wholegrains
Tropical fruits such as bananas	Temperate climate fruits such as apples and stone fruit

low-GI diets were usually designed to be similar in macronutrient composition, in some studies the low-GI diet contained more fibre. Indeed in one outpatient study, dietary education with emphasis on low-GI foods resulted in higher carbohydrate and fibre intakes and less saturated fat intake than achieved by patients given 'traditional' dietary counselling (43). However, on the whole, studies comparing high- and low-GI diets have contained much less fibre (< 50 g per day) than the earlier studies that provided the basis for recommending high-carbohydrate diets in diabetes (> 75 g per day). Lastly, low-GI, high-fibre diets may be the *only* strategy (diet or drug) that enables HbA_{1c} to be improved while simultaneously reducing the incidence of hypoglycaemic episodes in Type 1 diabetes (44).

These findings suggest that any adverse effect of high-carbohydrate diets on blood lipids is almost certainly linked to the high GI of most such diets. Indeed, any strategy that slows down the rate of digestion and absorption of carbohydrate (e.g. nibbling versus gorging, alpha-glucosidase therapy or purified supplements of viscous fibre, as well as low-GI diets) has been shown to improve glucose and lipid metabolism in diabetes (45).

WHICH DIET IS BEST FOR IMPROVING INSULIN SENSITIVITY?

The body's sensitivity to the hormone insulin predicts how well it handles a meal containing carbohydrate, i.e. how easily and quickly it restores normal glucose levels after consumption. In insulin-resistant states, large amounts of insulin are needed to restore euglycaemia and glucose and/or insulin levels may still be high 2 h later. In Type 2 diabetes, insulin resistance is often severe and is combined with impairments in insulin secretory capacity. Obesity, particularly abdominal obesity, is known to worsen insulin resistance and increase the risk of Type 2 diabetes (46).

The degree of insulin sensitivity is also affected by the energy content and macronutrient composition of the diet. Epidemiological and dietary intervention studies in humans indicate that a high-fat, energy-dense diet promotes weight gain and the development of obesity (47), impairs insulin sensitivity and increases the risk of developing Type 2 diabetes (48). Relatively high intakes of saturated fat appear to worsen insulin resistance and are also associated with higher blood levels of LDL-cholesterol and a greater risk of atherosclerosis (49,50).

Questions still remain about the optimal diet for improving insulin sensitivity in Type 2 diabetes. It is well recognised that higher carbohydrate intakes are related to improved insulin sensitivity in non-diabetic individuals (26). This is likely to be true in the early stages of Type 2 diabetes, but as pancreatic beta-cell function declines, higher carbohydrate intakes could compromise remaining insulin secretory capacity. There are few studies that document changes in insulin sensitivity directly in diabetic subjects and these tend to be inconclusive. Low-GI diets appear to improve insulin sensitivity in coronary heart disease patients (51,52) and animal models (53).

Indirect evidence suggests that the fibre content and GI of the diet may influence insulin sensitivity, weight gain and the risk of developing Type 2 diabetes. In the CARDIA study of young adults, low fibre consumption predicted 10-year weight gain and fasting insulin levels (a measure of insulin resistance) more strongly than did total or saturated fat consumption (54). Fibre but not amount and type of fat was associated with 2-h insulin levels. Two other large-scale prospective studies in healthy subjects showed that diets based on low-fibre, high-GI foods doubled the risk of developing Type 2 diabetes, after controlling for known risk factors such as age and body mass index (55,56). Importantly, the total carbohydrate and refined sugar content of the diet, and the amount and type of fat consumed, were *not* found to be independent risk factors in these studies.

DIETS FOR WEIGHT CONTROL: IS THE AMOUNT AND TYPE OF CARBOHYDRATE IMPORTANT?

Weight loss is usually a major treatment goal in Type 2 diabetes, but the ideal dietary composition for weight control is still the subject of debate. Many health professionals are concerned that high-fat diets, irrespective of the type of fat, might promote weight gain. The prevalence of obesity is often lower in people with high carbohydrate consumption (expressed as a percentage of energy) than in those with high fat intakes (but this is not always true). In animal studies, high-fat diets induce faster weight gain and greater insulin resistance compared with high-carbohydrate diets, whether fed *ad libitum* or isocalorically (50). In humans, several studies have shown that *ad libitum*

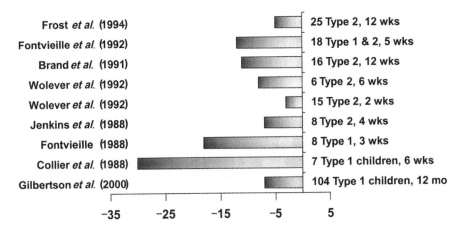

Frost *et al.* (1994) — 25 Type 2, 12 wks
Fontvieille *et al.* (1992) — 18 Type 1 & 2, 5 wks
Brand *et al.* (1991) — 16 Type 2, 12 wks
Wolever *et al.* (1992) — 6 Type 2, 6 wks
Wolever *et al.* (1992) — 15 Type 2, 2 wks
Jenkins *et al.* (1988) — 8 Type 2, 4 wks
Fontvieille (1988) — 8 Type 1, 3 wks
Collier *et al.* (1988) — 7 Type 1 children, 6 wks
Gilbertson *et al.* (2000) — 104 Type 1 children, 12 mo

−35 −25 −15 −5 5

Figure 11.3 Reduction in glycosylated proteins (glycosylated haemoglobin or fructosamine) on low GI in nine studies comparing high-carbohydrate, low- versus high-GI diets
Source: Redrawn from Brand-Miller *et al.* (38).

consumption of high-carbohydrate diets, even one high in refined sugar, was more effective in promoting long-term weight loss than higher fat diets (47,57,58).

Despite this, results from several recent intervention trials have indicated that high-MUFA diets are just as effective as high-carbohydrate diets in producing weight loss in diabetic subjects (59,60). However, in these studies MUFA was used in the context of a strictly controlled low-energy diet. By directly controlling energy intake, any spontaneous reduction in energy intake and body weight associated with the high-carbohydrate or high-fibre diet was unlikely. The long-term effect of *ad libitum* consumption of Western diets enriched in MUFA is currently not known. There is concern that the promotion of energy-dense, high-MUFA foods to diabetic subjects [as recommended by the American Diabetes Association (20)] may lead to gradual weight gain.

THE SATIETY VALUE OF HIGH-CARBOHYDRATE DIETS

The satiating capacity of high-carbohydrate diets may be the major explanation for weight control benefits. The energy density of foods strongly influences the amount of food people consume and consequently influences body weight (61). High-fat foods are energy dense, very palatable and less satiating, a combination which makes them easy to 'passively overconsume'

(62). On the other hand, less refined, 'natural' high-carbohydrate foods (legumes, wholegrains, fruits and starchy vegetables) are more bulky and difficult to overeat. In laboratory studies comparing the short-term filling powers of equal-calorie portions of different foods, the weight of food per 1000 kJ was the strongest determinant of short-term satiety (63). However, many new reformulated low-fat foods on the market (e.g. snack products, biscuits, ice cream, yoghurt) are as energy dense as their full-fat counterparts and unlikely to offer weight control benefits.

Low-GI diets may be particularly beneficial for weight control in people with diabetes. Low-GI foods are more satiating, calorie for calorie, than their high-GI counterparts [reviewed by Ludwig (64)]. Low-fat, energy-restricted diets based on low-GI foods have been found to result in greater weight loss in overweight people than conventional reduced-fat diets with a higher GI rating (64,65). Higher satiety resulting from the prolonged digestion and absorption of carbohydrate in the small intestine and the reduced post-prandial insulin secretion may explain these findings. In animal studies, high-GI diets promoted faster weight gain, higher body fat, higher adipocyte volume and hyper-triglyceridaemia than low-GI diets providing similar amounts of energy and macronutrients (66,67). High-GI diets were also associated with increased myocardial infarction in the Nurses' Health Study (68).

EVIDENCE FOR SUCROSE RESTRICTION IN DIABETIC DIETS

Many randomised, controlled trials have shown that the isocaloric substitution of moderate amounts of refined sucrose for starch in diabetic diets has no adverse effects on blood glucose or lipid levels in people with diabetes (69–71). In fact, several studies show *improved* glycaemic control, especially in children with Type 1 diabetes (72). This makes sense when we consider that most foods containing sugar have a GI less than 60, while that of most modern starchy foods is over 70 (37,73). Many diabetes associations now officially recognise that sucrose restriction is not necessary in diabetic diets, although some put an upper limit of 30 g per day (the average intake in the non-diabetic population is about 60 g per day). Unfortunately, the dietary dogma of sucrose avoidance in diabetic diets is so well entrenched in the mind of the public and most health professionals that little change has occurred in practice. Intense sweeteners and low-joule soft drinks are almost universally recommended in diabetic diets in the belief that this will enhance both glycaemic control and weight loss. This often detracts from more important dietary messages for people with diabetes (e.g. reduced saturated fat, increased high-fibre and low-GI foods).

The belief that sucrose facilitates excessive energy intake is one reason for continued use of intense sweeteners. However, there is little evidence that the long-term use of artificial sweeteners is particularly useful for weight loss – reducing sugar intake saves fewer calories than reducing dietary fat by the same amount (74). Some large-scale dietary surveys have shown that people who consume higher amounts of sugar and less fat tend to have lower body weights (75–77). Refined sucrose consumption correlates inversely with fat intake in both non-diabetic and diabetic populations. In addition, research shows that a moderate–high intake of sugar is not associated with a reduced intake of vitamins and minerals (78). One of the reasons for this is that sucrose increases the palatability and intake of nutritious foods such as cereals and dairy products. Sucrose also satisfies an instinctual desire for sweetness and has many functional roles in foods that extend beyond its sweetening power, including preservative, textural and flavour-modifying qualities.

Fructose has also been used as a sweetener in diabetic diets because it has a smaller blood glucose (GI = 20) and insulin-raising effect than isocaloric amounts of sucrose. Concerns about its potential to raise TG and LDL-cholesterol levels have limited its use (20), but in amounts up to 12% of energy, no untoward effects have been seen in subjects with diabetes (79).

Other nutritive/calorie-containing sweeteners such as maltodextrins, corn syrup, fruit juice/concentrate, honey, molasses, dextrose and maltose do not offer any advantage over sucrose in terms of energy content or glycaemic response. Indeed, post-prandial glycaemia is higher after maltodextrins and corn syrup than after sucrose. Sugar alcohols (sorbitol, mannitol, xylitol) and isomalt used as sweeteners in sugar-free confectionery produce a lower glycaemic response than sucrose and inhibit dental caries formation. Excessive consumption (> 20–30 g per day) should be avoided because of their laxative effect.

REALISTIC DIET PRESCRIPTIONS

Weight loss and weight control are arguably the most challenging aspects of managing diabetes, yet are likely to offer the most immediate and obvious benefit. People with diabetes find it more difficult to lose weight and maintain the loss compared with those without the disease. Fortunately, it is now clear that they do not need to reach their ideal body weight in order to improve their metabolic status; as little as a 5–10% reduction in body weight is sufficient to result in clinically relevant benefits (80).

Long-term weight control requires a comprehensive approach involving lifestyle changes, *not just food and energy restriction*. A modest reduction in energy intake (about 250 to 500 calories from the daily energy intake) and an increase in daily physical activity by 250 to 500 calories are realistic. A combination of strategies may help promote weight loss:

- Emphasis on low saturated fat, low-GI, high-carbohydrate foods – to promote satiety and reduce hyperinsulinaemia.
- Modest caloric restriction not extreme – to prevent excessive hunger.
- Distribution of carbohydrate intake throughout the day – smaller more frequent meals to reduce post-prandial hyperglycaemia.
- Increased physical activity – even incidental activity – to promote higher energy expenditure.
- Behaviour modification techniques and relaxing activities – to reduce stress-related eating.
- Support from family and other professionals – to increase compliance.

No single dietary approach will be suitable for all patients. Meal plans and dietary modifications need to be tailor-made to suit each patient's needs and lifestyle. Current medical status (HbA$_{1c}$, blood lipid levels, home blood glucose monitoring results, nutritional status, body weight, medication) needs to be assessed before any dietary modifications are recommended. Dietitians should reinforce that the dietary and exercise 'prescription' is an essential component of diabetes management, irrespective of medication.

THE FUTURE

Currently, many health professionals on both sides of the carbohydrate debate tend to believe that there is an ideal diet for everyone with diabetes – the 'one diet fits all' approach. But the future is likely to see the percentage of carbohydrate in the diabetic diet 'individualised' to increase compliance and take account of usual food habits. Emphasis on changes in the *types* of carbohydrate foods and *types* of oils and margarines may be more important to overall diabetes control than the amount of carbohydrate versus fat *per se*. While there is consensus that type of fat is important, there is less recognition of the major effects of fibre and rate of digestion of carbohydrate on glucose and lipid metabolism. There is sufficient evidence to say that a high-carbohydrate diet based on high-glycaemic index foods (even wholemeal versions) is probably not desirable in the management of diabetes. The *glycaemic load* (GI of the diet × carbohydrate content) of the diet needs to be considered and evaluated in intervention and observational studies, particularly in relation to insulin sensitivity, HbA$_{1c}$ and risk of complications.

Post-prandial elevations in the level of blood glucose appear to be a major determinant of HbA$_{1c}$ levels and therefore rates of complications of diabetes. But there is generally little recognition at present that post-prandial blood glucose values can be improved by diet, not just by drug therapy. If we are to recommend major changes to diet in the management of diabetes, then evidence-based medicine requires proof that they are safe and effective in the long term. Randomised, controlled trials in free-living populations should be the standard of evidence and outcomes should be measured in terms of changes in HbA_{1c} and rates of complications rather than surrogate measures such as fasting and 2 h post-prandial blood glucose and insulin responses, lipid concentrations and blood pressure. Unfortunately, current dietary recommendations are often based on results from dietary intervention studies as short as two to four weeks, some better controlled than others, using surrogate measures of glucose and lipid metabolism. Taken as a whole, at the present time there is better evidence favouring high-carbohydrate, high-fibre, low-GI diets in the overall management of diabetes.

REFERENCES

1. Turner RC, Cull CA, Frighi V, Holman RR. Glycemic control with diet, sulfonylurea, metformin, or insulin in patients with type 2 diabetes mellitus: progressive requirement for multiple therapies. UK Prospective Diabetes Study (UKPDS) Group. *J Am Med Assoc* 1999; 281 (12): 2005–2012.
2. The Diabetes Control and Complications Trial Research Group: The effect of intensive treatment of diabetes on the development and progression of long-term complications in insulin-dependent diabetes mellitus. *New Engl J Med* 1993; 329: 977–986.
3. UK Prospective Diabetes Study (UKPDS) Group: intensive blood-glucose control with sulfonylureas or insulin compared with conventional treatment and risk of complications in patients with type 2 diabetes (UKPDS 33). *Lancet* 1998; 352: 837–853.
4. Gavin JR. The importance of postprandial hyperglycaemia. *Int J Clin Pract* 1999: (Suppl 107): 14–17.
5. LeFèbvre PJ, Scheen AJ. The postprandial state and risk of cardiovascular disease. *Diabet Med* 1998; 15 (Suppl 4): S63–S68.
6. Coutinho M, Gerstein HC, Wang Y, Salim Y. The relationship between glucose and incident cardiovascular events: a metaregression analysis of published data from 20 studies of 95,783 individuals followed for 12.4 years. *Diabetes Care* 1999; 22: 233–240.
7. De Vegt F, Dekker JM, Ruhé HG *et al.* Hyperglycaemia is associated with all-cause and cardiovascular mortality in the Hoorn population: the Hoorn study. *Diabetologia* 1999; 42: 926–931.
8. Bastyr EJ, Stuart CA, Brodows RG *et al.* Therapy focused on lowering postprandial glucose, not fasting glucose, may be superior for lowering HbA_{1c}. *Diabetes Care* 2000; 23: 1236–1241.
9. The Diabetes Control and Complications Trial Research Group: The relationship of glycemic exposure (HBA_{1c}) to the risk of development and progression of retinopathy in the Diabetes Control and Complications Trial. *Diabetes* 1995; 44: 968–983.
10. Temelkova-Kurktshiev TS, Koehler C, Henkel E *et al.* Postchallenge plasma glucose and glycemic spikes are more strongly associated with atherosclerosis than fasting glucose or HBA_{1c} level. *Diabetes Care* 2000; 23: 1830–1834.

11. Truswell AS. Glycaemic index of foods. *Eur J Clin Nutr* 1989; 46 (Suppl 2): S91–S101.
12. Weinsier RL, Seeman A, Herrera MG *et al*. High- and low-carbohydrate diets in diabetes mellitus. Study of effects on diabetic control, insulin secretion, and blood lipids. *Ann Intern Med* 1974; 80: 332–341.
13. Anderson JW, Ward K. Long-term effects of high-carbohydrate, high-fiber diets on glucose and lipid metabolism: a preliminary report on patients with diabetes. *Diabetes Care* 1978; 1: 77–82.
14. Simpson HC, Simpson RW, Lousley S *et al*. A high carbohydrate leguminous fibre diet improves all aspects of diabetic control. *Lancet* 1981; 1 (8210): 1–5.
15. American Diabetes Association. Nutritional recommendations and principles for individuals with diabetes mellitus. *Diabetes Care* 1987; 10: 126–132.
16. The Diabetes and Nutrition Study Group of the European Association for the Study of Diabetes. Nutritional recommendations for individuals with diabetes mellitus. *Metabolism* 1988; 1: 145–149.
17. Nutrition Subcommittee of the British Diabetic Association's Professional Advisory Committee. Dietary recommendations for people with diabetes: an update for the 1990s. *Diabet Med* 1992; 9: 189–202.
18. Reaven GM. Dietary therapy for non-insulin-dependent diabetes mellitus. *New Engl J Med* 1988; 319: 862–864.
19. Garg A. High-monounsaturated-fat diets for patients with diabetes mellitus: a meta-analysis. *Am J Clin Nutr* 1998; 67 (Suppl.): 577S–582S.
20. American Diabetes Association. Nutritional recommendations and principles for individuals with diabetes mellitus. *Diabetes Care* 2001; 24 (Suppl 1): S44–S47.
21. Karlstrom B, Vessby B, Asp NG *et al*. Effects of an increased content of cereal fibre in the diet of Type 2 (non-insulin-dependent) diabetic patients. *Diabetologia* 1984; 26: 272–277.
22. Kinmonth AL, Angus RM, Jenkins PA *et al*. Whole foods and increased dietary fibre improve blood glucose control in diabetic children. *Arch Dis Child* 1982; 57: 187–194.
23. Ney D, Hollingsworth DR, Cousins L. Decreased insulin requirement and improved control of diabetes in pregnant women given a high-carbohydrate, high-fiber, low-fat diet. *Diabetes Care* 1982; 5: 529–533.
24. Howard BV, Abbott WGH, Swinburn BA. Evaluation of metabolic effects of substitution of complex carbohydrates for saturated fat in individuals with obesity and NIDDM. *Diabetes Care* 1991; 14: 786–795.
25. Story L, Anderson JW, Chen WJ *et al*. Adherence to high-carbohydrate, high-fiber diets: long-term studies of non-obese diabetic men. *J Am Diet Assoc* 1985; 85: 1105–1110.
26. Himsworth HP. The dietetic factor determining the glucose tolerance and sensitivity to insulin of healthy man. *Clin Sci* 1935; 2: 67.
27. Simpson RW, Mann JI, Eaton J *et al*. High-carbohydrate diets and insulin-dependent diabetes. *Br Med J* 1979; 2: 523–525.
28. Christiansen MP, Linfoot PA, Neese RA, Hellerstein MK. Effect of dietary energy restriction on glucose production and substrate utilization in type 2 diabetes. *Diabetes* 2000; 49: 1691–1699.
29. Mensink RP, Katan MB. Effect of dietary fatty acids on serum lipids and lipoproteins. A meta-analysis of 27 trials. *Arterioscler Thromb* 1992; 12: 911–919.

30. Parks EJ, Krauss RM, Christiansen MP *et al.* Effects of a low-fat, high-carbohydrate diet on VLDL-triglyceride assembly, production, and clearance. *J Clin Invest* 1999; 104: 1087–1096.

31. Frost G, Leeds AA, Dore CJ *et al.* Glycaemic index as a determinant of serum HDL-cholesterol concentration. *Lancet* 1999; 353: 1045–1048.

32. Liu S, Manson JE, Stampfer M *et al.* Dietary glycemic load assessed by food frequency questionnaire in relation to plasma high-density cholesterol and fasting triglycerides among postmenopausal women. *Am J Clin Nutr* 2001; 73: 560–566.

33. Vessby B, for the KANWU Study Group. Effect of dietary fat on insulin sensitivity and insulin action. *Diabetologia* 1999; 42 (Suppl 1): A46 (abstract).

34. Wolever TM, Jenkins DJ, Jenkins AL, Josse RG. The glycemic index: methodology and clinical implications. *Am J Clin Nutr* 1991; 54: 846–854.

35. Bornet FRJ, Costagliola D, Rizkalla SW *et al.* Insulinemic and glycemic indexes of six starch-rich foods taken alone and in a mixed meal by type 2 diabetics. *Am J Clin Nutr* 1987; 45: 588–595.

36. Wolever TMS, Jenkins DJA. The use of glycemic index in predicting the blood glucose response to mixed meals. *Am J Clin Nutr* 1986; 43: 167–172.

37. Foster-Powell K, Miller JB. International tables of glycemic index. *Am J Clin Nutr* 1995; 62: 871S–890S.

38. Brand-Miller J, Foster-Powell K. Diets with a low glycaemic index: from theory to practice. *Nutr Today* 1999; 34: 64–72.

39. Brand-Miller JC. Importance of glycemic index in diabetes. *Am J Clin Nutr* 1994; 59 (Suppl): 747S–752S.

40. Jarvi AE, Karlstrom BE, Granfeldt YE *et al.* Improved glycemic control and lipid profile and normalized fibrinolytic activity on a low-glycemic-index diet in type 2 diabetic patients. *Diabetes Care* 1999; 22: 10–18.

41. Wolever TMS, Mehling C. Long-term effect of varying the source or amount of dietary carbohydrate on postprandial plasma glucose, insulin, triacylglycerol, and free fatty acid concentrations in subjects with impaired glucose tolerance. *Am J Clin Nutr* 2003; 77: 612–621.

42. Luscombe ND, Noakes M, Clifton P. Diets high and low in glycemic index versus high monounsaturated fat diets: effects on glucose and lipid metabolism in NIDDM. *Eur J Clin Nutr* 1999; 53: 473–478.

43. Frost G, Wilding J, Beecham J. Dietary advice based on the glycaemic index improves dietary profile and metabolic control in type 2 diabetic patients. *Diabet Med* 1994; 11: 397–401.

44. Giacco R, Parillo M, Rivellese AA *et al.* Long-term dietary treatment with increased amounts of fiber-rich low-glycemic index natural foods improves blood glucose control and reduces the number of hypoglycemic events in type 1 diabetic patients. *Diabetes Care* 2000; 23: 1461–1466.

45. Chiasson JL, Josse RG, Hunt JA *et al.* The efficacy of acarbose in the treatment of patients with non-insulin-dependent diabetes mellitus. A multicenter controlled clinical trial. *Ann Intern Med* 1994; 121: 928–935.

46. Scheen AJ. From obesity to diabetes: why, when and who? *Acta Clin Belg* 2000; 55: 9–15.

47. Astrup A, Ryan L, Grunwald GK *et al.* The role of dietary fat in body fatness: evidence from a preliminary meta-analysis of *ad libitum* low-fat dietary intervention. *Br J Nutr* 2000; 83 (Suppl 1): S25–S32.

48. Vessby B. Dietary fat and insulin action in humans. *Br J Nutr* 2000; 83 (Suppl 1): S91–S96.

49. Kromhout D. Fatty acids, antioxidants, and coronary heart disease from an epidemiological perspective. *Lipids* 1999; 34 (Suppl): S27–S31.
50. Storlien LH, Higgins JA, Thomas TC *et al*. Diet composition and insulin action in animal models. *Br J Nutr* 2000; 83 (Suppl 1): S85–S90.
51. Frost G, Keogh B, Smith D, Akinsanya K, Leeds A. The effect of low-glycemic carbohydrate on insulin and glucose response in vivo and vitro in patients with coronary heart disease. *Metab Clin Exp* 1996; 45: 669–672.
52. Frost G, Leeds A, Trew G, Margara R, Dornhorst A. Insulin sensitivity in women at risk of coronary heart disease and the effect of a low glycemic index diet. *Metabolism* 1998; 47: 1245–1251.
53. Higgins JA, Brand Miller JC, Denyer GS. Development of insulin resistance in the rat is dependent on the rate of glucose absorption from the diet. *J Nutr* 1996; 126: 596–602.
54. Ludwig DS, Pereira MA, Kroenke CH *et al*. Dietary fiber, weight gain and cardiovascular disease risk factors in young adults. *J Am Med Assoc* 1999; 282: 1539–1546.
55. Salmeron J, Ascherio A, Rimm EB *et al*. Dietary fiber, glycemic load, and risk of NIDDM in men. *Diabetes Care* 1997; 20: 545–550.
56. Salmeron J, Manson JE, Stampfer MJ *et al*. Dietary fiber, glycemic load, and risk of non-insulin-dependent diabetes mellitus in women. *J Am Med Assoc* 1997; 277: 472–477.
57. Klem ML. Successful losers. The habits of individuals who have maintained long-term weight loss. *Minn Med* 2000; 83: 43–45.
58. Duncan KH, Bacon JA, Weinsier RL. The effects of high and low energy density diets on satiety, energy intake, and eating time of obese and nonobese subjects. *Am J Clin Nutr* 1983; 37: 763–767.
59. Walker KZ, O'Dea K, Nicholson GC, Muir JG. Dietary composition, body weight and NIDDM. *Diabetes Care* 1995; 3: 401.
60. Heilbronn LK, Noakes M, Clifton PM. Effect of energy restriction, weight loss and diet composition on plasma lipid and glucose in patients with type 2 diabetes. *Diabetes Care* 1999; 6: 889–895.
61. Poppitt SD, Prentice AM. Energy density and its role in the control of food intake: evidence from metabolic and community studies. *Appetite* 1996; 26: 153–174.
62. Blundell JE, MacDiarmid JI. Fat as a risk factor for overconsumption: satiation, satiety, and patterns of eating. *J Am Diet Assoc* 1997; 97 (Suppl 7): S63–S69.
63. Holt SH, Miller JC, Petocz P, Farmakalidis E. A satiety index of common foods. *Eur J Clin Nutr* 1995; 49: 675–690.
64. Ludwig DS. Dietary glycemic index and obesity. *J Nutr* 2000; 130 (Suppl): 280S–283S.
65. Slabber M, Barnard HC, Kuyl JM *et al*. Effects of a low-insulin-response, energy-restricted diet on weight loss and plasma insulin concentrations in hyperinsulinemic obese females. *Am J Clin Nutr* 1994; 60: 48–53.
66. Pawlak DB, Bryson JM, Denyer GS, Brand-Miller JC. High glycemic index starch promotes hypersecretion of insulin and higher body fat without affecting insulin sensitivity. *J Nutr* 2001; 130: 99–104.
67. Kabir M, Rizkalla SW, Champ M *et al*. Dietary amylose–amylopectin starch content affects glucose and lipid metabolism in adipocytes of normal and diabetic rats. *J Nutr* 1998; 128: 35–43.
68. Liu S, Willett WC, Stampfer MJ *et al*. A prospective study of dietary glycemic load, carbohydrate intake, and risk of coronary heart disease in US women. *Am J Clin Nutr* 2000; 71: 1455–1461.

69. Marchini JS, Faccio JR, Unamuno MR *et al*. Effect of local diets with added sucrose on glycemic profiles of healthy and diabetic Brazilian subjects. *J Am Coll Nutr* 1994; 13: 623–628.

70. Malerbi DA, Paiva ES, Duarte AL, Wachenberg BL. Metabolic effects of dietary sucrose and fructose in type II diabetic subjects. *Diabetes Care* 1996; 11: 1249–1256.

71. Wolever TMS, Brand-Miller JC. Sugars and blood glucose control. *Am J Clin Nutr* 1995; 62 (Suppl): 212S–227S.

72. Rickard KA, Loghmani ES, Cleveland JL *et al*. Lower glycemic response to sucrose in the diets of children with type 1 diabetes. *J Pediat* 1998; 133: 429–434.

73. Brand-Miller JC, Pang E, Broomhead L. The glycaemic index of foods containing sugars: comparison of foods with naturally-occurring vs added sugars. *Br J Nutr* 1995; 73: 613–623.

74. Mela D. Impact of macronutrient-substituted foods on food choice and dietary intake. *Ann N Y Acad Sci* 1997; 819: 96–107.

75. Lissner L, Heitmann BL. The dietary fat:carbohydrate ratio in relation to body weight. *Curr Opin Lipidol* 1995; 6: 8–13.

76. Bolton-Smith C. Intake of sugars in relation to fatness and micronutrient adequacy. *Int J Obes Rel Metab Disord* 1996; 20 (Suppl 2): S31–S33.

77. Gibson SA. Are high-fat, high-sugar foods and diets conducive to obesity? *Int J Food Sci Nutr* 1996; 47: 405–415.

78. Gibney M, Sigman-Grant M, Stanton JL, Keast DR. Consumption of sugars. *Am J Clin Nutr* 1997; 65: 1572–1574.

79. Uusitupa MIJ. Fructose in the diabetic diet. *Am J Clin Nutr* 1994; 59 (Suppl); 753S–757S.

80. Weinstock RS, Dai H, Wadden T. Diet and exercise in the treatment of obesity. Effects of three interventions on insulin resistance. *Arch Intern Med* 1998; 158: 2477–2483.

12

Effect of Variations in Amount and Kind of Dietary Fat and Carbohydrate in the Dietary Management of Type 2 Diabetes

GERALD M. REAVEN
Stanford University, Stanford, CA, USA

INTRODUCTION

Treatment of patients with Type 2 diabetes must focus on the prevention of the long-term vascular complications of this syndrome. The results (1) of the United Kingdom Prospective Diabetes Study (UKPDS) have clearly shown that improved glycaemic control will decrease the development of micro-vascular disease in patients with Type 2 diabetes. Therefore, consideration of the role of energetic macronutients of dietary fat and carbohydrate (CHO) in the management of patients with Type 2 diabetes must evaluate the impact of any recommendations in light of their effect on glycaemic control.

The results of the UKPDS were less encouraging concerning the ability of improved glycaemic control to reduce macrovascular disease (1). Indeed, neither lowering plasma glucose concentration (1), nor blood pressure (2), decreased myocardial infarction to the same degree as reported for the microangiopathic endpoints. The reason for this disparity between micro-vascular and macrovascular disease incidence in the UKPDS is not fully understood, but is at least partly due to the importance of abnormal lipoprotein metabolism in the genesis of coronary heart disease (CHD) in

Nutritional Management of Diabetes Mellitus. Edited by G. Frost, A. Dornhorst and R. Moses
© 2003 John Wiley & Sons, Ltd. ISBN 0 471 49751 7

patients with Type 2 diabetes. Consequently, recommendations concerning the CHO content of diabetic diets must take into account how they might affect dyslipidaemia in patients with Type 2 diabetes.

Although Type 2 diabetes is defined by hyperglycaemia, an increase in ambient glucose concentration is not the only metabolic abnormality in patients with Type 2 diabetes. In addition to diabetic dyslipidaemia, there is a cluster of abnormalities related to insulin resistance and circulating plasma insulin concentrations in patients with Type 2 diabetes (3–5). Since these changes may contribute to the increased prevalence of CHD, they must also be taken into account when dietary guidelines are proposed.

Finally, it is important to distinguish between the fat and CHO content of weight loss versus weight maintenance diets. The metabolic impact of variations in macronutrient content will vary enormously in these two situations, and this important difference cannot be ignored.

In this chapter an attempt will be made to discuss how variations in relative amount and kind of CHO could affect both microvascular and mascrovascular outcome in patients with Type 2 diabetes, taking into account the considerations discussed above, and results of clinical studies of patients with Type 2 diabetes.

CALORIE-RESTRICTED DIETS

There is little doubt that weight loss in response to calorie-restricted diets will improve both glycaemic control and dyslipidaemia in patients with Type 2 diabetes (6–11). However, there are two questions concerning this issue that deserve some attention. In the first place, do variations in the relative proportion of macronutrients have any effect on the ability of patients with Type 2 diabetes to lose weight? Three relevant papers bearing on this issue have been published in the last few years, comparing weight loss in response to calorie-restricted diets, varying only in terms of relative proportions of CHO and fat. The results showed that weight loss was identical when dietary CHO varied from 10% to 70% of daily calories, with proportionate changes in fat content (9–11). Since the longest of these studies only lasted for 12 weeks (8), it could be argued that differences in rate of weight loss might have emerged if the patients had been followed for longer. On the other hand, there is no evidence that relatively large variations in the relative amounts of dietary CHO and fat present in energy-restricted diets have a discernible effect on the ability of patients with Type 2 diabetes to lose weight.

Variations in relative amounts of dietary CHO and fat did not prevent the improvement in glycaemic control associated with weight loss, but in two of the studies (9,10) the fall in plasma glucose concentration was significantly greater on a higher monounsaturated fat (MUF)–lower CHO diet. Plasma triglyceride

(TG) and high-density lipoprotein (HDL) cholesterol concentrations fell with weight loss, irrespective of macronutrient content, but the decrement in TG concentration was greater, and the fall in HDL cholesterol attenuated, in response to calorie-restricted diets relatively high in MUFA and low in CHO. Low-density lipoprotein (LDL) cholesterol concentration decreased when either MUFA or CHO replaced saturated fat (SF) in the diet, but the improvement in LDL cholesterol concentration did not take place if dietary intake of SF was not decreased. Finally, improvement in all of these variables in response to a diet relatively high in MUFA and lower in CHO persisted several weeks after a period of weight maintenance with the test diets.

In summary, weight loss in overweight patients with Type 2 diabetes is of substantial clinical benefit, and is almost certainly the most powerful lifestyle modification to improve clinical outcome in this population. Although variations in relative proportion of dietary fat and CHO in energy-restricted diets do not seem to affect the amount of weight loss, the metabolic benefit associated with weight loss was somewhat greater when the diet was relatively higher in MUFA and lower in CHO.

METABOLIC EFFECTS OF VARIATIONS IN THE RELATIVE AMOUNTS OF DIETARY CARBOHYDRATE AND FAT CONTENT IN ISOCALORIC DIETS

As emphasised in the introduction, dietary recommendations for patients with Type 2 diabetes must take into account the impact of variations in macronutrient content on both microvascular and macrovascular disease. In this section attention will be focused on the effect of changes in the relative amount of CHO and fat in weight maintenance diets, evaluating the impact of such variations on the metabolic abnormalities characteristic of patients with Type 2 diabetes.

INSULIN RESISTANCE

The ability of insulin to stimulate muscle glucose disposal is decreased in the vast majority of patients with Type 2 diabetes (12,13). Although weight loss will enhance insulin-mediated glucose disposal in patients with Type 2 diabetes (6), there appears to be no evidence in patients with Type 2 diabetes that the frequently recommended relatively low fat–high CHO diets have any beneficial effect on insulin-mediated glucose disposal (14–16). Indeed, there is evidence from one study (16) that insulin resistance is accentuated in response to low fat–high CHO diets as compared to diets higher in MUFA and lower in CHO.

PLASMA GLUCOSE AND INSULIN CONCENTRATIONS

Several studies have been published describing the effect of reciprocal increases in CHO and decreases in fat intake on plasma glucose and insulin concentration in patients with Type 2 diabetes (15,17–20). Furthermore, the results have been remarkably similar, given the differences in the experimental protocols, and quite consistent with what would have been predicted in view of the pathophysiology of this syndrome. If CHO intake is increased in patients with Type 2 diabetes, plasma glucose concentrations will tend to rise, stimulating the pancreas to secrete more insulin. If patients with Type 2 diabetes retain significant B-cell reserve, more insulin will be secreted in this situation, attenuating any rise in plasma glucose concentrations at the expense of higher plasma insulin concentrations. Conversely, the less able the patient is to secrete additional amounts of insulin in response to an increase in CHO intake, the greater will be the rise in plasma glucose concentration, with minimal increases in ambient insulin concentration. Obviously, these are two extreme examples of an almost infinite series of possible combinations of the changes in plasma glucose and insulin concentrations that will result from increasing the relative proportion of CHO in the diet. In fact, most published data show that both plasma glucose and insulin concentrations increase in response to diets relatively low in fat and high in CHO. Perhaps the best example of this general conclusion is the publication of Parillo and colleagues (21) showing that postprandial plasma glucose concentrations did not increase significantly when diet-treated patients with Type 2 diabetes consumed relatively more CHO, presumably due to the fact that the low fat–high CHO diets were associated with higher postprandial insulin concentrations. The situation was reversed in sulphonylurea-treated patients, with higher post-prandial glucose and unchanged insulin concentrations, in response to increases in dietary CHO intake.

Based upon the above, there seems to be substantial evidence that postprandial glucose and/or insulin concentrations will increase when dietary fat content is decreased and CHO intake increased. The best one can hope for is that low fat–high CHO diets *may not* lead to decreased glycaemic control. However, even this can only be accomplished at the expense of increases in plasma insulin concentrations. The role of endogenous hyperinsulinaemia as a risk factor for CHD in patients with Type 2 diabetes is still unclear, but it may not be prudent to ignore the possibility that this, or abnormalities associated with it, may contribute to the accelerated atherogenesis that characterises these patients (22,23).

DYSLIPIDAEMIA

Diabetic dyslipidaemia is characterised by high plasma TG and low HDL cholesterol concentrations (22). Although less commonly measured, LDL particle diameter tends to be decreased in patients with Type 2 diabetes (23), and the postprandial accumulation of TG-rich lipoproteins accentuated (24). The close association of the latter two abnormalities with hypertriglycerid-aemia makes it less necessary to directly measure LDL particle diameter or postprandial lipaemia; if the plasma TG concentration of a patient with Type 2 diabetes exceeds 2 mM, it is almost certain that the individual will have smaller and denser LDL particles and day-long increases in remnant lipoprotein (RLP) concentration.

The fact that LDL cholesterol concentrations are not higher in patients with Type 2 diabetes than in non-diabetic individuals (22) does not preclude the need to consider how dietary recommendation would affect LDL cholesterol concentrations. Indeed, there is evidence that lowering of LDL cholesterol concentrations by pharmacological means will decrease risk of CHD (25,26).

Based on the above considerations, it seems clear that dietary recommenda-tions for patients with Type 2 diabetes, above and beyond weight loss, must take into account the effects of a given intervention on both LDL cholesterol metabolism, and the atherogenic lipoprotein phenotype of hypertriglycerid-aemia, low HDL cholesterol concentration, smaller and denser LDL particles, and an exaggerated degree of postprandial lipaemia. The goal is to maximally decrease CHD risk factors attributed to both forms of abnormal lipoprotein metabolism.

LDL Cholesterol

There is abundant evidence in non-diabetic individuals that replacing SF with either unsaturated fat or CHO will lower LDL cholesterol concentrations to a similar degree (27,28), and this appears to be the case in patients with Type 2 diabetes (15,17–20). Given the evidence that pharmacological lowering of LDL cholesterol decreases CHD risk in patients with Type 2 diabetes (25,26), the intake of SF should be limited to less than 10% of total calories in these individuals.

TG-rich Lipoproteins

The decision to replace SF with either unsaturated fat or CHO will have an enormous impact on the circulating concentration of TG-rich lipoproteins. There is substantial evidence in patients with Type 2 diabetes that diets low in SF and high in CHO will increase fasting plasma TG concentration as compared to substitution of SF with MUFA/PUFA (15,17–20). Evidence has recently been published that fasting RLP concentrations are also increased in patients with Type 2 diabetes (29), and the postprandial accumulation of RLPs of both endogenous (hepatic) and exogenous (intestine) origin are increased in patients with Type 2 diabetes (30). This latter observation is not simply a function of the increase in fasting TG-pool size characteristic of patients with Type 2 diabetes, but appears to also involve a decrease in the removal rate from plasma of TG-rich lipoproteins following a mixed meal.

HDL Cholesterol

Although a low HDL cholesterol concentration in patients with Type 2 diabetes is usually associated with a high plasma TG concentration, the difficulty in raising HDL cholesterol concentration with dietary manipulation is in marked contrast to the relative responsiveness of plasma TG concentrations. The reason for the difference is not clear. There is evidence that HDL cholesterol concentrations are inversely related to the fractional catabolic rate (FCR) of apo lipoprotein A-1 in patients with Type 2 diabetes (31), the more rapid the FCR of apo A-1, the lower the HDL cholesterol concentration. Furthermore, the higher the plasma insulin response to an oral glucose challenge, the faster the apo A-1 FCR (31). Perhaps the changes in circulating insulin concentration resulting from relatively minor variations in macro-nutrient composition in patients with Type 2 diabetes are not sufficient to modulate the FCR of apo A-1. Irrespective of the explanation, it appears that dietary manipulations have relatively little effect on HDL cholesterol concentrations in patients with Type 2 diabetes.

Dyslipidaemia and CHD Risk

As discussed above, there is evidence that drug-induced decreases in LDL cholesterol concentration decrease risk of CHD. Although there is ongoing debate as to whether or not hypertriglyceridaemia is an 'independent' risk factor in non-diabetic individuals (32), the importance of increases in plasma TG for predicting CHD in patients with Type 2 diabetes seems less controversial (32–34). There is little reason to question the importance of a low HDL cholesterol as a CHD risk factor, and there is increasing evidence in non-diabetic subjects of the atherogenic potential of postprandial lipaemia (the accumulation of RLPs throughout the day), and the appearance of smaller and denser LDL particles (35–37). Thus, it seems prudent to suggest that dietary recommendations for patients with Type 2 diabetes should take into account the predictable effects on lipoprotein metabolism.

METABOLIC EFFECTS OF VARIATIONS IN THE KIND OF CARBOHYDRATE IN ISOCALORIC DIETS

Evidence presented to this point has focused on the effects of variations in the relative amounts of dietary fat and CHO in isocaloric diets, and emphasised the untoward effects of replacing SF with CHO versus PUFA/MUFA. Another possible approach to this issue would be to continue the practice of replacing SF with CHO, but doing this with the *kind* of CHO that would maintain the beneficial effects of low SF–high CHO diets on LDL cholesterol concentration, without leading to the harmful impact on glucose, insulin and lipoprotein metabolism that has been observed with CHO-enriched diets. In this context, two different, but somewhat related, approaches have been evaluated – emphasising either the glycaemic index of the high CHO diets, or their fibre content.

VARIATIONS IN GLYCAEMIC INDEX

Perhaps the best example of the ability of differences in glycaemic index of CHO-enriched diets to modify glycaemic control and lipoprotein metabolism in patients with Type 2 diabetes is the report by Jarvi and colleagues (38). These investigators compared the metabolic effects of two diets, each containing 55% of total calories as CHO, in 20 patients, consuming each of the test diets for 24 days. The glycaemic indices were calculated to vary from 57 to 83 as compared to white wheat bread. The two test diets were compared to each other, as well as to baseline values obtained on an uncontrolled diet. Of considerable interest was the observation that fasting plasma glucose, TG, and LDL cholesterol concentrations fell on both diets, supporting the general belief that essentially any prescribed diet is better than no diet plan. On the other hand, the degree of improvement in all of these variables was the same, irrespective of the difference in glycaemic index of the diet. Furthermore, the improvements in day-long plasma glucose and insulin concentration appeared to be of somewhat lesser magnitude than in the study in which the CHO intake was reduced, and unsaturated fat intake increased (20). Brand and associates (39) conducted a somewhat similar study in 16 patients with Type 2 diabetes, comparing the metabolic effects of two diets, differing in their glycaemic index from 77 to 91. However, both of the diets were relatively low in CHO (~45%). The fasting plasma glucose concentrations were similar after the high glycaemic index and low glycaemic index diets, as were the fasting concentrations of plasma insulin, TG, LDL cholesterol and HDL cholesterol. However, the total integrated postprandial plasma glucose response following the low glycaemic index breakfast and lunch was lower by 14% as compared to the high glycaemic meals.

Two other papers are often cited as showing the benefits of differences in the glycaemic index of CHO-rich foods: in one of these (40), only six patients with Type 2 diabetes were studied, and their data were not presented separately; while in the other paper the patients were only followed for two weeks (41).

VARIATIONS IN FIBRE CONTENT

In the most general sense, it is deemed useful for patients with Type 2 diabetes to increase their dietary fibre intake, particularly of soluble fibre. At the same time, the clinical utility of this intervention is not clear. For example, the recommendation of the American Diabetes Association is for patients to increase their dietary fibre intake to 20–35 g/day, without clear evidence of the importance of this amount of fibre on glycaemic control (42). Chandalia and associates (43) have pursued this issue further, and evaluated the metabolic effect of essentially doubling the daily fibre intake of 13 patients with Type 2 diabetes. In this study they compared two diets, each containing $\sim 55\%$ of daily calories as CHO, with one test diet having twice as much total fibre (50 vs 24 g/day), and threefold the soluble fibre content (25 vs 8 g/day). The patients were studied at the end of two randomly assigned diet periods of six weeks in duration. Even if it is assumed that patients will be willing to consume diets made up almost entirely of oranges (300 g/day), green peas (110 g/day), zucchini (195 g/day), papaya (250 g/day), peaches (300 g/day), fruit cocktail (200 g/day) and cherries (100 g/day), the improvement in day-long plasma glucose concentrations was no greater, and the decline in plasma TG concentration of lesser magnitude, than when the low fat–high CHO diet was compared to a diet in which MUFA was increased and CHO decreased (20).

When put into the context of results of earlier studies evaluating variations in fibre content, it appears that the clinical benefit is closely related to the increment in daily fibre intake. More specifically, increases in fibre intake of ~ 15 g/day did not lead to any significant metabolic changes (44,45), whereas dietary increases up to 23 g/day (46) and 30 g/day (47) resulted in a modest improvement in glycaemic control, without any decrease in plasma TG concentration. Thus, there appears to be no study in which the untoward metabolic effects of CHO-enriched diets have been shown to be attenuated to the degree seen when MUFA/PUFA fat is used to replace SF (20), and the only instance in which the effects were even comparable involved the daily intake of 50 g fibre (43).

SUMMARY AND SUGGESTIONS

The most useful dietary intervention, by far, is the initiation of a calorie-restricted diet in patients with Type 2 diabetes who are overweight: the beneficial effects of weight loss on both glucose and lipid abnormalities in patients with Type 2 diabetes are both unequivocal and dramatic. Although there may be something to be gained by avoiding the use of low fat–high CHO diets in this context, the major benefits will depend upon the decrease in total calories, not in variations in kind of macronutrient.

There is also substantial evidence in support of the view that SF should be decreased in patients with Type 2 diabetes. The major lifestyle variable regulating total and LDL cholesterol is the intake of SF, and the lower the SF intake, the lower the LDL cholesterol concentration.

Given the above considerations, the only unresolved question that remains in dietary recommendations for patients with Type 2 diabetes is what to substitute for SF. It is difficult to find any scientific justification for continuing to recommend the continued use of low SF–high CHO diets in patients with Type 2 diabetes. As discussed in this chapter, several alternative approaches are possible. Based on published data, it is suggested that replacing SF with MUFA/PUFA is the simplest and most effective way to maximally improve glycaemic control, and attenuate the lipoprotein abnormalities characteristic of patients with Type 2 diabetes. In this context a diet containing (as per cent of total calories) approximately 15% protein, 45% CHO and 40% fat, with SF intake < 10% of total calories, does not require a substantial change in eating habits, while effectively minimising abnormalities of CHO and lipid metabolism. However, there are alternative approaches that have as their goal the continued use of CHO-enriched diets, but minimising the untoward manifestation of such a diet by increasing fibre intake and/or decreasing the glycaemic index of CHO-rich foods. The view that these dietary manipulations do not seem to be as effective as simply increasing the MUFA/PUFA content does not mean that recommendations to increase dietary fibre intake should be ignored, or that efforts to decrease the glycaemic index of CHO-rich foods have no utility. On the other hand, there seems to be little justification for placing entire reliance on these more complicated, and seemingly less effective, solutions for overcoming the untoward metabolic effects of CHO-enriched diets.

REFERENCES

1. UK Prospective Diabetes Study (UKPDS) Group. Intensive blood-glucose control with sulphonylureas or insulin compared with conventional treatment and risk of complications in patients with Type 2 diabetes. UKPDS 33. *Lancet* 1998; 352: 837–853.
2. UK Prospective Diabetes Study (UKPDS) Group. Tight blood pressure control and risk of macrovascular and microvascular complications in Type 2 diabetes. UKPDS 38. *Br Med J* 1998; 317: 703–713.
3. Niskanen L, Laakso M. Insulin resistance is related to albuminuria in patients with type II (non-insulin-dependent) diabetes mellitus. *Metabolism* 1993; 42: 1541–1545.
4. Ceriello A, Falleti E, Bortolotti N, Motz E, Cavarape A, Russo A, Gonano F, Bartoli E. Increased circulating intercellular adhesion molecule-1 levels in type II diabetic patients: the possible role of metabolic control and oxidative stress. *Metabolism* 1996; 45: 498–500.

5. Meigs JB, Mittleman MA, Nathan DM, Tofler GH, Singer DE, Murphy-Sheehy PM, Lipinska I, D'Agostino RB, Wilson PWF. Hyperinsulinemia, hyperglycemia, and impaired homeostasis. The Framingham Offspring Study. *J Am Med Assoc* 2000; 283: 221–228.

6. Henry RR, Wallace P. Olefsky JM. Effects of weight loss on mechanism of hyperglycemia in obese non-insulin dependent diabetes mellitus. *Diabetes* 1986; 35: 990–998.

7. Wing RR, Koeske R, Epstein LH, Nowalk MP, Gooding W, Becker D. Long-term effects of modest weight loss in Type 2 diabetic patients. *Arch Int Med* 1987; 147: 1749–1753.

8. Kelley DE, Wing RR, Bounocore C, Sturis J, Polonsky K, Fitzsimmons M. Relative effects of calorie restriction and weight loss in non insulin-dependent diabetes mellitus. *J Clin Endocrinol Metab* 1993; 77: 1287–1293.

9. Low CC, Grossman EB, Gumbiner B. Potentiation of effects of weight loss by monounsaturated fatty acids in obese NIDDM patients. *Diabetes* 1996; 45: 569–575.

10. Gumbiner B, Low CC, Reaven PD. Effects of a monounsaturated fatty acid-enriched hypocaloric diet on cardiovascular risk factors in obese patients with Type 2 diabetes. *Diabetes Care* 1998; 21: 9–15.

11. Heilbronn LK, Noakes M, Clifton PM. Effect of energy restriction, weight loss, and diet composition on plasma lipids and glucose in patients with Type 2 diabetes. *Diabetes Care* 1999; 22: 889–895.

12. Reaven GM. Insulin resistance in noninsulin-dependent diabetes mellitus: does it exist and can it be measured? *Am J Med* 1983; 74: 3–17.

13. Reaven GM. Role of insulin resistance in human disease. *Diabetes* 1988; 37: 1595–1607.

14. Borkman M, Campbell LV, Chisholm DJ, Storlien LH. High carbohydrate low-fat diets do not enhance insulin sensitivity in normal subjects. *J Clin Endocrinol Metab* 1991; 72: 432–437.

15. Garg A, Grundy SM, Unger RH. Comparison of effects of high and low carbohydrate diets on plasma lipoproteins and insulin sensitivity in patients with mild NIDDM. *Diabetes* 1992; 41: 1278–1285.

16. Parillo M, Rivellese AA, Ciardullo EV, Capaldo B, Giacco A, Benovese S, Riccardi G. A high monounsaturated-fat diet improves peripheral insulin sensitivity in non-insulin-dependent diabetic patients. *Metabolism* 1992; 41: 1371–1378.

17. Coulston AM, Hollenbeck CB, Swislocki ALM, Chen Y-DI, Reaven GM. Deleterious metabolic effects of high-carbohydrate, sucrose-containing diets in patients with non-insulin-dependent diabetes mellitus. *Am J Med* 1987; 82: 213–220.

18. Coulston AM, Hollenbeck CB, Swislocki ALM, Reaven GM. Persistence of hypertriglyceridemic effect of low-fat high-carbohydrate diets in NIDDM patients. *Diabetes Care* 1989; 12: 94–101.

19. Fuh MM-T, Lee MM-S, Jeng C-Y, Ma F, Chen Y-DI, Reaven GM. Effect of low fat–high carbohydrate diets in hypertensive patients with non-insulin-dependent diabetes mellitus. *Am J Hypertens* 1990; 3: 527–532.

20. Garg A, Bantle JP, Henry RR, Coulston AM, Griver KA, Raatz SK, Brinkley L, Chen Y-DI, Grundy SM, Huet BA, Reaven GM. Effects of varying carbohydrate content of diet in patients with non-insulin dependent diabetes mellitus. *J Am Med Assoc* 1994; 271: 1421–1428.

21. Parillo M, Giacco R, Ciardullo AV, Rivellese AA, Riccardi G. Does a high-carbohydrate diet have different effects in NIDDM patients treated with diet alone or hypoglycemic drugs. *Diabetes Care* 1996; 19: 498–500.

22. Reaven GM. Abnormal lipoprotein metabolism in non-insulin-dependent diabetes mellitus. *Am J Med* 1987; 83: 31–40.
23. Feingold KR, Grunfeld C, Doerrler W, Krauss RM. LDL subclass phenotypes and triglyceride metabolism in non-insulin dependent diabetes. *Arterioscler Thromb* 1992; 12: 1496–1502.
24. Chen Y-DI, Swami S, Skowronski R, Coulston A, Reaven GM. Differences in postprandial lipemia between patients with normal glucose tolerance and noninsulin-dependent diabetes mellitus. *J Clin Endocrinol Metab* 1993; 76: 172–177.
25. Sacks FM, Pfeffer MA, Moye LA, Rouleau JL, Rutherford JD, Cole TG, Brown L, Warnica JW, Arnold JM, Wun CC, Davis BR, Braunwald E, for the Cholesterol and Recurrent Events Trial Investigators. The effect of pravastatin on coronary events after myocardial infarction in patients with average cholesterol levels. *N Engl J Med* 1996; 335: 1001–1009.
26. Pyorala K, Pedersen TR, Kjeksus J, Faergerman O, Olsson AG, Thorgeirsson G. Cholesterol lowering with simvastatin improves prognosis of diabetic patients with coronary heart disease: a subgroup analyses of the Scandinavian Simvastatin Survival Study. *Diabetes Care* 1997; 20: 614–620.
27. Mensink RP, Katan MB. Effect of dietary fatty acids on serum lipids and lipoproteins. *Arterioscler Thromb* 1992; 12: 911–919.
28. Gardner CD, Kraemer HC. Monounsaturated versus polyunsaturated dietary fat and serum lipids – a meta-analysis. *Arterioscler Thromb Vasc Biol* 1995; 15: 1917–1927.
29. Watanabe N, Taniguchi T, Taketoh H, Kitagawa Y, Namura H, Kurimoto Y, Yamada S, Ishikawa Y. Elevated remnant-like lipoprotein particles in impaired glucose tolerance and Type 2 diabetic patients. *Diabetes Care* 1999; 21: 152–156.
30. Chen Y-DI, Swami S, Skowronski R, Coulston A, Reaven GM. Differences in postprandial lipemia between patients with normal glucose tolerance and noninsulin-dependent diabetes mellitus. *J Clin Endocrinol Metab* 1993; 76: 172–177.
31. Golay A, Zech L, Shi M-Z, Chiou Y-AM, Reaven GM, Chen Y-DI. High density lipoprotein (HDL) metabolism in noninsulin-dependent diabetes mellitus: measurement of HDL turnover using tritiated HDL. *J Clin Endocrinol Metab* 1987; 65: 512–518.
32. Austin MA, Hokanson JE, Edwards KL. Hypertriglyceridemia as a cardiovascular risk factor. *Am J Cardiol* 1998; 81: 7B–12B.
33. Fontbonne A, Eschwege E, Cambien F, Richard J-L, Ducimetiere P, Thibult N, Warnet J-M, Claude J-R, Rosselin G-E. Hypertriglyceridaemia as a risk factor of coronary heart disease mortality in subjects with impaired glucose tolerances or diabetes. *Diabetologia* 1989; 32: 300–304.
34. Taskinen M-R. Triglyceride is the major atherogenic lipid in NIDDM. *Diabetes Metab Rev* 1997; 13: 93–98.
35. Zilversmit DB. Atherogenic nature of triglyceride, postprandial lipidemia, and triglyceride-rich remnant lipoproteins. *Clin Chem* 1995; 41: 153–158.
36. Miesenbock G, Patsch JR. Postprandial hyperlipidemia: the search for the atherogenic lipoprotein. *Curr Opin Lipidol* 1992; 3: 196–201.
37. Karpe F, Hamsten A. Postprandial lipoprotein metabolism and atherosclerosis. *Curr Opin Lipidol* 1995; 6: 123–129.
38. Jarvi AE, Karlstrom BE, Granfeldt YE, Bjorck IE, Asp N-GL, Vessby BOH. Improved glycemic control and lipid profile and normalized fibrinolytic activity on a low-glycemic index diet in Type 2 diabetic patients. *Diabetes Care* 1999; 22: 10–18.

39. Brand JC, Colagiuri S, Crossman S, Allen A, Roberts DCK, Truswell AS. Low-glycemic index foods improve long-term glycemic control in NIDDM. *Diabetes Care* 1991; 14: 95–101.
40. Fontvieille AM, Rizkalla SW, Penfornis A, Acosta M, Bornet FRJ, Slama G. The use of low glycemic index foods improves metabolic control of diabetic patients over five weeks. *Diabet Med* 1992; 9: 444–450.
41. Wolever TMS, Jenkins DJA, Vuksan V, Jenkins AL, Buckley GC, Wong GS, Josse RG. Beneficial effect of a low glycemic index diet in type 2 diabetes. *Diabet Med* 1992; 9: 451–458.
42. American Diabetes Association. Nutrition recommendations and principles for people with diabetes mellitus. *Diabetes Care* 2000; 23: 543–546.
43. Chandalia M, Garg A, Lutjohann D, von Bergmann D, Grundy SM, Brinkley LJ. Beneficial effects of high dietary fiber intake in patients with Type 2 diabetes mellitus. *N Engl J Med* 2000: 342; 1392–1398.
44. Hollenbeck CB, Coulston AM, Reaven GM. To what extent does increased dietary fiber improve mellitus (NIDDM)? *Am J Clin Nutr* 1986; 43: 16–24.
45. Manhire A, Henry CL, Hartog M, Heaton KW. Unrefined carbohydrate and dietary fibre in treatment of diabetes mellitus. *J Human Nutr* 1981; 35: 99–101.
46. Karlstrom B, Vessby B, Asp N-G, Boberg M, Gustafsson I-B, Lithell H, Werner I. Effects of an increased content of cereal fibre in the diet of Type 2 (non-insulin-dependent) diabetic patients. *Diabetologia* 1984; 26: 272–277.
47. Hagander B, Asp NG, Efendic S, Nilsson-Ehle P, Schersten B. Dietary fiber decreases fasting blood glucose levels and plasma LDL concentration in noninsulin-dependent diabetes mellitus patients. *Am J Clin Nutr* 1988; 47: 852–858.

13

Diabetes and Alcohol

LINDA CARTER AND JOANNE BOYLE
Charing Cross Hospital, London, UK

INTRODUCTION

Studies in the general population show an improvement in mortality and morbidity from light to moderate ingestion of alcohol. This improved mortality was greatest amongst those individuals with the highest risk of ischaemic heart disease (1). The definition of light to moderate intake is, however, confusing and varies between researchers from one to three drinks per day, 3–4 units for men and 2–3 units for women per day, 0.5–1.0 g/kg body weight, or 'moderate drinking is the level below which overall net harmful effects are seen in population surveys, about three drinks per day. Thus less than three drinks per day is moderate or lighter drinking and heavy drinking is three or more drinks per day' (2).

Recommendations have generally been determined from epidemiological and retrospective data where the problem of evaluating thresholds is complicated by the underestimation of alcohol consumption. Drinking more frequently or larger measures than reported can lead to a lower apparent threshold of alcohol-related effects.

For people with diabetes, recommendations for alcohol intakes are complicated by the well-established risks of alcohol ingestion such as increasing blood pressure, increasing triglycerides and contributing to obesity versus the benefits of reducing the risk of ischaemic heart disease through increasing HDL cholesterol, increasing insulin sensitivity and the contribution of antioxidant nutrients. (The effect of alcohol ingestion on these individual risks and benefits is discussed later in this chapter.)

Nutritional Management of Diabetes Mellitus. Edited by G. Frost, A. Dornhorst and R. Moses
© 2003 John Wiley & Sons, Ltd. ISBN 0 471 49751 7

NUTRITIONAL RECOMMENDATIONS

For the general adult population 'sensible' limits are 21 units per week or 2–3 units per day for men and 14 units per week or 1–2 units per day for women. This remains the recommendation by the Royal College of Physicians despite the Department of Health increasing the recommended number of units to 28 and 21 units per week, respectively (3).

The current European nutritional recommendations for people with diabetes (1999) state 'For those who choose to drink alcohol, intakes of up to 15 g for women and 30 g for men are acceptable' per day (4,5). This equates to one small (125 ml) glass of wine (12% abv) or 1.5 units for women per day and two small glasses of wine (12% abv) for men, which equates to 3 units. However, many wines have a higher alcohol content and many people would regularly drink a larger measure. The present consensus outlined in the European and American nutritional recommendations for people with diabetes concludes that there are benefits (unless medically contraindicated) from light to moderate alcohol intakes taken with a carbohydrate-containing meal. Moderate intakes of wine, especially red wine, which contains non-nutrient flavonoid and phenolic compounds, which have antioxidant properties, may confer greater benefit than consumption of spirits or beer (6). Much of the evidence from studies is based on weekly intakes of alcoholic drinks, but considering that the beneficial effects of moderate drinking on fibrinolytic factors (7) and blood pressure (8) are transient, it is most beneficial to have light to moderate daily intakes. Health professionals should be cautious when advising on intakes because many people underestimate their alcohol consumption. Practical recommendations should be explained in terms of drinks and units to avoid confusion. Table 13.1 shows the alcoholic content and number of units contributed by commonly consumed alcoholic beverages.

PRACTICAL RECOMMENDATIONS

Provided alcohol intakes are not contraindicated (see below), for most people with diabetes it is healthiest for men to drink 2–3 units and women to drink 1–2 units per day. Higher intakes, even taken occasionally, will have an impact on blood pressure and triglycerides and will increase the risk of hypoglycaemia and ketoacidosis.

It is especially important that people with diabetes who are treated with insulin or sulphonylureas should eat a carbohydrate-containing meal and take their medication before drinking and have a bedtime snack (and long-acting insulin if prescribed) before going to sleep. They should also be aware that prolonged and severe hypoglycaemia can occur up to 36 h after binge drinking and this can be mistaken for intoxication. For those inclined to drink more

Table 13.1 The alcoholic content and number of units contributed by commonly consumed alcoholic drinks

Drink	Measure	No. of units	Alcohol (g)
Beers, lagers and cider			
3–5% abv	250 ml (0.5 pt)	0.75–1.25	7.5–12.5
	500 ml (1 pt)	1.5–2.5	15–25
6–8% abv	250 ml (0.5 pt)	1.5–2.0	15–20
	500 ml (1 pt)	3.0–4.0	30–40
Wine			
9–11% abv	Sm glass (125 ml)	1.0–1.4	10–14
	Med glass (175 ml)	1.1–2.0	11–20
	Lg glass (250 ml)	2.25–2.75	22.5–27.5
	1 bottle (750 ml)	6.75–8.25	67.5–82.5
12–14% abv	Sm glass (125 ml)	1.5–1.75	15–17.5
	Med glass (175 ml)	2.1–2.45	21–24.5
	Lg glass (250 ml)	3.0–3.5	42–49
	1 bottle (750 ml)	9.0–10.5	90–105
Fortified wines (sherry/port)			
16% abv	50 ml glass	0.8	8
Spirits (vodka/gin/rum, etc.)			
40% abv	25 ml	1.0	10

than the recommended intakes advice should be given on how to minimise the risk of hypoglycaemia. This might include eating carbohydrate-containing snacks that might not be particularly healthy, e.g. savoury snacks like crisps and peanuts or alternating alcoholic drinks with sugar-containing soft drinks or fruit juice.

The normal precautions for alcohol intakes still apply with regard to drinking and driving, but it is obviously very important to minimise the risk of hypoglycaemia.

There is no specific benefit for people with diabetes to consume low-carbohydrate beers/lagers or low-alcohol drinks; it is total alcohol intake, how rapidly it is consumed and whether it is consumed with or after food that will determine its effect.

CONTRAINDICATIONS

People with diabetes who should abstain from drinking alcohol include those with a history of alcohol abuse, pancreatitis, liver disease, gastritis and women during pregnancy. Also intakes should be restricted for those who have hypertriglyceridaemia, hypertension, neuropathy and frequent hypoglycaemia and hyperglycaemia.

People with DM who also take antiepileptics and tranquillisers should seek advice from their doctor or pharmacist before drinking alcohol because of possible drug interactions.

METABOLISM OF ALCOHOL

The liver metabolises alcohol at an average rate of 0.1 g/kg body weight per hour. Thus an average 70 kg man will require 2 h to metabolise 24 g alcohol, the equivalent of 1.5 small glasses of wine. The total quantity and the rate of alcohol ingestion determines its effect (9). Some of the alcohol in the stomach is metabolised by the enzyme alcohol dehydrogenase, which is present in the gastric mucosa. Women have less gastric alcohol dehydrogenase activity than men, so their blood alcohol concentration rises more markedly. Once absorbed the alcohol spreads rapidly into the body water and the smaller size and greater fat content of women amplifies the rise.

Alcohol is metabolised in a series of reactions to acetyl Co A which, in most extra-hepatic tissues, is then channelled into the TCA cycle. Here, it is oxidised and this generates most of the ATP from ethanol oxidation. A small proportion of the acetyl Co A that remains in the liver and that is present in the adipose tissue may act as a precursor for the biosynthesis of fatty acids and glycerol.

OXIDATION OF ETHANOL TO ETHANAL (ACETALDEHYDE)

Most of the absorbed alcohol is taken up by the liver. Here, three separate enzyme reactions oxidise the ethanol to ethanal.

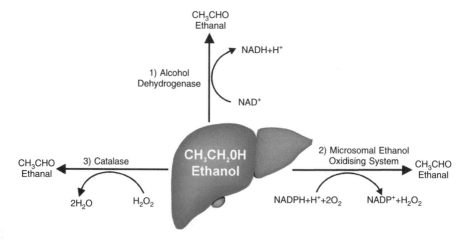

Figure 13.1 Pathway as described by Newsholme and Leech 1990. Reproduced with permission of John Wiley & Sons Limited

Alcohol Dehydrogenase

The reaction catalysed by alcohol dehydrogenase is the most widely known. This enzyme is also present in much smaller amounts in the gastric mucosa, kidney and adipose tissue.

Microsomal Ethanol Oxidising System

This enzyme system uses NADPH and oxygen to catalyse the reaction to ethanal. The enzyme cytochrome P450 is involved in this reaction and also in the detoxification of many drugs. Alcohol competes with these drugs for the enzyme site and its presence, therefore, can lead to higher circulating levels of drugs which may reach toxic levels (10).

Catalase

In the liver peroxisomes, the enzyme catalase reduces H_2O_2 to H_2O concomitantly as it oxidises ethanol to ethanal.

OXIDATION OF ETHANAL TO ACETATE

This reaction is catalysed by aldehyde dehydrogenase:

$$CH_3CHO + NAD^+ + H_2O \rightarrow CH_3COO^- + NADH + 2H^+$$

CONVERSION TO ACETYL Co A

Most of the acetate escapes from the liver and is converted to acetyl Co A in extra-hepatic tissues by the enzyme acetyl Co A synthetase:

$$CH_3COO^- + ATP^{4-} + CoASH \rightarrow CH_3COSCoA + AMP^{3-} + PPi^{3-}$$

The acetyl Co A is then oxidised via the TCA cycle which generates ATP.

REOXIDATION OF NADH AND REDUCTION OF NADPH

NADH is generated in the first two reactions of alcohol metabolism as outlined above. It is necessary for NADH to then be reoxidised to NAD^+ so that it can be involved in further oxidation reactions in the cytosol:

$$NADH \xrightarrow{\text{Reoxidation by the mitochondrial electron transport system}} NAD + H^+$$

The cytosolic NADH is reoxidised by the mitochondrial electron transport system, so substrate shuttles need to be used to transport the H atoms to the mitochondria.

Under some conditions, the rate of transfer of H atoms by these shuttles is less than the rate of NADH generation, so that the concentration of NAD^+ becomes greatly reduced. This low concentration of NAD^+ also restricts the conversion of lactate to pyruvate in the liver. This is one element by which alcohol increases the concentration of lactate in the blood.

The low NAD^+ level limits the rate of ethanol oxidation by alcohol dehydrogenase (the first step in alcohol metabolism). Alcohol decreases the ratio of NAD^+ to NADH within the hepatocyte while it is being oxidised.

METABOLIC AND CLINICAL EFFECTS OF ALCOHOL CONSUMPTION

Evidence suggests that some of the clinical effects of alcohol ingestion are not due to ethanol itself but to its metabolites NADH and ethanal (acetaldehyde). The NAD^+/NADH concentration ratio in the cytosol is maintained at a value of 1000 (11). The administration of alcohol can lower this ratio by at least 10-fold (12). The concentration of all substrates and products which thus use dehydrogenase enzymes will be affected by a change in the NAD^+/NADH concentration ratio. Therefore a reduction of this concentration ratio will lower the concentration of the oxidised reactant and increase that of the reduced reactant. If either of these reactants has an important metabolic role, marked changes in their concentration could produce abnormal effects.

The increased ethanal levels which are seen after alcohol ingestion are further raised if the activity of aldehyde dehydrogenase is inhibited. Inhibitors of the enzyme include the higher aliphatic aldehydes which are known to be present in alcoholic beverages.

The following physiological effects can be, in part, explained by the changes in the NAD^+/NADH ratio.

FATTY LIVER, HEPATITIS AND CIRRHOSIS

Chronic alcohol consumption can cause the deposition of excess triglycerol in the liver leading to a condition known as 'fatty liver'. This damage can lead to hepatitis and, if severe enough, to cirrhosis. The damage is thought to be due to the high concentrations of ethanal within the cell and if severe enough will result in cell death. Cell damage and death trigger an inflammatory response, i.e. infiltration of lymphocytes and activation of an immune response. If this is not treated it will lead to the formation of fibrous tissue and a severe reduction in the functioning of the liver.

HYPOGLYCAEMIA

In the fasted state, hepatic gluconeogenesis is essential for the production of glucose and maintenance of the blood sugar level. Ethanol is a potent inhibitor of gluconeogenesis. The suppression of gluconeogenesis, even at relatively low alcohol intakes, with low serum insulin and high serum glucagon, results in a decreased ratio of NAD^+ to NADH which inhibits the entry of the precursors of gluconeogenesis (i.e. glycerol, lactate, alanine and other amino acids) into the hepatocyte (13). This can lead to severe and prolonged hypoglycaemia when large volumes of alcohol are ingested rapidly and may occur up to 36 h after alcohol ingestion. The major problem of alcohol ingestion in the person with diabetes is induction and masking of hypoglycaemia, causing hypoglycaemia unawareness.

Hypoglycaemia most commonly occurs in the fasting state in people with Type 1 and Type 2 diabetes but also in non-diabetics, especially when hepatic glycogen stores are depleted or exhausted. Alcohol-induced hypoglycaemia may not be effectively treated by glucagon administration because it is related to depleted glycogen stores. Alcohol consumption leads to delayed glucose recovery from insulin-induced hypoglycaemia in people with Type 1 diabetes, and occurs despite normal adrenalin, nor-adrenalin and glucagon responses, however growth hormone and cortisol are reduced (14).

Hypoglycaemia in alcoholics can be exacerbated by a reduced ability to secrete some of the hormones involved in the control of lipolysis (e.g. cortisol and growth hormone) and results in a decrease in the rate of fatty acid release in starvation. Alcohol-induced severe hypoglycaemia can also result in irreversible neurological changes by causing irrecoverable damage to neurons and persistent disruption of cerebral functions (15).

Ketoacidosis

Alcohol ingestion can cause ketoacidosis in people with diabetes and non-diabetics, as a result of relative insulin deficiency. Starvation, causing a depletion of glycogen stores and alcohol metabolism, leads to an increase in $NADH/NAD^+$ ratio which inhibits gluconeogenesis. This is responsible for causing an increased glucagon/insulin ratio, which increases ketogenesis (16,17). Diabetic ketoacidosis is a potentially life-threatening condition and requires prompt diagnosis and treatment of dehydration and metabolic abnormalities. Alcohol-induced ketoacidosis can be further complicated by hypoglycaemia (however it more commonly presents with hyperglycaemia).

LACTIC ACIDOSIS

The metabolism of alcohol increases the ratio of NADH to NAD^+ which inhibits the entry of the precursors of gluconeogenesis, i.e. glycerol, lactate, alanine and other amino acids into the hepatocyte (13). The accumulation of lactate increases the risk of lactic acidosis, which is especially serious and potentially life-threatening for those people with diabetes who are treated with a biguanide.

ENDOCRINE DISTURBANCES

Chronic alcoholism can also affect gonadal function and lead to testicular atrophy, gynaecomastia (enlargement of male breasts) and sterility. It is not known what the exact mechanism for these changes is, but it is thought to be a result of reduced liver function. This reduced liver function decreases the rate of metabolism of female sex hormones, thereby leading to an increased level of circulating oestrogens. A second mechanism is thought to be that alcohol reduces synthesis of testosterone (18). Testosterone synthesis involves many steps and some of the intermediates may be dependent on the $NAD^+/NADH$ concentration ratio which, as has already been discussed, is affected by alcohol consumption.

HYPERTENSION

The UK Prospective Diabetes Study underlined the importance of well-controlled hypertension for people with Type 2 diabetes to reduce the risk of microvascular complications. There is a direct/empiric relationship between alcohol intake and blood pressure. Some researchers have found this relationship to be J-shaped (19), others U-shaped, but there is agreement that light to moderate drinkers have lower blood pressure than those who abstain and blood pressure rises steeply with heavier intakes. In heavy drinkers ingesting > 300 g or 30 units per week there is a four times greater risk of stroke than in non-drinkers (20), whereas moderate alcohol consumption, up to two drinks per day, is protective for ischaemic stroke (21). Alcohol consumption showed a clear positive correlation with the subsequent development of haemorrhagic stroke but did not show a correlation with the thromboembolic variety (22). Although blood pressure is important in thrombotic stroke, alcohol's metabolic effects may exert a counterbalancing protective influence against the occlusive atherosclerotic process, as might be the case for coronary heart disease (19). So although moderate alcohol intake is cardioprotective, greater alcohol intake can neutralise the effect by having an adverse effect on blood pressure (23). The INTERSALT and British Heart Study found that the effect on blood pressure from alcohol is similar to that of obesity and greater than that for salt in the populations studied.

A reduction in systolic blood pressure of 5 mmHg achieved by favourable lifestyle changes would reduce coronary mortality by 9%. Epidemiological evidence suggests that light to moderate drinkers who stop drinking may increase their coronary mortality by up to 10% compared to heavier drinkers who stop drinking, who may experience a 4 mmHg fall in systolic pressure and possibly a 27% reduction in coronary mortality [Klatsky, 1992, cited in Bulpitt (24)].

Studies show a link between increasing alcohol intakes and higher blood pressure. Klatsky (19) cites the Framingham Study as showing that the prevalence of hypertension ($\geqslant 160$ mmHg systolic or $\geqslant 95$ mmHg diastolic) was about two times higher among persons drinking 60 ounces or more of alcohol per month (57 g/day) than among those drinking less than 30 ounces per month (28.5 g/day). Also the Los Angeles Heart Study showed a significant increase in blood pressure for men who drank alcohol three or more times weekly compared to those who drank less than three times weekly or who were non-drinkers. Blood pressure is acutely affected and hypertension is resolved in those who stop drinking (6).

The 'Kaiser Permanente' investigation looked at the effect of ethnicity and found African–American men reached a maximum blood pressure at a lower alcohol intake. Among women of all races, blood pressure was lower in light to moderate drinkers than non-drinkers (25,26). All these studies were carried out in the general population not in people with diabetes, however considering the link between diabetes and hypertension and the importance of tight blood pressure control in reducing the risk of complications, recommendations regarding alcohol intakes should be cautious.

CORONARY HEART DISEASE

Light to moderate alcohol consumption is associated with a similar reduction in CHD risk among diabetic and non-diabetic men and women (27,28). Among the mechanisms accounting for the risk reduction are increased circulating concentrations of HDL cholesterol, inhibition of blood coagulation and the presence of antioxidant substances which reduce oxidative damage (Table 13.2). However, it is also well established that alcohol increases plasma triglyceride. Alcoholic hyperlipaemia results primarily from increased hepatic secretion of VLDL and secondarily from impairment in the removal of triglyceride-rich lipoproteins from the plasma. Raised triglycerides are also a feature of the

Table 13.2 Potential benefits of moderate alcohol intake

Increase in total HDL cholesterol
Increased fibrinolytic activity
Decreased platelet aggregation
Reduced incidence of myocardial infarction
Reduced insulin resistance – lower risk of developing Type 2 DM

Source: Adapted from Bell (37). Copyright © 1996 American Diabetes Association. From *Diabetes Care*, Vol. 19, 1996: 509–513. Reprinted with permission from The American Diabetes Association.

Table 13.3 Risks of heavy alcohol intake

Short term	Long term
Decreased gluconeogenesis	Increased risk of neuropathy
Hypoglycaemia	Increased risk of obesity and malnutrition
Increased insulin resistance	Increased frequency of accidents, gastritis, psychiatric problems
Hyperglycaemia	Liver disease
Increased free fatty acids, ketones, ketoacidosis and lactic acidosis (if treated with metformin)	Increased risk of breast and other cancers
Increased triglycerides	Pancreatitis
Hypertension	Cardiomyopathy/heart failure
Pancreatitis	

Source: Adapted from Bell (37). Copyright © 1996 American Diabetes Association. From *Diabetes Care*, Vol. 19, 1996; 509–513. Reprinted with permission from The American Diabetes Association.

metabolic profile of Type 2 diabetes, together with small dense LDL and low concentrations of HDL cholesterol. Hypertriglyceridaemia is an independent risk factor for coronary artery disease especially for people with Type 2 diabetes; reduction of alcohol intakes; tight glycaemic control and weight loss can help to reduce this risk (29). In subjects with alcohol-induced hypertriglyceridaemia, alcohol withdrawal has beneficial effects on the LDL profile by shifting the particle size from small to large, thus reducing susceptibility to oxidation.

With moderate alcohol consumption the increase in HDL becomes the predominant feature in the reduction of CHD risk and maximal benefit appears to be at the level of one drink per day (30). In irregular binge drinkers the increase in HDL cholesterol is not seen, adverse changes in LDL are acquired (31) and cardiovascular risk increases (Table 13.3).

Antioxidants in alcoholic beverages, especially polyphenolic compounds in red wine, have been proposed as an important contributory factor to the protective effect of regular alcohol use against atherosclerotic cardiovascular disease, by reducing oxidative damage to LDL, reducing its potential atherogenicity. The unique cardioprotective properties of red wine reside in the action of flavonoids which are minimal in white wine (except champagne). These flavonoids, especially resveratrol and quercetin, confer more potent antioxidant properties than alpha-tocopherol (32). These phenolic compounds found in wine are also thought to decrease platelet aggregation and prevent thrombus formation.

INSULIN SENSITIVITY

Moderate alcohol consumption among healthy subjects may be associated with increased insulin sensitivity and a reduced risk of diabetes (28). Reaven and co-workers (33) found that light to moderate alcohol consumption is associated with enhanced insulin-mediated glucose uptake, lower plasma glucose and insulin concentrations in response to oral glucose in healthy men and women. For people with diabetes, light to moderate alcohol intakes with meals do not substantially alter the blood glucose concentration (34,35). However, heavy intakes may be associated with an increase in glucose intolerance. So the effect on insulin sensitivity depends on the amount of alcohol consumed (36).

OBESITY

Whether or not the consumption of alcohol constitutes a risk for weight gain and 'whether alcohol calories count' has been widely debated. Alcohol is utilised as an energy substrate by the body, contributing 7 kcal/g to energy intakes, however, unlike other energy sources, there is no immediate storage mechanism in the body. The net efficiency of energy utilisation is lower from alcohol than for fat and carbohydrate and its thermogenic effect has been assessed as 15% from acute doses (38). Lieber (39), when proposing the microsomal ethanol oxidising system (MEOS) for metabolising alcohol, hypothesised that in heavy drinkers this is uncoupled and energy from alcohol is dissipated.

Another major issue for body-weight regulation is the extent to which alcohol spares other energy substrates from oxidation (40). As alcohol cannot be stored readily it is oxidised at a steady rate in preference to other substrates, thus being carbohydrate- and fat-sparing.

There is no evidence that consuming alcohol under isoenergetic conditions, i.e. replacing carbohydrate or fat calories with alcohol calories, increases the risk of obesity. Indeed some researchers have found an inverse relationship between alcohol intake and BMI and adiposity, despite an increase in total energy intake (41). Further research is needed to investigate the extent to which alcohol calories taken in addition to 'normal' diet increase the risk of weight gain.

NEUROLOGICAL EFFECTS

The acute neurological effects of alcohol include a lowering or removal of inhibition, stimulation, an antidepressant effect and increased aggressiveness. Longer-term effects include brain damage, physical dependence (on alcohol) and sleep disturbances. It is thought that these effects are mediated through the involvement of biogenic amines (dopamine, noradrenaline, 5-hydroxy-tryptamine).

NEUROPATHY

Neuropathy is any disease of the peripheral nerves, usually causing weakness and numbness. Neuropathy is a complication of both diabetes and excessive alcohol intakes. Therefore the risk of neuropathy increases when diabetics regularly drink more than the recommended levels of alcohol (42), and there is a direct and linear relationship between increasing alcohol intakes and worsening symptoms of neuropathy.

IMPOTENCE

There is some evidence of a correlation between heavy alcohol intakes and an increased risk of impotence in men with diabetes compared to those who report moderate intakes (43). In people with diabetes and non-diabetics there is an increased risk of functional loss of peripheral sensory and motor nerves and autonomic neuropathy with chronic heavy alcohol intakes.

SUMMARY

Evidence from many studies in the general population points to beneficial effects of small to moderate daily intakes of alcoholic drinks, but there is also strong evidence of the risks of heavier intakes. For the person with diabetes perhaps the most concerning of these risks is the impact on blood pressure, particularly for African–Caribbean men (at lower intakes), dramatically increasing the risk of stroke.

For people with Type 2 diabetes small to moderate daily intakes can improve their metabolic profile and reduce CHD risk by raising HDL cholesterol, increasing insulin sensitivity, increasing fibrinolytic activity, reducing platelet aggregation, improving antioxidant status and improving blood pressure.

For people with Type 1 diabetes the benefits of small to moderate intakes are similar to those for the general population, but the risks from heavier intakes are severe hypoglycaemia (which can be mistaken for intoxication) or ketoacidosis.

There is a need for further work to accurately evaluate at what level of alcohol intake the risks outweigh the benefits, as most of the studies use self-reported data, which because of underestimation could mean there is a lower apparent threshold of alcohol-related effects.

BIBLIOGRAPHY

Newsholme EA and Leech AR. 1990. *Biochemistry for the Medical Sciences*. John Wiley & Sons Ltd.

REFERENCES

1. Fuchs CS, Stampfer MJ, Colditz GA, Giovannucci EL, Manson JE, Kawachi I, Hunter DJ, Hankinson SE, Hennekens CH, Rosner B, Speizer FE, Willett WC. Alcohol consumption and mortality among women. *N Engl J Med* 1995; 332: 1245–1250.
2. Klatsky AL. Alcohol and hypertension. *Clin Chim Acta* 1996; 246: 91–105.
3. Royal College of Physicians, Royal College of Psychiatrists, Royal College of General Practitioners. Alcohol and the heart in perspective – sensible limits reaffirmed. London: RCP, RCPsych, RCGP, 1995.
4. Ha TKK, Lean MEJ. Technical review. Recommendations for the nutritional management of patients with diabetes mellitus. *Eur J Clin Nutr* 1998; 52: 467–481.
5. The Diabetes and Nutrition Study Group (DNSG) of the European Association for the Study of Diabetes (EASD). Recommendations for the nutritional management of patients with diabetes mellitus. *Eur J Clin Nutr* 2000; 54: 353–355.
6. Gronbaek M, Deis A, Sorensen TA, Bedier U, Schriohr P, Jensen G. Mortality associated with moderate intakes of wine, beer or spirits. *Br Med J* 1995; 310: 1165–1169.
7. Hendricks HFJ, Venstra J, Velthius-te Wierik EJM, Schaafsma G, Kluff C. Effect of moderate dose of alcohol with evening meal on fibrinolytic factors. *Br Med J* 1994; 308: 1003–1006.
8. Maheswaran R, Gill JS, Davis P, Beevers DG. High blood pressure due to alcohol. A rapidly reversible effect. *Hypertension* 1991; 17: 787–792.
9. Franz MJ, Horton ES Sr, Bantle JP, Beebe CA, Brunzell JD, Coulston AM, Henry RR, Hoogwerf BJ, Stacpoole PW. Nutritional principles for the management of diabetes and related complications (technical review). *Diabetes Care* 1994; 17: 490–518.
10. Chakraborty J. Alcohol and its metabolic interactions with other drugs. *Metabolism* 1978; 7: 273–296.
11. Krebs HA. Pyridine nucleotides and rate control. *Exp Biol* 1973; 27: 299–318.
12. Krebs HA. The effects of ethanol on the metabolic activities of the liver. *Adv Enzym Regul* 1968; 6: 467–480.
13. Arky RA, Veverbrants E, Abramson EA. Irreversible hypoglycaemia: a complication of alcohol and insulin. *J Am Med Assoc* 1968; 206: 575–578.
14. Avogaro A, Beltramello P, Gnudi L. Alcohol intake impairs glucose counter-regulation during acute insulin-induced hypoglycemia in IDDM patients: evidence for a critical role of free fatty acids. *Diabetes* 1993; 42: 1626–1634.
15. Arky RA, Freinkel N. Alcohol hypoglycaemia. *Arch Intern Med* 1964; 114: 501–507.
16. Wrenn KD, Slovis CM, Minion GE, Rutkowski R. The syndrome of alcoholic ketoacidosis. *Am J Med* 1991; 91: 119–128.
17. Halperin ML, Hammeke M, Josse RG, Jungas RL. Metabolic acidosis in the alcoholic: a pathophysiologic approach. *Metabolism* 1983; 32: 308–315.
18. Ellingboe J, Varanelli CC. Ethanol inhibits testosterone biosynthesis by direct action on Leydig cells. *Res Commun Chem Pathol Pharm* 1979; 24: 87–102.
19. Klatsky AL. Blood pressure and alcohol intake. In: *Hypertension, Pathophysiology, Diagnosis and Management*, eds JH Laragh and BM Brenner. New York: Raven Press, 2nd edition, 1995.
20. Gill JS, Zezulka AV, Shipley MJ, Gill SK, Beevers DG. Stroke and alcohol consumption. *New Engl J Med* 1986; 315: 1041–1046.

21. Sacco RL, Elkind M, Boden-Albala B, Lin IF, Kargman DE, Hauser WA, Shea S, Paik MC. The protective effect of moderate alcohol consumption on ischaemic stroke. *J Am Med Assoc* 1999; 281 (1): 53–60.

22. Donahue RP, Abbott RD, Reed DW, Yano K. *J Am Med Assoc* 1986; 255: 2311–2314.

23. Marmot MG, Elliot P, Shipley MJ, Dyer AR, Ueshima HU, Beevers DG, Stamler R, Kesteloot H, Rose G, Stamler J. Alcohol and blood pressure: the INTERSALT study. *Br Med J* 1994; 308: 1263–1267.

24. Bulpitt CJ. Letter, Alcohol and blood pressure. *Br Med J* 1994; 309: 275–276.

25. Klatsky AL, Friedman GD, Siegelaub AB. Alcohol and hypertension. *Comp Ther* 1978; 4: 60–68.

26. Harburg E, Ozgoren F, Hawthorne VM, Schork MA. Community norms of alcohol usage and blood pressure: Tecumseh, Michigan. *Am J Public Health* 1980; 70: 813–820.

27. Ajani UA, Gaziano JM, Lotufo PA, Lui S, Hennekens CH, Buring JE, Manson JE. Alcohol consumption and risk of CHD by DM status. *Circulation* 2000; 102 (5): 489–490.

28. Solomon CG, Hu FB, Stampfer MJ, Colditz GA, Speizer FE, Rimm EB, Willett WC, Manson JE. Moderate alcohol consumption and risk of CHD among women with type 2 diabetes. *Circulation* 2000; 102 (5): 487–488.

29. Gotto AM. Triglyceride as a risk factor for coronary artery disease. *Am J Cardiol* 1998; 82 (9A): 22–25.

30. Gaziano JM, Manson JE. Diet and heart disease. The role of fat, alcohol and antioxidants. *Cardiol Clin* 1996; 14 (1): 69–83.

31. McKee M, Britton A. The positive relationship between alcohol and heart disease in eastern Europe: potential physiological mechanisms. *J R Soc Med* 1998; 91 (8): 402–407.

32. Constant J. Alcohol, ischaemic heart disease and the French paradox. *Coron Art Dis* 1997; 8 (10): 645–649.

33. Facchini F, Ida Chen YD, Reaven GM. Light to moderate alcohol intake is associated with enhanced insulin sensitivity. *Diabetes Care* 1994; 17 (2): 15–19.

34. Christiansen C, Thomsen C, Rasmussen O. Effect of alcohol on glucose, insulin, free fatty acid and triacylglycerol responses to a light meal in non-insulin dependent diabetic subjects. *Br J Nutr* 1994; 17: 449–454.

35. Gin H, Morlat P, Raynaud JM, Aubertin J. Short-term effect of red wine (consumed during meals) on insulin requirements and glucose tolerance in diabetic patients. *Diabetes Care* 1992; 15: 546–548.

36. Razey G, Heaton KW, Bolton CH, Hughes AO. Alcohol consumption and its relation to cardiovascular risk factors in British women. *Br Med J* 1992; 304: 80–83.

37. Bell SH. Alcohol and the NIDDM patient. *Diabetes Care* 1996; 19 (5): 509–513.

38. Suter PM, Jequier E, Schutz Y. Effect of ethanol on energy expenditure. *Am J Physiol* 1994; 266: R1204–R1212.

39. Lieber CS. Metabolism and metabolic actions of ethanol. In: *The Year in Metabolism*, ed. N Freinkel. New York: Plenum Press, 1976: 317–342.

40. Schutz Y. Role of substrate utilization and thermogenesis on body-weight control with particular reference to alcohol. *Proc Nutr Soc* 2000; 59: 511–517.

41. Kleges RC, Mealer CZ, Kleges LM. Effect of alcohol intake on resting energy expenditure in young women social drinkers. *Am J Clin Nutr Apr* 1994; 59 (4): 805–809.

42. McCulloch DK, Campbell IW, Prescott RJ, Clarke BF. Effect of alcohol intake on symptomatic peripheral neuropathy in diabetic men. *Diabetes Care* 1980; 3: 245–247.

43. McColloch DK, Young RJ, Prescott RJ, Campbell IW, Clarke BF. The natural history of impotence in diabetic men. *Diabetologia* 1984; 26: 437–440.

14

Inpatient Nutritional Support of Sick Patients with Diabetes

HILARY PEAKE

Hammersmith Hospital, London, UK

INTRODUCTION

This chapter discusses the nutritional management of hospitalised adult patients with diabetes. It covers the aetiology of hyperglycaemia, the effects of diabetes on nutritional status, the metabolic consequences of stress and specific nutrient mixes.

Artificial nutritional support can cause significant hyperglycaemia in individuals with pre-existing diabetes mellitus or pre-diabetes conditions like impaired glucose tolerance and impaired fasting glucose. Artificial nutritional support can also exaggerate the hyperglycaemic response to stress caused by injury or illness unmasking glucose intolerance in the previously glucose-tolerant. Parenteral nutrition (PN), for example, can result in approximately 30% of patients developing transient diabetes (1).

AETIOLOGY

Patients with hyperglycaemia form a heterogeneous group. It is vital to identify the aetiology of the hyperglycaemia in order to tailor appropriate clinical care with clear medical and nutritional management aims and objectives. At any time approximately 10% of hospitalised patients have diabetes, with 85% of these having Type 2 diabetes (2). The stress response to trauma/illness

Nutritional Management of Diabetes Mellitus. Edited by G. Frost, A. Dornhorst and R. Moses
© 2003 John Wiley & Sons, Ltd. ISBN 0 471 49751 7

commonly exacerbates hyperglycaemia in patients with pre-existing diabetes and not infrequently produces significant hyperglycaemia in previously euglycaemic patients (3). The hyperglycaemic response to stress is due to the increase in circulating counter-regulatory hormones (glucagon, cortisol, growth hormone and adrenaline) which together result in an increase in hepatic glucose production, a decrease in peripheral glucose uptake (4) and an increase in insulin resistance.

THE IMPORTANCE OF ACHIEVING GOOD GLYCAEMIC CONTROL IN HOSPITAL

Out of hospital the focus for good glycaemic control is to minimise long-term microvascular and macrovascular diabetic complications. In hospital, over the short term, the rationale for good glycaemic control is to ensure a metabolic environment that promotes the best possible immune activity and wound healing. Hyperglycaemia has a detrimental effect on the immune system, adversely affecting chemotaxis, granulocyte adhesion, phagocytosis, intra-cellular killing and complement function (5,6). The increased risk of infection in diabetic patients may well be explained by the operation of some or all of these effects. An increase in the rate and/or severity of infection is likely to contribute to the increased length of stay of diabetic patients in hospital (7). In unconscious patients or those with difficult-to-assess neurological function, there is a real danger of unrecognised hypoglycaemia and the benefits of tight control need to be balanced against this risk.

PRACTICALITIES OF FEEDING HOSPITALISED PATIENTS

The optimal blood glucose level for ill patients receiving nutritional support is unclear and the literature provides many different blood glucose targets and approaches to avoid both hyper- and hypoglycaemia. The specific targets for glycaemic control for each patient must take into consideration some of the following variables: age, prognosis, aetiology of the hyperglycaemia, level of consciousness, severity of any infection, degree of metabolic stress and immune status.

Achieving tight control may be less relevant when nutritional support is to be given over a short period of time. The potential benefits of tight glycaemic control during nutritional support may only be apparent when feeding is given for three weeks or more.

Although the metabolic consequences of diabetes are known to involve fat metabolism resulting in a significant dyslipidaemia, there are few defined management targets for serum lipids when giving nutritional support to diabetic patients. The degree of dyslipidaemia is frequently disproportional to the degree of hyperglycaemia and requires monitoring and control separate to the diabetes (8). Some of the clinical consequences of hyperlipidaemia include: impairment of the immune response, endothelial dysfunction, an increased tendency to develop a coagulopathy and an exacerbation of insulin resistance.

NUTRITIONAL ASSESSMENT

Before nutritional support is initiated the indications, aims/objectives and ideal route of nutritional support need to be determined based on both the nutritional assessment of the patient and the clinical features of the condition being treated. There is no clinically applicable gold standard for assessing nutritional status (9) and, of necessity, assessment is commonly based on subjective parameters.

The initial nutritional assessment is vital as it will influence an important aspect of the patient's care. The variable parameters which can be used for this assessment are listed in Table 14.1. The nutritional assessment is very similar regardless of whether the patient is hyperglycaemic or not. However, when assessing a patient with diabetes for nutritional support, their recent glycaemic control and treatment are highly relevant as poor glycaemic control can compromise the patient's overall nutritional status.

IS ARTIFICIAL NUTRITIONAL SUPPORT NECESSARY?

Artificial nutritional support is only indicated for patients who are malnourished or who would become malnourished if not given artificial nutritional support. Artificial nutritional support has no clinical benefit if given for less than five days. In order to obtain benefit patients need to be fed for seven days or more (10).

The major aims and objectives of nutritional support for patients with diabetes are:

1. To maintain or improve nutritional status.
2. To promote wound healing.
3. To optimise glycaemic control.
4. To achieve optimal lipid control.
5. To avoid hyper- or hypoglycaemia.

NUTRITIONAL REQUIREMENTS

The presence of hyperglycaemia does not influence the need or requirements for nutritional support and these remain similar to those of glucose-tolerant

Table 14.1 Nutritional assessment parameters

	Assessment parameter	Level indicating depletion	Comments
Anthropometry	Height (m) Weight (kg)	Not applicable	Calculate body mass index
	Usual weight	Not applicable	Weight history from patients or notes
	Body mass index (kg/m²)	$<19\,kg/m^2$ (10% of healthy population)	Affected by frame size. To assess whether malnourished use BMI, usual weight and % weight loss
	Recent unintentional weight loss (20)	2% (1–2 weeks) 5% (1 month) 7.5% (3 months) 10% (>6 months)	To assess weight loss over a short period check urea and fluid balance status to ensure weight changes are reliable. Reported weight loss can be very inaccurate
	Triceps skinfold thickness (TSF)	Male: <9.5 mm Female: <18.5 mm 80% of normal value (21)	Use percentiles for age and sex. Readings affected by oedema
	Mid-arm muscle circumference (MAMC)	Male: <23 cm Female: <17.8 cm 80% of normal value (21)	Use percentiles for age and sex. Readings affected by oedema
	Grip strength	Single spring handgrip dynamometer using non-dominant arm (highest reading of 3). Protein malnutrition indicated if <85% reference range	Functional assessment. Poor specificity. Unsuitable for unconscious or physically disabled patients
Dietary intake	Dietary assessment Inadequate oral intake identified by full diet history/record charts	Nutritional intake 500 kcal <requirements NBM for 5 days 1/3 meals consumed for one week 2/3 meals consumed for two weeks	Only applicable if patient previously well nourished. With previously malnourished patient start nutritional intervention sooner. Phosphate, chromium and trace element deficiencies can cause hyperglycaemia by decreasing insulin sensitivity

Category	Indicator	Value	Comment
SGA (subjective global assessment)	Subjective assessment (22)	Square shoulders Limbs evidence of muscle and fat loss Loss of fat pads under eyes Denting of temples	Very subjective. Not sensitive at monitoring changes in nutritional status. Useful to use in conjunction with objective parameters
Laboratory indicators	Serum albumin	<30 g/l	Underlying disease is the usual cause of a low albumin. Nutritional support usually required when CRP high and albumin low. Use pre- not post-up albumin for assessment. Check human albumin solution is not being administered
	Urea	<2.0 mmol/l	Very low levels can indicate malnutrition or over-hydration. Interpret in conjunction with creatinine
	Creatinine	<55 mmol/l	Below normal range may indicate decreased muscle bulk
	Total lymphocyte count	<1200 mm^3 (= % lymphocytes × WBC/100)	Likely to reflect disease state rather than nutritional status. Sensitivity and specificity low
	Glycaemic control Laboratory/ward glucose testing	HbA$_{1c}$ >8 mmol/l Fasting pl. glucose >8 mmol/l 2 h post-prandial >12 mmol/l	Poor glycaemic control increases energy expenditure, adversely affecting weight, muscle bulk, wound healing and immune function (23). Causes pseudo-hyponatraemia. For every 0.34 mmol/l rise in glucose, sodium falls 1 mmol/l
Clinical condition	Age Organ failure Cancer	Elderly Renal Except breast	
Socio-economic status	Poor Socially isolated Dementia	Housing Housebound, less than one visitor per week High alcohol intake	

patients. Special consideration needs to be given to the following circumstances.

UNDERNOURISHED PATIENTS (BMI < 19 kg/m²)

If a patient is undernourished additional energy, protein and electrolytes are required to restore their nutritional status. Additional nutrition should only be provided to patients who are not catabolic and who are increasing their physical activity to allow the repletion of muscle mass.

OBESE PATIENTS (BMI > 30 kg/m²)

Obese patients should receive nutritional support based on their actual body weight. It is usually inappropriate to give calorie-reducing diets during illness, with the following exceptions:

1. Morbid obesity (BMI > 50 kg/m²);
2. Obesity-related life-threatening conditions, e.g. sleep apnoea.

ROUTE OF NUTRITIONAL SUPPORT

Once the decision has been made that nutritional support is required, the optimal route needs to be determined. Enteral nutrition should be used whenever possible. There are many advantages of enteral over parenteral nutrition, including economic considerations, the avoidance of infections associated with parenteral nutrition and a more physiological impact on the intestinal bacterial milieu.

METHODS OF NUTRITIONAL SUPPORT

Enteral nutrition is particularly suited to patients with diabetes due to a more physiological delivery of nutrients. Although enteral feeding may have some complications, they are generally less severe than those associated with parenteral nutrition. The anticipated length of feeding and the perceived nutritional requirements will influence the route of nutritional support to be chosen. The first line of nutritional support is oral diet, with or without nutritional supplements, and only if the patient is at risk of aspiration or cannot meet their nutritional requirements orally should other routes be considered. The decision of how best to feed enterally or when to instigate parenteral nutrition requires a consensus from the clinical team and, if possible, the agreement of the patient and/or carers. Options for enteral nutrition routes are:

1. Oral diet
2. Nutritional oral supplements
3. Tube feeding
   - Pre-pyloric
     (a) nasogastric
     (b) gastrostomy (surgical or endoscopic)
   - Post-pyloric
     (a) nasoduodenal
     (b) jejunal
     (c) jejunostomy (gastrostomy with an extension jejunostomy)

ORAL DIET

The standard dietary recommendation for diabetic patients may not be appropriate for anorexic or ill patients who have a poor oral intake. If a patient is eating very little, then providing palatable sugar-containing food may help stimulate the appetite. The inclusion of high-fat food is valuable in helping the patient maximise their energy intake in smaller portions. Conversely the inclusion of high-fibre diets (complex carbohydrates) may limit food intake by causing early satiety. The provision of extra high-protein and energy snacks may be sufficient to meet a patient's nutritional requirement. These dietary modifications are likely to increase the intake of simple sugar and the glycaemic index of the diet, but these potentially adverse changes need to be offset against the risks of malnutrition. There are some foods with a high energy content that have a low glycaemic index, and it may be advantageous to encourage foods like ice cream, custard, yoghurt, sponge cake and muffins to minimise the glycaemic response.

NUTRITIONAL ORAL SUPPLEMENTS

If the nutritional requirements cannot be met with snacks and the hospital diet, food supplements may be required. Oral supplements can come in a range of savoury and sweet flavours. There are a variety of presentations including powder, pre-made carton sip feeds, glucose polymers (powders and syrups) and protein powders. These products may be nutritionally complete, i.e. suitable as a sole source of nutrition. The recommendation as to which oral supplements are to be chosen should be guided by the patient's preferences. The sugar content of the supplement is often offset by the patient's reduced dietary carbohydrate intake and can be invaluable in preventing hypoglycaemia during periods of poor oral intake.

ENTERAL TUBE FEEDING

Enteral tube feeding can be continuous, intermittent or overnight. The method chosen will depend on a number of factors and should be determined in conjunction with the management goals of the clinical team.

Once the regimen has been decided the type of enteral tube feed needs to be selected. The choice of feed should be individualised and based on the nutritional and fluid requirements. The approximate composition of UK generic feeds is outlined below. There are some small changes that relate to the different manufacturers and, where this is the case, information is presented as ranges.

Standard Enteral Tube Feeds (1 kcal/ml, osmolarity 201–250 moso/l)

These contain 15–16% of energy as whole protein (milk protein), 30–35% of energy as a mixture of long- and medium-chain fats (40% MUFA and 30% SFA and PUFA), e.g. linseed, sunflower, safflower oil, rapeseed and may also contain fish oil. Carbohydrates provide 50–56% of the energy content of the feed. Carbohydrate is mainly present as maltodextrins, but may also contain sucrose, oligosaccharides, polysaccharides, corn syrups and starches.

High-energy Feeds (1.5 kcal/ml, osmolarity 300 moso/l)

These have the same percentage energy from macronutrients on a per kcal basis. The osmolarity of these products is increased to 300 moso/l due to the reduced volume of this product.

Fibre feeds

The amount of fibre per 100 ml is usually between 1–2 g. The type of fibre ranges from soy, inulin wheat fibre, fructo-oligosaccharides, oat fibre and gums. The feed may contain fibre from a mixed or single source. The ratio of soluble to insoluble fibre in the mixed fibre source feeds varies, with some products having equal proportions whilst others contain 75% insoluble and 25% soluble fibre.

Specialist Feeds

Additional feeds are also available for the management of patients with special needs, e.g. renal failure, malabsorption, electrolyte restrictions, milk protein intolerance and inflammatory bowel disease. As a general rule elemental or semi-elemental feeds have an osmolarity between 300–500 moso/l.

Specialist feeds for people with diabetes are available and aim to reduce the usual high liquid carbohydrate content of standard feeds ($>50\%$ of the calories as carbohydrate). A high liquid carbohydrate content tends to exacerbate hyperglycaemia and often necessitates the initiation of, or an increase in, insulin therapy (7). Tube feeding is associated with a more rapid increase in post-prandial glucose than solid diets of similar nutritional composition. High post-prandial glucose levels have the disadvantage of predisposing to hypertriglyceridaemia (11,12).

COMPOSITION OF SPECIALIST FEEDS FOR THE MANAGEMENT OF HYPERGLYCAEMIA

Coulston has recently reviewed the clinical experience of modified enteral formulas for managing diabetic patients. Most of the evidence used to support the use of specialised enteral feeds in diabetic management has been extrapolated from the general diabetic literature and is aimed at avoiding hyperglycaemia (11). Promotional literature from the different nutritional companies is primarily based on dietary guidelines and not based on clinical studies. Although some studies have looked at the glycaemic effect of different liquid formulas given as oral test meals (high-fibre, low-carbohydrate, standard formula) (13), long-term studies are lacking. Only short-term studies have been carried out using specialised oral diets in which carbohydrate content is reduced by increasing MUFA content. These short-term studies have been undertaken either as single test meals or over short periods of time involving relatively few subjects.

One of the longer studies examining the metabolic effects and clinical outcomes of a modified versus a standard formula for enteral tube feeding in diabetic patients was by Craig et al. (14). This pilot study was a prospective randomised double group parallel trial in which 34 patients with diabetes were randomised to receive either modified (55% fat, 33% CHO) or standard enteral tube feeds (35% fat, 53% CHO) for up to three months. Glycaemic control was judged to be significantly better following the modified feed during weeks 1, 5 and 7. However this occurred despite any significant differences being found in the HbA_{1c} level, fasting glucose and lipid profile!

Devising a tube feed for people with diabetes based on dietary nutrients known to improve glycaemic control is not a precise science. Many of the nutrients included in tube feeds need to be chemically modified to enable delivery from a tube. As the glycaemic response of a food is dependent on its physical properties, changing nutrients from their solid phase to a liquid phase can radically change the glycaemic properties. With respect to glycaemic control, while there is good evidence of the beneficial effect of fibre in the solid diet, the addition of fibre in the liquid diet has not been shown to be of benefit (12). In addition, fibre supplementation to tube feeding can be problematic as optimal fibre blends increase feed viscosity, making formula flow through fine-bore feeding tubes extremely difficult. The lack of improvement in glycaemic control with tube feeds containing fibre is probably related to the biophysical properties of fibre in a liquid. For tube feeds the post-prandial insulin and glucose responses are related to the carbohydrate load and not to its fibre content.

COMPLICATIONS OF ENTERAL NUTRITIONAL SUPPORT

Gastrointestinal symptoms are the most frequent side-effects of tube feeding with gastroparesis and diarrhoea being the most common complications.

Gastroparesis is extremely common among patients with diabetes and affects 30–75% of all patients undergoing nutritional enteral feeding (7). Gastroparesis reduces the tolerance to enteral nutritional support as well as causing bloating, satiety, nausea and vomiting. The irregular and unpredictable rate of gastric emptying associated with gastroparesis can result in poor glycaemic control. This poor control can, in turn, cause an exacerbation of gastroparesis. In addition to changing the enteral formula, a number of pro-kinetic drugs are available that can improve gastric emptying. If these strategies are unsuccessful then a change to jejunal feeding may be helpful.

Chronic diarrhoea occurs in 20–85% of people with diabetes receiving enteral feeding and can be a difficult management problem. The management of diarrhoea requires a systematic approach including the following:

1. Be aware of bowel history and any altered bowel habits prior to tube feeding.
2. Consider all possible contributory factors for the diarrhoea.
3. Take note of all prescribed and non-prescribed medications being taken, particularly broad-spectrum antibiotics.
4. Consider bacterial overgrowth and specific infections (e.g. *Clostridium difficile*).

Consider other bowel pathology. Also bear in mind that enteral feeding itself may be a cause of diarrhoea due to the use of hyperosmolar feeds or feeds with an inadequate sodium content as well as rapid administration, e.g. bolus feeding.

PARENTERAL NUTRITION

Parenteral nutrition provides no added value over enteral feeding in patients with a functioning gastrointestinal tract and is associated with an increased risk of complications. It is also more expensive (15,16). Parenteral nutrition is only indicated when enteral nutrition is contraindicated, and this usually occurs when the gastrointestinal tract is either non-functioning or not accessible. The decision to instigate PN should ideally be made by the clinical team with consumer involvement if practical.

Parenteral nutrition is associated with hyperglycaemia in at least 15% of patients (7). The presence of hyperglycaemia in patients receiving PN is important as it is associated with a marked increase in infection risk. Intravenous catheter-related infections are five times higher in patients receiving central PN (5), and this figure is higher still in the presence of hyperglycaemia.

ROUTES USED FOR PARENTERAL NUTRITION

Parenteral nutrition is hyperosmolar and requires a large central vein. Central access can be achieved either by a peripherally inserted central catheter (PICC) threaded up into a larger central vein or by direct access to a central vein. Patients who are only receiving parenteral nutrition short term are more suitable for a PICC.

1. Central access
   (a) Short term, multilumen lines
   (b) Long term, e.g. Hickman line or Portacath
   (c) PICC > 15 cm long
2. Peripheral access (at or below the antecubital fossa)
   (a) PICC > 15 cm long
      (length of parenteral nutrition > 5 days and < 4 weeks)
   (b) Midline, e.g. PICC ≈ 15 cm long
      (length of parenteral nutrition > 5 days and < 2 weeks)

The energy content in PN is provided by a mixed source of fat and carbohydrate (usually 50% non-protein energy from CHO and fat). Mixed energy provision is important. The inclusion of fat improves substrate utilisation, enables the delivery of fat-soluble vitamins and reduces the osmolarity of feeds which may be used for simultaneous peripheral feeding. The protein component in PN is made up of essential amino acids and soluble non-essential amino acids. PN is usually administered in an all-in-one bag.

A variety of PN pre-compounded bags (i.e. standard bags) are available, designed to meet the nutritional requirements for most patients. Some hospital pharmacies are able to compound PN bags for individual patients when required. Parenteral nutrition should always be administered continuously over 24 h with a suitable infusion pump to minimise infusion errors. These pumps ensure a constant controlled infusion rate to prevent marked swings in blood glucose and electrolyte values or rapid changes in fluid balance.

All diabetic patients will require insulin during PN administration for glycaemic control as oral hypoglycaemic agents are unsuitable for a variety of reasons. Individuals with stress-induced glucose intolerance (3) will also usually require insulin treatment during PN feeding.

The glycaemic management during parenteral nutrition needs to be tailored and adapted to the nutritional support required. Blood glucose levels usually reflect the underlying illness rather than the route of nutritional support. Irrespective of this, parenteral nutrition support can be optimised to help minimise both hyper- and hypoglycaemia by adhering to the following points:

1. Prevent overfeeding;
2. Ensure infusion rate of CHO in the PN does not exceed the patient's glucose oxidation rate;
3. Optimise the fat to CHO ratio;
4. Reduce the rate of the PN to prevent rebound hypoglycaemia before stopping PN.

Although the optimal substrate provision for intravenous nutrition has not been elucidated, the amount of energy provided by glucose should not exceed the patient's glucose oxidation rate (6–7 mg/kg/min) (17). Exceeding the glucose oxidation rate may increase the metabolic rate and worsen glucose tolerance (18).

Some authorities advocate increasing the fat component to 60–70% of non-protein energy in parenteral nutrition in order to reduce the CHO component to 30–40%. However there are concerns regarding high fat intakes. These include possible adverse effects on immune function and the generation of free radicals from the polyunsaturated fat. There are insufficient antioxidants in PN to neutralise any excess in free radical production. A high fat content in PN increases the possibility of hyperlipidaemia and this has the potential in septic or critically ill patients to precipitate pancreatitis and renal failure.

Reducing the carbohydrate component in patients with hyperglycaemia will reduce the glucose load of the feed, but this may not be sufficient to allow the withdrawal of insulin. Alternative sugars other than glucose have been tried experimentally as potential CHO substitutes and these include fructose, sorbitol, xylitol and glycerol. To date these alternative sugars have not been found to successfully prevent or improve hyperglycaemia.

AIMS AND OBJECTIVES FOR ACHIEVING OPTIMAL GLYCAEMIC CONTROL AND NUTRITIONAL SUPPORT

All patients receiving nutritional support need to be carefully monitored to prevent possible complications. Each hospital should have clearly stated monitoring protocols for nutritional support, reflecting national guidelines. The frequency of monitoring depends on the clinical situation and needs to be individualised.

Patients with hyperglycaemia and those who are severely malnourished should be monitored closely to prevent metabolic complications, including the potential life-threatening re-feeding syndrome. This syndrome is associated with profound electrolyte disturbances and fluid overload. During re-feeding there is a switch from fat to carbohydrate metabolism with an increase in insulin release. During carbohydrate repletion, insulin-stimulated glucose uptake is accompanied by an increased cellular uptake of potassium, phosphorus and water. Insulin also stimulates the sodium-potassium adenosinetriphosphatase (ATPase) pump, which uses magnesium as a co-factor and magnesium requirements increase as a consequence.

MEDICAL MANAGEMENT FOR ACHIEVING OBJECTIVES OF GLYCAEMIC CONTROL

ORAL HYPOGLYCAEMIA AGENTS

OHAs are relatively contraindicated during critical illness. Metformin is not usually a suitable drug for ill patients. It is contraindicated for patients undergoing any form of imaging that requires contrast media. It is also not suitable for patients with a moderate degree of renal or hepatic disease. The OHAs most suitable for hospital use are the short-acting insulin secretagogues, e.g. repaglinide or nateglinide. Long-acting sulphonlyurea drugs should be avoided as they are a potent cause of hypoglycaemia, particularly in the elderly.

OHAs may be suitable in clinically stable patients receiving enteral (gastric administration) feeds. OHAs may be crushed when the patient's level of consciousness is reduced or when there are difficulties with swallowing. Care must be taken to crush the tablets properly and flush after administration in order to reduce the risk of blocking the enteral feed tube. The use of OHAs is really only suitable when the enteral tube is pre-pyloric.

INSULIN

Insulin is required for all patients with Type 1 diabetes and those with Type 2 diabetes with significant hyperglycaemia or critical illness. The type of insulin regimen used will be tailored to the particular circumstances of the patient. The choices range from a continuous infusion to the use of subcutaneous, intermittent, quick-acting insulin on a background of once or twice daily long-acting insulin. The timing of insulin administration should, whenever possible, relate to the type and timing of the feed.

If adding insulin to a PN bag then some of the insulin will be adsorbed onto the plastic of the parenteral nutrition bag and giving sets. Under some circumstances up to 80% of the insulin added to a PN bag can be 'lost' in this way. The exact figure will vary according to the bag surface area, volume of solution, length of administration set, its temperature and electrolyte content (19).

CONCLUSION

When considering the principles underlying nutritional assessment and the design of nutrition programmes for patients with hyperglycaemia or diabetes, there are a number of useful questions to bear in mind:

1. What is the nutritional status of the patient?
2. Is artificial nutritional support indicated?
3. Can the patient's requirements be met by oral nutritional support?
4. Should enteral or parenteral feeding be used?
5. What will be the best formula?
6. What is an acceptable blood glucose range?
7. What insulin regimen will be most effective?
8. Are there any disorders of gastrointestinal motility?

REFERENCES

1. Hongsermeier T, Bistrian BR. Evaluation of a practical technique for determining insulin requirements in diabetic patients receiving total parenteral nutrition. *J Parenter Enteral Nutr* 1993; 17: 16–19.
2. Panser LA, Naessens JM, Noberga FT, Palumbo PJ, Bailard DJ. Utilisation trends and risk factors for hospitilisation in diabetes mellitus patients. *Mayo Clin Proc* 1990; 65: 1171–1184.
3. Wright J. Total parenteral nutrition and enteral nutrition in diabetes. *Curr Opin Clin Nutr Metab Care* 2000; 3: 5–10.
4. Coulston AM. Enteral nutrition in the patient with diabetes mellitus. *Curr Opin Clin Nutr Metab Care* 2000; 3: 11–15.
5. McMahon MM, Rizza RA. Nutrition support in hospitalized patients with diabetes mellitus. *Mayo Clin Proc* 1996; 71: 587–594.
6. Pomposelli JJ, Baxter JK, Babineau TJ, Pomfret EA, Driscoll DF, Forse RA, Bistrain BR. Early post operative glucose control predicts nosocomial infection rate in diabetes patients. *J Parenter Enteral Nutr* 1998; 22: 77–81.
7. Pitts DM, Kilo KA, Pontious SL. Nutritional support for the patient with diabetes. *Crit Care Nurs Clin North Am* 1993; 5: 47–56.
8. Wright J. Effect of high-carbohydrate versus high-monounsaturated fatty acid diet on metabolic control in diabetes and hyperglycemic patients. *Clin Nutr* 1998; 17 (Suppl 2): 35–45.
9. Plester C. Position Paper: Malnutrition in Hospital. British Dietetic Association. January 1996, 1–7.

10. Sandstrom R, Drott C, Hyltander A, Arfvidsson B, Schersten T, Wickstrom I, Lundholm K. The effect of postoperative intravenous feeding (TPN) on outcome following major surgery evaluated in a randomized study. *Ann Surg* 1993; 217: 185–195.
11. Schrezenmeir J. Rationale for specialized nutrition support for hyperglycemic patients. *Clin Nutr* 1998; 17 (Suppl 2): 26–34.
12. Cashmere KA. Effects of defined formulas diet with and without fibre, on blood glucose, insulin and GIP in patients with type II diabetes mellitus. *Diabetes* 1983; 32 (Suppl 1): 85A.
13. Sanz-Paris A, Calvo L, Guallard A, Salazar I, Albero R. High-fat versus high-carbohydrate enteral formulae: effect on blood glucose, C-peptide, and ketones in patients with type 2 diabetes treated with insulin or sulfonylurea [see comments]. *Nutrition* 1998; 14: 840–845.
14. Craig LD, Nicholson S, Silverstone FA, Kennedy RD. Use of a reduced-carbohydrate, modified-fat enteral formula for improving metabolic control and clinical outcomes in long-term care residents with type 2 diabetes: results of a pilot trial. *Nutrition* 1998; 14: 529–534.
15. Woodcock NP, Zeigler D, Palmer D, Buckley P, Mitchell CJ, MacFie J. Enteral versus parenteral nutrition: a pragmatic study. *Nutrition* 2001; 17: 1–12.
16. Lipman TO. Grains or veins: is enteral nutrition really better than parenteral nutrition? A look at the evidence. *J Parenter Enteral Nutr* 1998; 22: 167–182.
17. Wolfe RR, O'Donnell TF Jr, Stone MD, Richmand DA, Burke JF. Investigation of factors determining the optimal glucose infusion rate in total parenteral nutrition. *Metabolism* 1980; 29: 892–900.
18. Orr ME. Hyperglycemia during nutritional support. *Crit Care Nurs* 1992; 12: 64–70.
19. Trissel LA. *Handbook of Injectable Drugs*, 11th edn. Bethesda, MD: American Society of Health System Pharmacists, 2001; 747–748.
20. A.S.P.E.N. Board of Directors. Guidelines for the use of Parenteral and Enteral Nutrition in Adult and Paediatric Patients. *Parenteral and Enteral Nutrition* 1993; 17: 4, suppl.
21. Bishop CW, Bowen PE, Ritchley SI. Norms for nutritional assessment of American adults by upper arm anthropometry. *Am J Clin Nutr.* 1981; 34: 2530–2539.
22. Detsky AS, McLaughlin JR, Baker JP, Johnson N, Whittaker S, Mendelson RA, Jeejeebhoy KN. What is subjective global assessment of nutritional status? *J Parenter Ent Nutr* 1987; 11: 8–13.
23. Park RH, Hansell DT, Davidson LE, Henderson G, Legge V, Gray GR. Management of diabetic patients requiring nutritional support. *Nutrition* 1992; 8: 316–320.

15

Diabetes and Renal Replacement Therapy

MARIE KELLY AND THUSHARA DASSANAYAKE

Hammersmith Hospital, London, UK

INTRODUCTION

The renal dietitian is an important member of the clinical team looking after patients with diabetes and end stage renal failure (ESRF). An understanding of the metabolic and nutritional changes that occur prior to and during ESRF is essential in order to provide nutritional advice to these patients. This is applicable irrespective of whether they are treated with haemodialysis (HD), peritoneal dialysis (PD) or renal transplantation.

PREVALENCE

Diabetes has become the commonest cause of ESRF in Western countries. In the UK around 16% of patients starting renal replacement therapy (RRT) have ESRF due to diabetic nephropathy (1). This figure is considerably higher in areas of the country where there are ethnic populations with an increased susceptibility to diabetes (2).

DIALYSIS INITIATION

Ideally, all diabetic patients approaching ESRF should be involved in the development of their own personalised care plan. This will enable a negotiation

Nutritional Management of Diabetes Mellitus. Edited by G. Frost, A. Dornhorst and R. Moses
© 2003 John Wiley & Sons, Ltd. ISBN 0 471 49751 7

of the necessary dietary changes leading up to and extending to the initiation of elective dialysis (3).

Dialysis guidelines from the National Kidney Foundation promote the early initiation of RRT for diabetic patients, due to an increased susceptibility to uraemic symptoms at lower serum creatinine levels than non-diabetic subjects (4). Early RRT for diabetic renal failure not only relieves the symptoms of nausea, anorexia and vomiting but also helps reduce overall mortality. However, despite these recommendations, dialysis is frequently delayed due to either personal resistance or inadequate dialysis resources.

Some diabetic patients with already compromised renal function, will require the emergency initiation of dialysis during an intercurrent illness. However, this does not mean that all will require long-term RRT.

GLYCAEMIC CONTROL

Achieving good glycaemic control is important for all patients with ESRF as this can retard the progression of the microvascular and macrovascular complications (5). Good glycaemic control at the start of dialysis has also been shown to improve mortality risk. For patients on continuous ambulatory peritoneal dialysis (CAPD) hyperglycaemia increases circulating advanced glycation end products (AGE), which have been implicated in causing endothelium and peritoneal membrane damage with loss of ultrafiltration capacity. Good glycaemic control reduces thirst, which in turn helps to reduce fluid associated weight gain.

RENAL REPLACEMENT THERAPY

A brief outline on the principles of RRT is given below. Most patients with ESRF initially require dialysis, either haemodialysis or peritoneal dialysis. Only a minority of individuals, usually those with a suitable relative willing to donate a kidney, will have immediate access to a renal transplant.

DIALYSIS

While survival on dialysis continues to improve, diabetic patients still do less well than non-diabetic patients (6). Results from the Italian Cooperative Peritoneal Study Group Registry show the 10-year patient survival for the 301 diabetic patients to be less than half that of the 1689 non-diabetic subjects (20.6% vs 55.6%) (7). Higher mortality rates among diabetic patients receiving HD also occur (8), but with good glycaemic control these rates can be improved (9).

Peritoneal dialysis is the preferred mode of treatment for diabetic patients with microvascular and macrovascular co-morbidities. Continuous ambulatory peritoneal dialysis allows for a slow ultrafiltration process that provides greater cardiovascular stability than HD. Blood pressure control is easier and residual renal function is preserved for longer. It also provides incidentally for an alternative route of insulin administration. Initial concerns that diabetic CAPD patients may have higher dialysis-associated infection rates have not been confirmed (10,11).

DIALYSIS PROCEDURES

Continuous Ambulatory Peritoneal Dialysis

CAPD is a method of long-term dialysis that requires a permanent intra-peritoneal catheter. The peritoneum acts as a semi-permeable membrane that allows diffusion of solutes and facilitates the removal of water by ultrafiltration. The daily CAPD regimen comprises a drain-in period, followed by a dwell time of approximately 4 h and a drain-out period. This cycle is usually repeated four times each day (12,13).

Haemodialysis

Haemodialysis requires the surgical construction of an arterio-venous fistula that is usually sited in the non-dominant forearm using the cephalic vein and either the radial or brachial artery. After six to eight weeks the fistula has usually thickened sufficiently to allow it to be cannulated with two large-bore needles that take blood to and from the dialysis machine. Blood is pumped through a semi-permeable membrane filter in the dialysis machine allowing removal of excess solutes and fluid. Haemodialysis is repeated every two to three days with the time on dialysis dependent on the patient's body size and residual renal function. If a patient has no permanent access and requires emergency dialysis this can be done through a temporary neckline or a semi-permanent catheter in a central vein (14).

FACTORS INFLUENCING NUTRITIONAL STATUS IN DIALYSIS PATIENTS

Approximately 40% of dialysis patients exhibit some degree of protein and energy malnutrition and this is associated with an increased risk of morbidity and mortality. In the Modification in Renal Disease Feasibility Study (MDRD) in which 840 patients were prospectively studied, 42% of CAPD patients and 30% of HD patients were considered to be malnourished (15). Contributing factors to protein energy malnutrition occurring in dialysed patients are shown in Table 15.1.

Table 15.1 Factors implicated in protein–energy malnutrition in dialysis patients

Factors	Comments
Reduced nutritional intake	Energy and protein intakes consistently lower than requirements Uraemic symptoms can continue for upto three months after starting dialysis
Underdialysis	Nutritional intake deteriorates with inadequate dialysis
Gastroparesis	Abdominal distension Vomiting Early satiety
Dialysis-related effects	Abdominal discomfort with infusion of PD dialysate Protein losses, 6–12 g amino acids during one HD session Daily protein losses on CAPD of 5–15 g/day Peritonitis protein losses up to 20 g/day
Metabolic/endocrine factors	Hyperparathyroidism Hyperglucagonaemia Insulin resistance Vitamin D deficiency
Co-morbidity and infections	IHD and episodes of hypotension limiting dialysis time PVD can limit vascular access for HD Infections of vascular access in HD patients and peritonitis in PD

NUTRITIONAL ASSESSMENT/SCREENING

Ideally the nutritional status of patients approaching ESRF and starting dialysis should be monitored. As a single marker of nutritional status is unreliable, a number of nutritional parameters, as outlined in Chapter 14, can help identify those who are malnourished. Dual-energy X-ray absorptometry remains a useful method for assessment of lean body mass (15).

Nutrition scores such as subjective global nutrition assessment (SGA), based on clinical, physical and subjective measures are useful tools. The SGA is considered better suited to assessing study populations.

Serial biochemical flow charts are useful in assessing nutritional status (see Table 15.3). A decline in pre-dialysis serum urea, creatinine, potassium and phosphate may be indicative of a loss of lean body mass, rather than an improvement in nutritional status (17). Additional points to consider in the nutritional assessment of dialysis patients are given in Table 15.2.

Table 15.2 Additional factors in the nutritional assessment of dialysis patients

Factors	Comment
Anthropometry	Ensure measurements are taken at patient's dry weight: Post-dialysis for the HD patient After drained-out period for CAPD Adjust for oedema
Serum biochemistry	Serial biochemical measurements are useful in monitoring nutritional status
Protein catabolic rate (nPCR)	An indirect marker of protein intake in stable dialysis patients The nPCR for stable HD patients > 1.2 g/kg/day The nPCR for stable PD patients 1.3 g/kg/day Patients with nPCR < 0.8 g/kg/day require a dietary intake assessment

NUTRITIONAL REQUIREMENTS

Prior to dialysis most diabetic patients will have followed a diet that attempted to balance their carbohydrate intake with other aspects of their diabetes management. Many will already be on a diet that is low in phosphate and potassium and some will also be on a low-protein diet. Prior to dialysis, nutritional intake is usually inadequate with most patients having a negative energy balance (18). Intensive dietetic counselling is required for all patients starting dialysis to help them improve their dietary intake within the constraints of the combined diabetic/renal diet.

Energy Requirements for Dialysis Patients

Energy requirements to achieve neutral nitrogen balance in stable diabetic dialysis patients are similar to those of healthy non-diabetic adults (35 kcal/kg body weight), with lower requirements for subjects over 65 years of age (30–35 kcal/kg body weight) (19). Patients on CAPD receive part of their energy requirements from dialysate glucose (see below) (20).

If CAPD patients have difficulty in meeting their recommended dietary energy intakes due to early satiety, they should be encouraged to eat after 'drain-out' and to wait 20–30 min before commencing the next dialysate bag. Avoiding fluids at mealtimes can also improve appetite by minimising stomach distension. If energy requirements are not achieved despite dietetic input, nutritional supplements should be considered (21).

Table 15.3 A checklist for interpreting blood results of dialysis patients

Biochemistry (normal range)	Low	Good	Acceptable	High
Urea (mmol/l) (2.5–5.5)	< 20 vegetarian status poor appetite residual function	20–28 check dialysis adequacy or urea reduction ratio to ensure patient not underdialysed	28–32	> 32 high protein intake inadequate dialysate drugs, i.e. steroids catabolism acidosis
Creatinine (μmol/l) (55–125)	< 700 small muscle mass (check BMI) residual function	700–1200 normal levels in dialysis patients		> 1200 depends on size of patient. May be underdialysed
Potassium (mmol/l) (3.5–5.5)	< 3.5 residual function diarrhoea vomiting malnourished re-feeding	3.5–5.5 (PD) 3.5–6.00 (HD)	6.0 (PD), 6.5 (HD) check diet, drugs, blood transfusion underdialysed hyperglycaemic acidotic	
Phosphate (mmol/l) (0.8–1.4)	< 0.8 too many binders malnourished re-feeding	0.8–1.8	1.8–2.0	> 2.0 check diet and binders check Ca and PTH levels
Calcium (mmol/l) adjusted (2.15–2.6)	< 2.15 check adjusted for albumin	2.15–2.6	2.6–2.8	> 2.8 check $CaCO_3$ tablets bone disease active vitamin D high PTH
Albumin (g/l) (35–55)	< 30 infection (CRP) nephritic malnourished	33–45 NB: 30–34 may indicate malnutrition	45	> 45 underdialysed constipated acidotic

NB: Use pre-dialysis HD bloods. This information is not applicable to other groups of renal patients.

Energy Gains and Losses from Glucose Fluxes During Dialysis

Energy requirements for CAPD patients are partially met from absorbed dialysate glucose. Requirements from dietary intake are therefore lower at 30 kcal/kg body weight (25 kcal/kg if obese) and 25–30 kcal/kg body weight if older than 65 years (21).

Patients absorb approximately 70% of dialysate glucose, amounting to 300–600 kcal or 2.5–17 g of glucose per hour during dwell times (22) (See table 15.4). Bag volumes range from 1 to 3 litres, with higher dextrose concentrations and larger volumes used to maximize solute clearance and ultrafiltration. The exact amount of glucose absorbed will depend on the dialysate glucose concentration and volume, the number of exchanges, the dwell time between each exchange and the permeability of the patient's peritoneal membrane. Membrane permeability is likely to be increased in people with diabetes. Increasing glucose loads can predispose to hyperglycaemia, hyperinsulinaemia, hyper-lipidaemia, and obesity.

On the basis of a 70% absorption rate of glucose from dialysate fluid, between 2.5–17 g of glucose can be absorbed per hour during dwell times. This glucose load can predispose to hyperglycaemia, leading in turn to hyper-insulinaemia, hyperlipidaemia and obesity.

During HD blood values frequently fall below 4.0 mmol/l when patients are dialysed against a glucose-free dialysate (23).

Such patients should be advised to either eat a snack before or during dialysis. The choice of a slowly absorbed, low-glycaemia snack is ideal for this purpose.

Due to the metabolic problems associated with glucose as the main osmotic agent for inducing ultrafiltration in PD, alternative osmotic agents are now becoming available. High molecular weight glucose polymer solutions such as Icodextrin appear to be safe and effective. Icodextrin has the advantage of a reduced glucose and calorific load but requires dwell times of between 8–12 h and is therefore often left *in situ* overnight. No studies of use in diabetic patients have so far been published (24).

Table 15.4 Approximate energy provided by glucose-containing dialysate

Dialysate (1 l)	Grams of absorbed glucose	Energy provided (kcal)
1.36% dextrose	10	40
2.27% dextrose	16	60
3.86% dextrose	27	100

NUTRITIONAL REQUIREMENTS IN DIALYSIS PATIENTS

The general principles surrounding the nutritional requirements of patients with ESRF receiving dialysis are generally applicable to both diabetic and non-diabetic subjects and are briefly outlined below.

DIETARY PROTEIN

Protein requirements are increased in dialysis patients due to protein losses during dialysis (20) (see Table 15.5) and can be as high as 20 g albumin daily in CAPD with peritonitis. These losses are further increased in the diabetic patient (25) due to greater peritoneal membrane permeability. For non-diabetic stable dialysis patients daily protein intake recommendations based on NKF-KDOQI data (21) and supported by nitrogen balance studies are 1.2 g/kg/day for HD patients and 1.2–1.3 g/kg/day for CAPD patients. Adequate total energy intake is required to maximise the effectiveness of dietary protein utilisation (20).

MINERAL AND VITAMINS

Potassium

Hyperkalaemia in dialysis patients is a potential cause of sudden death. Recommendations to keep serum potassium levels between 3.5–6.5 mmol/l pre-dialysis for HD patients and 3.5–5.5 mmol/l for CAPD patients were published in 2002 (26). Potassium restrictions are usually unnecessary in CAPD patients due to the continuous nature of this form of dialysis. By way of contrast, HD patients accumulate potassium between dialysis sessions.

Phosphate

Hyperphosphataemia is very prevalent among patients with ESRD and is a cause of hyperparathyroidism, metastatic calcification (when the serum calcium–phosphate product exceeds 5.5 mmol/l) (27) and has been associated with excess cardiovascular mortality in HD patients (28). The recommended

Table 15.5 Amino acid and protein losses during dialysis

Dialysis Modality	Amino acids (g)	Proteins/peptides (g)
CAPD/day	2–3.5	5–15
HD/session	6–12	2–3

dietary intake of phosphorus for HD and PD dialysis patients is approximately 17 mg/kg/day. The removal of phosphate during dialysis is limited due to the high distribution volume for phosphate and the rapid rebound of serum phosphate following dialysis. Hyperphosphataemia is common and dietary restriction of dairy products, bony fish and offal meats combined with the use of phosphate buffers remains the best means of minimising hyper-phosphataemia. Medical and dietary treatment of hyperphosphataemia is aimed at keeping the parathyroid hormone level within two to three times the upper limit of the normal range and the alkaline phosphatase and calcium concentrations within the normal range.

Sodium

On starting dialysis sodium intake should be limited to below 100 mmol, equivalent to 6 g salt/day. When dialysis patients become anuric their fluid and sodium intake needs to be further restricted, to 1 litre fluid/day and 80–100 mmol sodium/day. In patients able to maintain a urinary output above 1 l/day, fluid restriction of 1.5–2 l/day and more flexible sodium intake may be appropriate. Residual urinary excretion is maintained for longer in PD than HD patients and hence fluid and sodium intake can initially be more liberal in PD patients.

Vitamins

The role of vitamin supplementation in dialysis patients is controversial. Vitamin status is compromised in dialysis patients due to poor nutritional intake and the cooking methods required for a low-potassium and low-phosphate diet. Fat-soluble vitamins other than vitamin D are not routinely prescribed due to the risk of vitamin A toxicity. Vitamin D is prescribed for bone protection and the prevention of hyperparathyroidism. Among the water-soluble vitamins 10 mg/day of pyridoxine and 60 mg/day of ascorbic acid are recommended as low concentrations can occur in dialysis patients. In addition folic acid may also be low and there may be a need for supplementation.

L-carnitine is an essential co-factor in fatty acid and energy metabolism and recent work suggests that it might be effective in reducing the erythropoetin requirements for controlling anaemia. The US Food and Drug Administration department have recently approved its use in the prevention and treatment of carnitine deficiency in HD patients. Currently, however, there is insufficient evidence to support its routine use in such patients (29).

NUTRITIONAL MANAGEMENT IN DIALYSIS PATIENTS

There are general principles regarding the nutritional management of patients on dialysis with ESRF. These are generally applicable to both diabetic and non-diabetic subjects (30,31) and are briefly covered below.

PREVENTION OF HYPERKALAEMIA

Hyperkalaemia in the HD patient may be due to dietary indiscretions, either as a result of unfamiliar foods of high potassium content or increased portion sizes of known potassium-containing foods. Patients on haemodialysis are usually advised to limit their potassium intake to less than 1 mmol/kg/day. Patients therefore need to avoid high-potassium foods, limit the intake of fruit and vegetables and cook using techniques to lower potassium levels.

Patients with residual urinary function can still excrete some urinary potassium and therefore may safely consume more fruit and vegetables provided there is close monitoring. Hyperkalaemia is less common in CAPD due to continuous potassium removal on dialysis.

In diabetic patients with poor glycaemic control, undergoing dialysis, hyperkalaemia can result from insulin insufficiency. Improving glycaemic control can reduce serum potassium levels. Insulin requirements can drop following the commencement of haemodialysis. In addition to poor glycaemic control, hyperkalaemia is also associated with a number of other non-dietary causes of hyperkalaemia.

PREVENTION OF HYPERPHOSPHATAEMIA

Patient awareness of phosphate-containing foods is essential in order to limit phosphate intake. Dairy products have two to three times more phosphate than equal quantities of protein derived from meat and therefore need to be limited. Milk intake should not exceed 1–3 pt/day and other dairy-containing foods such as chocolate, cheese and yoghurt should be restricted. Other high-phosphate foods such as offal and offal-containing products, veal and fish with edible bones, such as sardines, pilchards and shell fish also need to be limited.

Phosphate binders reduce the absorption of dietary phosphate but when they are comprised solely of calcium salts they can result in hypercalcaemia leading to metastatic calcification. For this reason phosphate binders made from non-calcium salts, such as Sevelamer, may be preferred for the prevention of hyperphosphataemia. To be effective, phosphate binders containing calcium carbonate should be taken before meals as the ability of this salt to bind with phosphate is pH-dependent. The calcium in the phosphate binders may have the added advantage of helping patients achieve the necessary daily calcium requirements.

SODIUM INTAKE

Restricting sodium intake helps minimise thirst and hypertension. In certain individuals this can be difficult as so many convenience foods have a high salt content. A diet history can usually help in eliminating the very high sodium sources.

Interdialytic weight gains should not exceed 3% of the patient's dry weight. This is particularly important in diabetic HD patients, as excessive weight gains have been linked with increased mortality, possibly due to increasing hypertensive and cardiovascular stress.

HYPOALBUMINAEMIA AND PROTEIN MALNUTRITION

Hypoalbuminaemia can cause fluid and sodium retention, and is also linked to increased mortality. Medical management includes further fluid restriction and increased dialysis ultrafiltration. The use of hypertonic CAPD solutions to stimulate ultrafiltration can result in hyperglycaemia and an increase in protein loss. Dietary management is aimed at increasing protein intake. This is particularly a problem in vegetarian patients who rely on pulses and dairy products. While these products are good for diabetic control, they do deliver a greater phosphate load and increase the need for phosphate binders. For malnourished dialysis patients with poor appetites, high-protein energy dense comfort foods can provide a valuable source of energy and protein. When patients are unable to meet their protein requirements due to factors such as a reduced appetite, an inability to prepare foods or a lack of sufficient funds, high protein sip feeds should be considered.

Amino acid-containing dialysates for CAPD patients provide a potential means to improve nitrogen balance in severely hypoalbuminaemic patients. Further benefits to the use of such solutions require further evaluation (32,33).

ADDITIONAL NUTRITIONAL SUPPORT

Haemodialysis patients who continue to report weight loss and poor nutritional intake and who are unable to take nutritional supplements should be considered for either enteral support or intradialytic parenteral nutrition (IDPN) (34). Nasogastric feeding is the preferred short-term option for hospitalised inpatients but this is not usually practical in the outpatient setting. The relatively recent introduction of Percutaneous Endoscopic Gastrostomy (PEG) feeding in HD patients has been shown to be successful in many cases. Balancing the patient's fluid allowance with their nutritional requirements is a major factor when prescribing the feed. The use of high energy dense (2 kcal/ml), low electrolyte feeds has made it possible to feed intermittently dialysed HD patients without causing fluid overload. However, not all patients will require this type of 'renal' feed. Patients with a low serum potassium and phosphate, i.e. CAPD patients, may require a high electrolyte feed of similar energy density. Continual review of serum biochemistry and fluid requirements is essential when prescribing this type of feed.

Interdialytic Parenteral Nutrition (IDPN) can be considered when nasogastric or PEG feeding in HD patients is not established. This consists of giving patients 1 l of a parenteral feed containing between 800–1000 kcals and 50 g amino acids via the venous return line during each dialysis session. Although the overall efficacy of IDPN is not well established, improvements in appetite, immune and nutritional status have been reported (35). A drawback to IDPN is that it can not be given during the dialysis-free days of the week.

SPECIFIC NUTRITIONAL MANAGEMENT IN DIABETIC DIALYSIS PATIENTS

The dietary management of diabetic patients receiving dialysis has to be adapted to achieve the best attainable glycaemic control. Dietary management also has to address any other aspects of the metabolic syndrome which may be present, such as obesity, dyslipidaemia and insulin resistance.

GLYCAEMIC CONTROL

Although it is a popular patient myth that the principles of a good diabetic diet cannot be achieved within the confines of dialysis dietary restrictions, in reality there is sufficient scope for dietary adjustments using lower glycaemic index food choices to prove this wrong. However, not all low glycaemic foods are suitable for dialysis patients; potatoes, yam, cassava, sweet potato and green banana all contain significant amounts of potassium. Suitable low glycaemic foods include porridge, pasta, basmati rice, couscous and granary breads. Boiling vegetables in large volumes of water can reduce the potassium content considerably. Hence, when an individual's staple diet includes carbohydrate foods with a high potassium content, suitable cooking methods can make many more of these foods available for inclusion in the diet.

Since there is a high prevalence of diabetic ESRF in ethnic minority populations, a number of cultural and religious factors that can influence glycaemic control need to be considered. The most important of these is a wish to fast for religious observance, even though exemptions can be obtained. For example, during Ramadan, fasting can last up to 18 h in the summer months with no foods or drinks being taken between dawn and sunset. Of necessity large meals are usually taken before dawn and after sunset and are likely to include fried foods and carbohydrate-rich meals including specially prepared sweet foods. During such periods, without expert adjustment of treatment regimens, large fluctuations in blood glucose can occur. Hypoglycaemia may also be a problem among haemodialysis patients who are not being dialysed against a glucose-containing dialysate. Dietary advice should be directed towards limiting sweet foods taken after sunset and promoting low glycaemic foods such as basmati rice, chapati or naan breads made with wholewheat flour and not besan flour (chick pea) which is high in potassium.

OBESITY

Weight reduction using dietary intervention is generally considered suitable within the general population when the BMI is above $30 \, kg/m^2$. A considerable number of CAPD patients are either obese or have a tendency to become so. The weight management of CAPD patients is difficult as many are receiving additional calories from the glucose absorbed during dialysis. Increasing physical activity is often unrealistic in a population confined to their house for much of the day.

DYSLIPIDAEMIA AND OTHER CARDIOVASCULAR RISK FACTORS

The dyslipidaemia of ESRF is characterised by raised plasma triglycerides with a normal cholesterol level. This form of dyslipidaemia becomes worse after starting CAPD. The lipid profile on CAPD is generally more atherogenic than with other dialysis modalities. A possible contributory factor for this atherogenic lipid profile is the glucose absorption from the dialysates giving rise to enhanced triglyceride synthesis. Chronic hyperinsulinaemia is a major component of the metabolic syndrome and a recognised risk factor for atherosclerosis (36). There is a preferential sieving of the smaller cardio-protective lipoprotein: HDL-cholesterol among the proteins lost into the dialysate rather than that of other lipoproteins (37).

The dyslipidaemia of ESRF is an independent risk factor for atherosclerosis in ESRD (38). To date there are no convincing trials to show that the 3-hydroxy-3-methylglutaryl coenzyme A reductase inhibitors (statin) are equally as effective as they are for non-renal-compromised patients, and although widely used, their benefits are not unequivocally established (39,40). Dietary management of glycaemic control for diabetic patients on PD improves hypertriglyceridaemia and overall dyslipidaemia. The effectiveness of dietary manipulation of plasma lipids in PD patients is limited and it could be argued that if adhered to, properly constructed dialysis diets are close to optimal lipid-lowering recommendations (41,42). General healthy eating advice given to patients with normal renal function may not be appropriate, as many PD patients are undernourished and advice to reduce saturated fat should not be at the expense of reducing total protein or energy intake. Current recommendations are that 35% of energy should be derived from fat (41), with emphasis placed on reducing the saturated to polyunsaturated fat ratios.

HYPOGLYCAEMIC AGENTS AND DIALYSIS

The diet for the diabetic patient on dialysis needs to reflect their diabetic treatment. An understanding of how ESRF and dialysis interacts with the action of hypoglycaemic agents and insulin is important for the renal dietitian if the prescribed diet is to minimise periods of hypo- and hyperglycaemia.

ORAL HYPOGLYCAEMIC AGENTS

Oral agents are rarely used in Type 2 diabetic patients undergoing dialysis. By the time diabetic patients have developed ESRF extensive β-cell failure will have occurred and most patients will have already been switched to insulin. During the pre-dialysis period metformin is contraindicated as are the longer acting sulphonylureas such as glibenclamide. An insulin secretagogue like repaglinide, whose metabolism is not dependent on renal function for clearance, is safe. The glitazone class of insulin sensitisers can also be used in subjects with moderate renal failure. However, in reality, by the time patients are requiring CAPD or HD, insulin provides not only the safest but also the most flexible and easiest way to optimise glycaemic control.

INSULIN

Insulin requirements in ESRD patients are difficult to predict as renal and extra-renal breakdown of insulin is diminished on the one hand and its half-life is prolonged on the other. With advancing renal failure this effect is antagonised by insulin resistance, which usually improves with regular dialysis. On initiation of CAPD, the timing of insulin doses should be adjusted to complement the pattern of glucose absorption. Very strict glycaemic control becomes increasingly difficult in dialysis patients because of the risk of intradialytic and nocturnal hypoglycaemia. A balance around optimising glycaemic control needs to be made as good glycaemic control reduces catabolism and improves nutritional status. One expert committee has suggested an HbA_{1c} target of below 8%.

Administering insulin via the intraperitoneal route can improve glycaemic control and lessen hyper- or hypoglycaemic episodes. Intraperitoneal insulin absorbed into the portal venous circulation results in a more physiological portal to peripheral insulin ratio of approximately 3:1 and lower systemic insulin levels (43). However this route of administration promotes a more atherogenic lipid profile and may cause focal hepatic fat accumulation, and there also remains a theoretical risk of peritonitis.

SUMMARY

As the prevalence of diabetes grows so will the need for renal replacement therapies. The dietary management of patients as they approach ESRF should focus on minimising uraemic symptoms while ensuring a sufficient protein and energy intake to prevent malnutrition. Both the nutritional status and the glycaemic control of an individual as they start dialysis are independent important predictors of their future morbidity and mortality. Achieving glycaemic control in patients undergoing regular dialysis requires a careful balance between the dialysis prescription and meal planning. While the nutritional requirements, constraints and demands are by and large similar for the diabetic and non-diabetic patient, the need to address atherosclerotic cardiovascular risk factors is still greater in the diabetic patient. Today many of the diabetic patients undergoing dialysis are malnourished with poor glycaemic, lipid and metabolic profiles. There is a real need for well-constructed nutritional studies in the diabetic dialysed population to formulate evidence-based dietary interventions that will help to extend the patient's life expectancy to that of a non-diabetic dialysed subject.

REFERENCES

1. UK Renal Registry. The Third Annual Report. http://www.renalreg.com/2000.
2. Roderick PJ, Raleigh VS, Hallam L, Mallick NP. The need and demand for renal replacement therapy in ethnic minorities in England. *J Epidemiol Community Health* 1996; 50: 334–339.
3. Stevens PR. Anticipating the impact of the renal national service framework. *Br J Renal Med* 2002; 7: 20–24.
4. National Kidney Foundation. Dialysis Outcome Quality Initiative (DOQI) guidelines. http://www.kidney.org/professionals/doqi/guidelines/2000.
5. Ibrahim HA, Vora JP. Diabetic nephropathy. *Baillières Best Pract Res Clin Endocrinol Metab* 1999; 13: 239–264.
6. Patient Mortality & Survival. United States Renal Data System. *Am J Kidney Dis* 1998; 32 (Suppl 1): S69–S80.
7. Rychlik I, Miltenberger-Miltenyi G, Ritz E. The drama of the continuous increase in end-stage renal failure in patients with type II diabetes mellitus. *Nephrol Dial Transplant* 1998; 13 (Suppl 8): 6–10.
8. Viglino G, Cancarini GC, Catizone L, Cocchi R, De Vecchi A, Lupo A, Salomone M, Segoloni GP, Giangrande A. Ten years experience of CAPD in diabetics: comparison of results with non-diabetics. Italian Cooperative Peritoneal Dialysis Study Group. *Nephrol Dial Transpl* 1994; 9: 1443–1448.

9. Bommer J. Attaining long-term survival when treating diabetic patients with ESRD by hemodialysis. *Adv Ren Replace Ther* 2001; 8: 13–21.

10. Holley JL, Bernardini J, Piraino B. Risk factors for tunnel infections in continuous peritoneal dialysis. *Am J Kidney Dis* 1991; 18: 344–348.

11. Vas SI. Infections of continuous ambulatory peritoneal dialysis catheters. *Infect Dis Clin North Am* 1989; 3: 301–328.

12. Ronco C, Bosch JP, Lew SQ, Feriani M, Chiaramonte S, Conz P, Brendolan A, La Greca G. Adequacy of continuous ambulatory peritoneal analysis: comparison with other dialysis techniques. *Kidney Int Suppl* 1994; 48: S18–S24.

13. Zappacosta AR, Perras ST. The process of prescribing CAPD. In: *CAPD: Continuous Ambulatory Peritoneal Dialysis*. Philadelphia, PA: Lippincott, 1984: 4–23.

14. Gokal R, Hutchison A. Dialysis therapies for end-stage renal disease. *Seminol Dial* 2002; 15: 220–226.

15. Locatelli F, Fouque D, Heimburger O, Drueke TB, Cannata-Andia JB, Horl WH, Ritz E. Nutritional status in dialysis patients: a European consensus. *Nephrol Dial Transpl* 2002; 17: 563–572.

16. The Modification of Diet in Renal Disease Study: design, methods, and results from the feasibility study. *Am J Kidney Dis* 1992; 20: 18–33.

17. Pifer TB, McCullough KP, Port FK, Goodkin DA, Maroni BJ, Held PJ, Young EW. Mortality risk in hemodialysis patients and changes in nutritional indicators: DOPPS. *Kidney Int* 2002; 62: 2238–2245.

18. Kopple JD. Dietary protein and energy requirements in ESRD patients. *Am J Kidney Dis* 1998; 32 (Suppl 4): S97–S104.

19. Ahmed KR, Kopple JD. Nutrition in maintenance hemodialysis patients, In: *Nutritional Management of Renal Disease*, eds JD Kopple and SG Massry. Baltimore, MD: Williams and Wilkins, 1998: 563–600.

20. Bergstrom J, Furst P, Alvestrand A, Lindholm B. Protein and energy intake, nitrogen balance and nitrogen losses in patients treated with continuous ambulatory peritoneal dialysis. *Kidney Int* 1993; 44: 1048–1057.

21. The National Kidney Foundation-Kidney Dialysis Outcome Quality Initiative (NKF-KDOQ). http://www.kidney.org/professionals/doqi/guidelines, 2002.

22. Grodstein GP, Blumenkrantz MJ, Kopple JD, Moran JK, Coburn JW. Glucose absorption during continuous ambulatory peritoneal dialysis. *Kidney Int* 1981; 19: 564–567.

23. Jackson MA, Holland MR, Nicholas J, Lodwick R, Forster D, Macdonald IA. Hemodialysis-induced hypoglycemia in diabetic patients. *Clin Nephrol* 2000; 54: 30–34.

24. Mistry CD, Gokal R, Peers E. A randomized multicenter clinical trial comparing isosmolar icodextrin with hyperosmolar glucose solutions in CAPD. MIDAS Study Group. Multicenter Investigation of Icodextrin in Ambulatory Peritoneal Dialysis. *Kidney Int* 1994; 46: 496–503.

25. Nakamoto H, Imai H, Kawanishi H, Nakamoto M, Minakuchi J, Kumon S, Watanabe S, Shiohira Y, Ishii T, Kawahara T, Tsuzaki K, Suzuki H. Effect of diabetes on peritoneal function assessed by personal dialysis capacity test in patients undergoing CAPD. *Am J Kidney Dis* 2002; 40: 1045–1054.

26. Renal Association. *Treatment of Adult Patients with Renal Failure. Recommended Standards and Audit Measures*, 3rd edition. London: Royal College of Physicians, 2002.

27. Delmez JA, Slatopolsky E. Hyperphosphatemia: its consequences and treatment in patients with chronic renal disease. *Am J Kidney Dis* 1992; 19: 303–317.

28. Ganesh SK, Stack AG, Levin NW, Hulbert-Shearon T, Port FK. Association of elevated serum phosphate, calcium/phosphate product, and parathyroid hormone

with cardiac mortality risk in chronic hemodialysis patients. *J Am Soc Nephrol* 2001; 12: 2131–2138.

29. Hurot JM, Cucherat M, Haugh M, Fouque D. Effects of L-carnitine supplementation in maintenance hemodialysis patients: a systematic review. *J Am Soc Nephrol* 2002; 13: 708–714.

30. Renal Disease. In: *Manual of Dietetic Practice*, 3rd edition, ed. B. Thomas. London: Blackwell Science, 2001: 420–434.

31. NKF K/DOQI NKF K/DOQI Guidelines, Nutrition in Chronic Renal Failure. http://www.kidney.org/professionals/doqi/guidelines/, 2000.

32. Brunori G, Leiserowitz M, Bier DM, Stegink L, Martis L, Algrim Boyle C, Serkes K, Vonesh E, Jones M. Treatment of malnourished CAPD patients with an amino acid based dialysate. *Kidney Int* 1995; 47: 1148–1157.

33. Jones M, Hagen T, Boyle CA, Vonesh E, Hamburger R, Charytan C, Sandroni S, Bernard D, Piraino B, Schreiber M, Gehr T, Fein P, Friedlander M, Burkart J, Ross D, Zimmerman S, Swartz R, Knight T, Kraus A Jr, McDonald L, Hartnett M, Weaver M, Martis L, Moran J. Treatment of malnutrition with 1.1% amino acid peritoneal dialysis solution: results of a multicenter outpatient study. *Am J Kidney Dis* 1998; 32: 761–769.

34. Foulks CJ. An evidence-based evaluation of intradialytic parenteral nutrition. *Am J Kidney Dis* 1999; 33: 186–192.

35. Chertow GM. Modality-specific nutrition support in ESRD: weighing the evidence. *Am J Kidney Dis* 1999; 33: 193–197.

36. Lindholm B, Norbeck HE. Serum lipids and lipoproteins during continuous ambulatory peritoneal dialysis. *Acta Med Scand* 1986; 220: 143–151.

37. Kagan A, Bar-Khayim Y, Schafer Z, Fainaru M. Kinetics of peritoneal protein loss during CAPD: II. Lipoprotein leakage and its impact on plasma lipid levels. *Kidney Int* 1990; 37: 980–990.

38. Wanner C, Quaschning T. Dyslipidemia and renal disease: pathogenesis and clinical consequences. *Curr Opin Nephrol Hypertens* 2001; 10: 195–201.

39. Mathur S, Devaraj S, Jialal I. Accelerated atherosclerosis, dyslipidemia, and oxidative stress in end-stage renal disease. *Curr Opin Nephrol Hypertens* 2002; 11: 141–147.

40. Massy ZA, Ma JZ, Louis TA, Kasiske BL. Lipid-lowering therapy in patients with renal disease. *Kidney Int* 1995; 48: 188–198.

41. Feriani M, Dell'Aquila R, La Greca G. The treatment of diabetic end-stage renal disease with peritoneal dialysis. *Nephrol Dial Transpl* 1998; 13 (Suppl 8): 53–56.

42. Saltissi D, Morgan C, Knight B, Chang W, Rigby R, Westhuyzen J. Effect of lipid-lowering dietary recommendations on the nutritional intake and lipid profiles of chronic peritoneal dialysis and hemodialysis patients. *Am J Kidney Dis* 2001; 37: 1209–1215.

43. Nevalainen PI, Kallio T, Lahtela JT, Mustonen J, Pasternack AI. High peritoneal permeability predisposes to hepatic steatosis in diabetic continuous ambulatory peritoneal dialysis patients receiving intraperitoneal insulin. *Perit Dial Int* 2000; 20: 637–642.

16

Nutritional Management of Diabetic Renal Transplant Recipients

BARBARA ENGEL

Charing Cross Hospital, London, UK

This chapter provides the necessary background information required for a health care professional to give dietary advice to a diabetic renal transplant recipient. The chapter covers the main causes of morbidity and mortality in diabetic renal transplant patients and examines whether dietary intervention can improve graft survival and clinical outcome.

INTRODUCTION

RENAL TRANSPLANTATION AND DIABETES

End stage renal failure (ESRF) from diabetes is increasing and the number of diabetic patients receiving a renal transplant is growing. Diabetes is also a common metabolic complication following a successful renal transplant, due partly to the steroids used to prevent graft rejection and to the associated weight gain they cause. In one study involving 114 patients with normal glucose tolerance, a week before transplantation, only 36 (32%) retained normal glucose tolerance 9 to 12 months post-transplant with 27 (24%) patients becoming frankly diabetic. Both β-cell dysfunction and insulin resistance contribute to the development of diabetes post-transplant (1,2).

Nutritional Management of Diabetes Mellitus. Edited by G. Frost, A. Dornhorst and R. Moses
© 2003 John Wiley & Sons, Ltd. ISBN 0 471 49751 7

MORBIDITY AND MORTALITY

Transplantation provides the best renal replacement option for diabetic patients with ESRF, improving the quality of life (3,4), and resulting in less neuropathy and anorexia. Unfortunately, renal transplantation does not improve pre-existing metabolic conditions such as dyslipidaemia or bone disease. These continue to progress and contribute to the long-term morbidity and mortality. The medications used to prevent graft rejection also contribute to metabolic risk factors, including weight gain and metabolic bone disease.

Five-year survival rates are higher following a renal transplant than with regular dialysis, especially for people with diabetes. Despite this, five-year survival rates for diabetic patients are still appreciably lower (66–75%) than for non-diabetic patients (90–95%) (5,6). Mortality rates are lower when diabetic patients receive a combined kidney–pancreas transplant than an isolated kidney (6,7). To what extent this is due to improved glycaemic control is uncertain, as patient selection criteria for a dual kidney–pancreatic transplant inevitably select patients with low co-morbidity scores. Diabetic microvascular disease, retinopathy and neuropathy improve initially following renal transplantation. The neuropathy improvement is however more sustained in patients receiving a combined kidney–pancreas transplant (8,9).

Ischaemic heart disease is present in 40% of diabetic patients prior to transplant (3,4), and when present carries a threefold risk of a further coronary event over the next four years (5). The higher mortality rate of diabetic compared to non-diabetic renal transplant recipients is mainly related to this high incidence of pre-existing coronary heart disease. In a four-year follow-up study of 101 transplant patients with Type 1 diabetes, the absolute mortality rate was 30%, with 57% of these deaths attributed to arterial disease (5). Peripheral vascular disease also progresses after a renal transplant, and the risk of ulcers and poor wound healing is increased in these immunocompromised patients.

DIETARY INTERVENTION STUDIES

A 20-year literature search identifies few dietary intervention studies in renal transplant patients. The number of subjects included in these intervention and observational studies is small and many of these short studies fail to adequately differentiate the effects of diet and medication, see Table 16.1.

KIDNEY SURVIVAL

A transplanted kidney is susceptible to hyperglycaemia and hypertension (3,4). Hypercholesterolaemia and hypertriglyceridaemia also influence graft survival

Table 16.1 Dietary intervention and observational studies in renal transplant recipients

Author	Study protocol	Outcome
Patel (30)	Four months' diet and lifestyle advice given to 11 new transplant patients compared to 22 patients previously transplanted in the previous four years receiving no dietary advice	There was a significantly lower weight gain at four months and one year in the group given dietary advice than in the historical controls receiving no dietary advice (5.5 kg vs 11.8 kg)
Tonstad et al. (26)	26 patients post-transplant given a Step 1 American Heart Association diet for 12 weeks <30% total calories from fat <300 mg cholesterol/day <10% total calories from saturated fat	Weighed dietary records showed a decrease in total fat (30 to 27%) and a fall in saturated fat (12 to 8% of total calories). Body weight and lipids profile remained unchanged, apart from a small fall in triglyceride values in patients with a BMI <26 kg/m^2
Hines (31)	$N = 43$. Step 1 American Heart Association diet prescribed for two to eight months	Total cholesterol decreased significantly by 0.54 mmol/l, LDL-cholesterol by 0.53 mmol/l. In all 20% of patients reached target levels of total cholesterol <5.2 mmol/l and 35% of patients reached the LDL-cholesterol target of <3.5 mmol/l. Total fat intake fell by 7.6% of total calories
Barbagallo et al. (32)	$N = 78$ normal and hyperlipidaemic subjects given a Step 1 American Heart Association diet for 12 weeks that was isocaloric with usual diet	Cholesterol reduced by 10% (6.02 to 5.41 mmol/l), triglyceride by 6.5% (1.81 to 1.7 mmol/l). Improvements in LDL-cholesterol occurred in patients with high starting LDL-cholesterol levels
Foldes et al. (24)	$N = 21$ diabetic transplant patients, given a diet for eight weeks and followed for one year	No change in lipid profile with diet, but significant decrease in total cholesterol after 12 weeks when patients were also given fluvastatin
Lal et al. (33)	Step I and 2 American Heart Association diet given to non-DM transplant patients	No significant change in total cholesterol or triglyceride
La Rocca et al. (25)	Dietary advice and lipid management in Type 1 diabetic patients receiving a kidney or a kidney and pancreatic transplant	There was a decrease in total fat and cholesterol intake in both groups and a significant decrease in plasma cholesterol in the kidney-pancreas transplant group from 5.3–4.9 mmol/L
Moore et al. (21)	18 patients (four diabetic) given an American Heart Association Step 1 diet (also weight reducing and low sodium) with a serum cholesterol > 200 mg/dl	Weight loss 2 lb. Cholesterol decreased from 262 to 241 mg/dl after eight weeks

(10–12). The benefits of good glycaemic control on graft survival may however require three or more years to become apparent. The rationale for optimising glycaemic control is based on the knowledge that prior to transplant poor glycaemic control influences glomerular filtration loss, and that long-term graft survival following a combined kidney and pancreas transplant (K-P) is better than for an isolated kidney (13,14). Improved lipoprotein concentrations are also observed after K-P transplantation and this again is attributable to better glycaemic control (15).

Low-protein diets in the diabetic patients with CRF have been shown to have a beneficial effect on disease progression and proteinuria. A number of studies in (mostly non-diabetic) transplant patients have shown that reducing protein intake may improve graft survival and slow the progression of renal disease in chronic rejection (16–18). Hyperlipidaemia prior to, and following, transplant is also associated with an increased risk of graft rejection (12).

There is a suggestion that fish oils can protect the kidney in cyclosporine-treated renal transplant recipients. However the role of omega-3 unsaturated fatty acid supplementation remains controversial. In one randomised prospective controlled trial early dietary supplementation post-transplant with daily 6 g fish oil for one month favourably influenced renal function in the recovery phase following a rejection episode in patients treated with cyclosporine (19,20). In another study although patients taking 6 g/day of fish oils did not show any improvement in rejection rates at one year they did have a non-significant improvement in their renal function (20). The role of dietary intervention with antioxidants and diets to decrease PAI-1 synthesis in renal transplant recipients requires further evaluation.

CARDIOVASCULAR DISEASE

Both renal disease and diabetes are associated with accelerated CVD. The sedentary lifestyle adopted by many renal patients exacerbates weight gain and many of the recognised metabolic risk factors attached to this. Dietary advice needs to address the usual modifiable CVD risk factors in this group. It could be argued that a diabetic with a functioning renal transplant should receive the same advice as other diabetics without renal failure. However, the response to diet therapy may not be similar due to the anti-rejection medications prescribed (21).

Obesity prior to a renal transplant is associated with higher five-year mortality rates. In one study of 127 obese ($BMI > 31 \, kg/m^2$) non-diabetic renal transplant recipients the five-year survival rate was 67%. This was significantly lower than the 89% observed in the 127 non-obese ($BMI < 27 \, kg/m^2$) non-diabetic renal transplant recipients (22). Most of this excess mortality can be attributed to cardiac disease. Even if weight loss cannot be achieved prior to transplantation, intensive dietary advice is required post-transplant to limit the usual weight gains that occur. In one study of non-diabetic patients the percentage of patients who had a $BMI > 25 \, kg/m^2$ increased from 22% to 36% post-transplantation (23).

There are a few dietary intervention studies that deal specifically with diabetic patients post-transplantation (15,24,25). However these studies only involve small numbers of patients followed for a relatively short period of time, and none adequately separate the effects of diet from the effects of medication. In non-diabetic transplant patients the effectiveness of the Step 1 American Heart Association diet to reduce weight gains and improve lipid profiles has been very variable. Even when significant weight loss is achieved, by six months, lipid profiles do not always improve. Hyperlipidaemia appears to be related more to renal impairment than dietary fat modification, especially if weight reduction does not occur (26). Population studies have shown that a reduced-fat diet is required for at least two years to achieve any reduction in cardiovascular events, and this possibly explains the disappointing results of shorter-term studies in post-transplantation patients (see Table 16.1).

Hyperhomocysteinaemia (tHcy) is another independent risk factor for coronary heart disease (27). Both Type 1 and Type 2 diabetic patients with renal failure have approximately fourfold higher tHcy levels than controls prior to transplantation. These levels can fall by a third after a successful renal transplant and further falls have been reported with folic acid, B6 and B12 supplements (28). The routine place of these dietary supplements in diabetic renal transplant patients awaits further studies.

TREATMENT STRATEGIES

For diabetic renal transplant recipients with pre-existing heart disease the lipid-lowering drugs, belonging to the class of HMG-CoA reductase inhibitors, and universally known as the 'statins', are thought to be more effective at reducing cholesterol levels than advocating a low-cholesterol diet. However there are no studies in the diabetic renal transplant population that allow us to judge whether these drugs are as effective at reducing cardiovascular disease as in the general diabetic population. Controlled studies on transplant patients examining 'healthy' eating, lifestyle changes, glycaemic control and the use of fish oils, vitamins and other 'functional foods' are required to determine their benefit in graft survival and long-term cardiovascular health.

BONE DISEASE

Metabolic bone disease continues to influence morbidity and mortality after a successful transplant. Despite normalisation of phosphate excretion and improved activation of vitamin D, parathyroid hormone levels can remain elevated. Bone resorption continues due to the adverse effects of corticosteroids on osteoblast function and calcium absorption from the gut. Type 1 diabetic transplant recipients have been reported to have a higher fracture rate than non-diabetic recipients (40% vs 11%) (29). This increased fracture rate is similar in the male and female diabetic subjects, and contrasts with results from the non-diabetic transplant recipients in whom the female fracture rate is approximately twice that of men. Increased intake of dietary calcium and the use of calcitriol and alendronate can help to neutralise the adverse effect of corticosteroids.

CONCLUSION

Renal transplantation offers diabetic patients an improved quality of life and longevity. Metabolic risk factors can be exacerbated by the immunosuppresion needed to minimise graft rejection. Dietary advice to limit post-transplant weight gain should be given along with advice aimed at meeting protein requirements, improving glycaemic control and hyperlipidaemia and reducing the risk of metabolic bone disease. The impact of this type of dietary advice on overall morbidity and mortality remains to be fully evaluated.

REFERENCES

1. Jindal RM, Hjelmesaeth J. Impact and management of posttransplant diabetes mellitus. *Transplantation* 2000; 70 (Suppl 11): S58–S63.
2. Hjelmesæth J, Midtvedt K, Jenssen T, Hartmann A. Insulin resistance after renal transplantation: impact of immunosuppressive and antihypertensive therapy. *Diabetes Care* 2001; 24: 2121–2126.
3. Ritz E, Stefanski A. Diabetic nephropathy in type II diabetes. *Am J Kidney Dis* 1996; 27: 167–194.
4. Ritz E, Keller C, Bergis K, Strojek K. Pathogenesis and course of renal disease in IDDM/NIDDM. *Am J Hypertens* 1997; 10 (9/2): 202S–207S.
5. Lemmers MJ, Barry JM. Major role for arterial disease in morbidity and mortality after kidney transplantation in diabetic recipients. *Diabetes Care* 1991; 14: 295–301.
6. Carlstrom J, Norden G, Mjornstedt L, Nyberg G. Increasing prevalence of cardiovascular disease in kidney transplant patients with Type 1 diabetes. *Transpl Int* 1999; 12: 176–181.
7. Biesenbach G, Margreiter R, Konigsrainer A, Bosmuller C, Janko O, Brucke P, Gross C, Zazgornik J. Comparison of progression of macrovascular diseases after kidney or pancreas and kidney transplantation in diabetic patients with end-stage renal disease. *Diabetologia* 2000; 43: 231–234.
8. Adang EM, Engel GL, van Hooff JP, Kootstra G. Comparison before and after transplantation of pancreas–kidney and pancreas–kidney with loss of pancreas – a prospective controlled quality of life study. *Transplantation* 1996; 62: 754–758.

9. Ekstrand A, Groop L, Pettersson E, Gronhagen-Riska C, Laatikainen L, Matikainen E, Seppalainen AM, Laasonen E, Summanen P, Ollus A *et al.* Metabolic control and progression of complications in insulin-dependent diabetic patients after kidney transplantation. *J Intern Med* 1992; 232: 253–261.
10. Dimeny E, Wahlberg J, Lithell H, Fellstrom B. Hyperlipidaemia in renal transplantation – risk factor for long-term graft outcome. *Eur J Clin Invest* 1995; 25: 574–583.
11. Dimeny E, Fellstrom B. Metabolic abnormalities in renal transplant recipients. Risk factors and predictors of chronic graft dysfunction? *Nephrol Dial Transplant* 1997; 12: 21–24.
12. Hamar P, Muller V, Kohnle M, Witzke O, Albrecht KH, Philipp T, Heemann U. Metabolic factors have a major impact on kidney allograft survival. *Transplantation* 1997; 64: 1135–1139.
13. Solders G, Tyden G, Persson A, Groth CG. Improvement of nerve conduction in diabetic neuropathy. A follow-up study 4 yr after combined pancreatic and renal transplantation. *Diabetes* 1992; 41: 946–951.
14. Manske CL, Wang Y, Thomas W. Mortality of cadaveric kidney transplantation versus combined kidney–pancreas transplantation in diabetic patients. *Lancet* 1995; 346: 1658–1662.
15. Georgi BA, Bowers VD, Smith JL, Wright FH, Corry RJ. Comparison of fasting serum cholesterol levels between diabetic recipients who undergo renal–pancreas transplants and renal transplantation only. *Transplant Proc* 1989; 21 (1/3): 2839–2840.
16. Bernardi A, Biasia F, Piva M, Poluzzi P, Senesi G, Scaramuzzo P, Garizzo O, Stoppa F, Cavallaro B, Bassini S, Bucciante G. Dietary protein intake and nutritional status in patients with renal transplant. *Clin Nephrol* 2000; 53: 3–5.
17. Biesenbach G, Zazgornik J, Janko O, Hubmann R, Syre G. Effect of mild dietary protein restriction on urinary protein excretion in patients with renal transplant fibrosis. *Wien Med Wochenschr* 1996; 146: 75–78.
18. Salahudeen AK, Hostetter TH, Raatz SK, Rosenberg ME. Effects of dietary protein in patients with chronic renal transplant rejection. *Kidney Int* 1992; 41: 183–190.
19. Homan van der Heide JJ, Bilo HJ, Donker AJ, Wilmink JM, Sluiter WJ, Tegzess AM. The effects of dietary supplementation with fish oil on renal function and the course of early postoperative rejection episodes in cyclosporine-treated renal transplant recipients. *Transplantation* 1992; 54: 257–263.
20. Kooijmans-Coutinho MF, Rischen-Vos J, Hermans J, Arndt JW, van der Woude FJ. Dietary fish oil in renal transplant recipients treated with cyclosporin-A: no beneficial effects shown. *J Am Soc Nephrol* 1996; 7: 513–518.
21 Moore RA, Callahan MF, Cody M, Adams PL, Litchford M, Buckner K, Galloway J. The effect of the American Heart Association step one diet on hyperlipidemia following renal transplantation. *Transplantation* 1990; 49: 60–62.
22. Modlin CS, Flechner SM, Goormastic M, Goldfarb DA, Papajcik D, Mastroianni B, Novick AC. Should obese patients lose weight before receiving a kidney transplant? *Transplantation* 1997; 64: 599–604.
23. Locsey L, Asztalos L, Kincses Z, Berczi C, Paragh G. The importance of obesity and hyperlipidaemia in patients with renal transplants. *Int Urol Nephrol* 1998; 30: 767–775.
24. Foldes K, Maklary E, Vargha P, Janssen J, Jaray J, Perner F, Gero L. Effect of diet and fluvastatin treatment on the serum lipid profile of kidney transplant, diabetic recipients: a 1-year follow up. *Transpl Int* 1998; 11 (Suppl 1): S65–S68.

25. La Rocca E, Ruotolo G, Parlavecchia M, Librenti MC, Secchi A, Caldara R, Bonfatti D, Bernardi M, Di Carlo V, Pozza G. Dietary advice and lipid metabolism in insulin-dependent diabetes mellitus kidney- and pancreas-transplanted patients. *Transplant Proc* 1992; 24: 848–849.
26. Tonstad S, Holdaas H, Gorbitz C, Ose L. Is dietary intervention effective in post-transplant hyperlipidaemia?. *Nephrol Dial Transplant* 1995; 10: 82–85.
27. Ducloux D, Motte G, Massy ZA. Hyperhomocysteinemia as a risk factor after renal transplantation. *Ann Transplant* 2001; 6: 40–42.
28. Socha MW, Polakowska MJ, Socha-Urbanek K, Fiedor P. Hyperhomocysteinemia as a risk factor for cardiovascular diseases. The association of hyperhomocysteinemia with diabetes mellitus and renal transplant recipients. *Ann Transplant* 1999; 4: 11–19.
29. Nisbeth U, Lindh E, Ljunghall S, Backman U, Fellstrom B. Increased fracture rate in diabetes mellitus and females after renal transplantation. *Transplantation* 1999; 67: 1218–1222.
30. Patel MG. The effect of dietary intervention on weight gains after renal transplantation. *J Ren Nutr* 1998; 8: 137–141.
31. Hines L. Can low-fat/cholesterol nutrition counseling improve food intake habits and hyperlipidemia of renal transplant patients? *J Ren Nutr* 2000; 10: 30–35.
32. Barbagallo CM, Cefalu AB, Gallo S, Rizzo M, Noto D, Cavera G, Rao Camemi A, Marino G, Caldarella R, Notarbartolo A, Averna MR. Effects of Mediterranean diet on lipid levels and cardiovascular risk in renal transplant recipients. *Nephron* 1999; 82: 199–204.
33. Lal SM, Trivedi HS, Van Stone JC, Ross G Jr. Effects of dietary therapy on post renal transplant hyperlipidemia. A prospective study. *Int J Artif Organs* 1994; 17: 461–465.

Index

Note. Abbreviations used in the index: GI = glycaemic index;
MUFA = monounsaturated fatty acids.

Nutritional Management of Diabetes Mellitus. Edited by Gary Frost, Anne Dornhorst and Robert Moses.
© 2003 John Wiley & Sons, Ltd: ISBN 0471497517